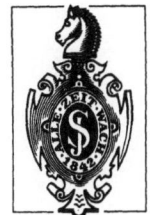

This work was awarded the "Jubiläumspreis"
of the Swiss Society of Radiology and Nuclear Medicine
upon its 75th anniversary

G. K. von Schulthess

Morphology and Function in MRI

Cardiovascular and Renal Systems

With a Foreword by
W. A. Fuchs and A. Margulis

With 155 Figures in 273 Separate Illustrations

Springer-Verlag
Berlin Heidelberg New York
London Paris Tokyo

Dr. med., Dr. rer. nat. GUSTAV KONRAD VON SCHULTHESS
Universitätsspital Zürich
Departement Medizinische Radiologie
Rämistrasse 100
CH-8091 Zürich

ISBN-13:978-3-642-73518-9   e-ISBN-13:978-3-642-73516-5
DOI: 10.1007/978-3-642-73516-5

Library of Congress Cataloging-in-Publication Data. Schulthess, Gustav Konrad von. Morphology and function in MRI. Cardiovascular and renal systems. G. K. von Schulthess; with a foreword by W. A. Fuchs and A. Margulis. p. cm. Includes bibliographies and index. ISBN-13:978-3-642-73518-9 1. Cardiovascular system - Magnetic resonance imaging. 2. Kidneys - Magnetic resonance imaging. 3. Cardiovascular system - Diseases - Diagnosis. 4. Kidneys - Diseases - Diagnosis. I. Title. [DNLM: 1. Cardiovascular Diseases - diagnosis. 2. Cardiovascular System - anatomy & histology. 3. Cardiovascular System - physiology. 4. Kidney - anatomy & histology. 5. Kidney Diseases - diagnosis. 6. Kidney - physiology. 7. Magnetic Resonance Imaging. WG 141 S3865m] RC670.5.M33S38 1988 616.1'0757-dc19 DNLM/DLC for Library of Congress 88-24780 CIP

© Springer-Verlag Berlin Heidelberg 1989
Softcover reprint of the hardcover 1st edition 1989

2121/3130-543210 - Printed on acid-free paper

To Verena, Alexandra,
Patrick, and Benjamin

Foreword

Magnetic resonance imaging (MRI) is an established technique for visualizing normal anatomy and morphological pathology. Current research in magnetic resonance is directed towards the evaluation of organ function by examining the physiology of motion and flow, studying the clearance pathways of paramagnetic contrast material, and elucidating biochemical processes with magnetic resonance spectroscopy. This book on the morphology and function of the cardiovascular and renal systems as studied by MRI provides the reader with a comprehensive overview of the functional and hemodynamic aspects of the cardiovascular system and their effects on MRI. Magnetic resonance morphology and function of the heart and vascular system are discussed in two separate chapters. Renal morphology and function are analyzed in great detail both in normal patients and in pathological conditions, particularly in relation to the excretion of contrast material. The introductory physics chapter provides the basic notions of the physics and technology of magnetic resonance, which are essential for understanding concepts of motion and flow in MRI.

Based on extensive personal experience, the author succeeds brilliantly in providing a comprehensive insight into the problems of functional MRI of the cardiovascular system and the kidney. This book describes the current state of the art and supplies an essential baseline for future research in MRI of cardiovascular disease. As the author rightly states, the crossroads of physics and medicine in this technique is proving to be the crossroads of morphological and functional imaging. The author himself is admirably suited to write on the synthesis of physics, anatomy, physiology, and pathology, having a Ph.D. in physics and an M.D., being a radiologist, and having published frequently in peer-review journals. He also represents in a true sense the product of the best in European and American education, having been schooled on both continents and absorbing the essence of the culture and science of both. We are proud to introduce this excellent piece of work by our colleague to the scientific community.

Zurich   W. A. FUCHS
San Francisco   A. MARGULIS

Preface

Magnetic resonance imaging (MRI) has become a clinical tool over the past few years and is now widely accessible for patient care. Thus, an increasing number of physicians are exposed to this new imaging modality. The phenomenon of nuclear magnetic resonance has proved to be an extremely versatile and powerful tool in physics, chemistry, and biology, and the same can be expected in medicine. The initial clinical experience with depicting morphological pathology has supported this expectation. However, in addition to depicting morphology, MRI has tremendous potential for yielding information on organ function, particularly in three areas: in the examination of the physiology and pathophysiology of motion and flow, in the evaluation of the handling and the observation of clearance pathways of injected paramagnetic "markers", and in observing biochemical processes with magnetic resonance spectroscopy (MRS).

The contents of this book are directed towards clinicians, radiologists, nuclear medicine, cardiovascular and renal specialists alike, who want to educate themselves on the present status and the potentials of MRI for gaining information on the morphology and function of the cardiovascular and renal systems. At first glance, the choice of the clinical subspecialities treated in this book, the cardiovascular and renal systems, may look somewhat arbitrary. In a sense this is true. As a single-author book, this treatise is more subjective than a standard textbook, in that it reflects the author's areas of prime research interests. However, at second glance, the choice to discuss the cardiovascular and renal systems may not be so arbitrary at all. It is in these two organ systems where MRI is currently pushed to new frontiers of clinical application, and where there is a heavy emphasis on the interrelations between data on morphology and function in clinical practice. MRI is extremely motion and flow sensitive. It thus promises to be an ideal tool for investigating the cardiovascular system. In fact, the great vessel/soft tissue contrast in MRI is a result of blood flow and thus of cardiovascular function. Blood flow (and related CSF flow) phenomena are present on almost every clinical MR image, and in a sense, most images contain information on the cardiovascular system. In the kidney, which is involved in the excretion of most soluble substances from the body, the clearing function of such substances can be examined. Application of renally excreted contrast media in MRI, the ones presently available for clinical use, make the kidneys the only organ system in which the temporal evolution of the distribution of a bolus of injected paramagnetic contrast medium can be studied. Since MRI is innocuous, and arbitrary slice orientations can be obtained, long axis slices through the renal parenchyma can be looked at repeatedly over time, and function information extracted. With these capabilities to depict function in addition to morphology, MRI will form an important link between radiology, which is more directed towards identifying pathomorphology, and nuclear medicine, which emphasizes its ability to examine function abnormalities of organ systems. Thus, not only the clinician, but also the basic researcher may find in this book interesting information on the interrelation between morphology and function obtainable by MRI in these two organ systems. MRS will not be discussed, because with this potentially very powerful method few relevant clinical data are available as yet.

Understanding MR function imaging requires a more thorough understanding of the physical basis of MRI than does the acquisition of standard MR images to depict morphology. Thus, an introductory chapter on physics cannot be avoided, and it is an important goal of this book to present the physics of MR in a way that makes it possible for the clinician to grasp the basic concepts underlying the newest MRI tools. On the other hand, MR technology is completely left out, as it is of no relevance to the understanding of the concepts and the clinical applications presented.

Thus, in summary, this book places itself at two crossroads, the crossroad of physics and medicine and the crossroad of morphological and function imaging in MRI.

Acknowledgements. A large number of people have made this work possible, both spiritually and technically. Professor Alois Rüttimann and Dr. Jean-Pierre Stucky are almost fully responsible for getting me started on the MR track. It is therefore apt that my gratitude go to them first. Special thanks also go to the minister of health of Zurich, Dr. Peter Wiederkehr, who sent me for one fully salaried year to San Francisco, where it was possible to gain clinical MR experience at an early stage of its development. To the "San Franciscans", Professors Alex Margulis, chairman of the department, Hedvig Hricak, Larry Crooks, and particularly Charles B. Higgins, I am indebted for my MR training. It is due to the creative environment of their department that many of the ideas contained in this book were conceived. Professor Josef Wellauer, former chairman of our department, is gratefully acknowledged for supporting and bearing with this enthusiastic US-trained physician and homecomer, and for tolerating his American views on medical science in general and on the role of research in the radiologic sciences in particular. Many thanks also go to Professor Sven Paulin, chairman of the Department of Radiology, Beth Israel Hospital, Harvard Medical School, Boston, who spent a few extremely fruitful and stimulating weeks of his sabbatical in Zurich and infused me with another dose of American optimism.

Responsible for my being able to complete this work, and in such a relatively short time, was Professor Walter A. Fuchs, whose support during the first year of his term as chairman of our department was invaluable. His genuine understanding of my views and hopes made work on this book and in his department a joy. Many thanks also go to the department staff, in particular to Drs. Borut Marincek, Niels Augustiny, Michael Langlotz, and Thomas Vollrath, who in one way or another had to work extra hard, to permit me to have some hours for writing without having to think of clinical responsibilities. Particular gratitude goes to my two young research associates, Drs. Stefan Duewell and Rudolf Wüthrich, whose input into this book in terms of data has been considerable, and whose interest in research and willingness to work nights and weekends have laid the foundations for a scientific hothouse in our department. Thanks also go to Dr. Ron Kikinis, a one-time collaborator, and Dr. Walter Kuoni. Stimulating discussions with Drs. Chris Boesch, Graeme McKinnon, Dieter Meier, and Ian Young, among others, are gratefully acknowledged.

Many thanks go to the referring physicians in our hospital, who, by their willingness to send interesting patients, have contributed to the images in this work. These are Professors Rudolf Ammann, Alfred Bollinger, Dieter Hauri, Hans-Peter Krayenbühl, and Marko Turina. On the other end, close and cordial collaboration with Professor Olaf Kübler and his group from the Institute for Communication Research at the Swiss Federal Institute of Technology has made possible our ventures into sophisticated data analysis.

Material and technical support for this work has come from institutions and many individuals. Generous research support by the Swiss National Science Foundation, the Krebsliga des Kantons Zürich, Switzerland, and the Radium Stiftung Zürich, Switzerland, as well as continuing technical support by the Philips corporation and its Swiss subsidiary, is gratefully acknowledged. Paramagnetic contrast media were kindly provided by Schering AG, Berlin (Gd-DTPA), Guerbet SA, Paris (Gd-DOTA), and Dr. H.H.Peter, CIBA-Geigy AG (ferrioxamine derivatives), Basel. People who have contributed their time and effort in helping to create this book at various stages of completion are Ms. Susanne Dittus, Anni Fischer, Caterina Giudici, and Hadwig Speckbacher. Particular thanks go to the two skillful and intelligent secretaries who worked over my drafts, Ms. Antoinette Schumacher and Margrit Wyder, and to our photographer, Sandra Barmettler, who single-handedly produced each photograph in this book; their help has been invaluable.

Zurich 1988   G. K. VON SCHULTHESS

Contents

Chapter 3   The Effects of Motion and Flow on Magnetic Resonance Imaging

Chapter 4   Cardiac Morphology and Function in Magnetic Resonance Imaging

Chapter 5 Vascular Morphology and Function in Magnetic Resonance Imaging

Chapter 6 Renal Morphology and Function in Magnetic Resonance Imaging

Appendices

Introduction

Magnetic resonance imaging (MRI) has rapidly evolved from its first experimental clinical trials in 1980 to become a method that is used routinely and that is the primary modality for diagnosing such diseases as cerebral tumors and many musculoskeletal disorders such as avascular necrosis of the hip. In general, imaging the morphology of non-moving parts of the human body is no longer a challenge to MRI. However, in the chest and the abdomen, where nonsuppressible, physiologic motion prevails, MRI still has to prove its advantages. Despite this, there is little doubt that MRI will be a very useful imaging method also in the chest and the abdomen. The advantages of MRI result from the versatility of the nuclear magnetic resonance (NMR) phenomenon, and this versatility is only now beginning to be explored for imaging purposes. There are two important qualities of MRI in addition to its high spatial resolution that are likely to dominate future developments. First, the NMR phenomenon is extremely sensitive to motion and flow, which makes it potentially an ideal tool for producing images of cardiovascular function in addition to depicting cardiovascular morphology. Second, MRI is considerably more sensitive to paramagnetic substances introduced into the body than, e.g., computed tomography (CT) to radiologic contrast agents. This, combined with the fact that MRI is harmless and thus makes it possible to obtain multiple scans at the same level of the body, permits the acquisition of information on the temporal evolution of the distribution of injected contrast agents. For example, high-resolution dynamic scanning of the kidneys after bolus injection of a contrast agent is possible, providing a combination of morphological and function images as in the cardiovascular system. Such function scanning has proven to yield useful information in nuclear medicine and in CT scanning. The contents of this book focus on the combination of morphological and functional data provided by MRI, which now is rapidly evolving from a tool for morphological data gathering into an imaging modality also capable of function imaging. These properties of MRI make it likely that it will take a role somewhere in between radiology and nuclear medicine.

Even early investigators were aware that the NMR phenomenon was a useful tool for studying motion. Shortly after the discovery of the phenomenon by Bloch et al. [1] and Purcell et al. [2] in 1946, Hahn [3] noted that pulsed NMR experiments were affected by diffusion in fluids, and the theoretical analysis of this problem was published by Purcell et al. in 1954 [2]. As early as 1959, Singer used NMR to measure blood-flow rates [4]. In the late 1960s, Stejiskal and Tanner [5] developed a method by which they could strongly amplify MR sensitivity to motion by applying additional magnetic fields. It is interesting to note that a present-day imaging apparatus uses precisely such fields for an entirely different purpose, namely the spatial localization of the signal, thus accidentally sensitizing images to motion.

Parallel to the exploration of MR flow sensitivity, researchers became aware of the fact that paramagnetic impurities in a sample strongly affected the outcome of NMR experiments, by introducing "additional" internal magnetic fields. A first theory for paramagnetic impurities in solids was formulated by Bloembergen [6]. Experimental and theoretical studies decribing their effect in fluids were performed thereafter. Summaries of the effects of paramagnetic substances in biology were published in the early 1970s [7, 8].

In 1973 Lauterbur [9] and Mansfield and Grannell [10] proposed methods with which MR images could be obtained. In 1972 Damadian had put forward a scheme by which relaxation of biologic tissues of a small area in the body could be achieved [11]. This latter method, measuring just a single point in space at a time, clearly was too slow to be used in routine clinical imaging. However, by measuring an entire projection of an object at once, it was at least theoretically possible to measure a body cross section in a few minutes. In 1975 the group around Ernst [12] proposed imaging schemes called two- and three-dimensional Fourier transformation methods (2DFT and 3DFT), variants of which form the mainstay of today's reconstruction algorithms used in clinical MRI. It was soon recognized that other data acquisition schemes were possible in principle, i.e., using gradient echoes rather than spin echoes and partial flip-angle schemes, permitting data acquisition for a slice in seconds [13] rather than in minutes. This type of imaging begins to be implemented clinically now [14]. The fastest, but technically most demanding imaging technique, echo planar imaging, which can produce images in milliseconds, has shown some early promise [15, 16], but its technology ist not yet mature enough for it to be used routinely.

References

1. Bloch F, Hansen WW, Packard ME (1946) Nuclear induction. Phys Rev 69: 127
2. Purcell EM, Torrey HC, Pound RV (1946) Resonance absorption by nuclear magnetic moments in a solid. Phys Rev 69: 37
3. Hahn EL (1950) Spin echos. Phys Rev 80: 580
4. Singer JR (1959) Blood-flow rates by NMR measurements. Science 130: 1652–1655
5. Stejiskal EO, Tanner JE (1965) Spin diffusion measurements: spin echoes in the presence of a time-dependent field gradient. J Chem Phys 42: 288–292
6. Bloembergen N (1949) On the interaction of nuclear spins in a crystalline lattice. Physica 15: 386
7. La Mar GN, De Horrocks W, Hom RH (1973) NMR of paramagnetic molecules. Academic Press, New York
8. Dwek RA (1973) NMR in Biochemistry. Clarendon Press, New York
9. Lauterbur PC (1973) Image formation by induced local interactions. Examples employing nuclear magnetic resonance. Nature 242: 190
10. Mansfield P, Grannell PK (1973) NMR 'diffraction' in solids. J Phys C6, L422
11. Damadian R (1974) Apparatus and method for detecting cancer in tissue. US Patent #3,789,832
12. Kumar A, Welti D, Ernst RR (1975) NMR Fourier zeugmatography. J Mag Resonance 18: 63–89
13. Haase A, Mattaei D, Hänicke W, Merboldt KD (1986) Flash imaging: rapid NMR imaging using low flip-angle pulses. J Magnetic Resonance 67: 258–266
14. Utz JA, Herfkens RJ, Heinsimer JA (1987) Cine MR determination of left ventricular ejection fraction. AJR 148: 839–843
15. Mansfield P, Morris PG (1982) NMR imaging in biomedicine. Academic Press, New York
16. Rzedzian RR, Pykett IL (1987) Instant images of the human heart using a new, whole-body MR imaging system. AJR 149: 245–250

Chapter 1   The Physical Basis of Magnetic Resonance Imaging

1.1 The Nuclear Magnetic Resonance Effect

With the term "spin" we characterize a property of elementary particles such as protons and electrons which can be understood only within the theoretical framework of quantum mechanics. Thus, the NMR phenomenon is quantum mechanical in na-

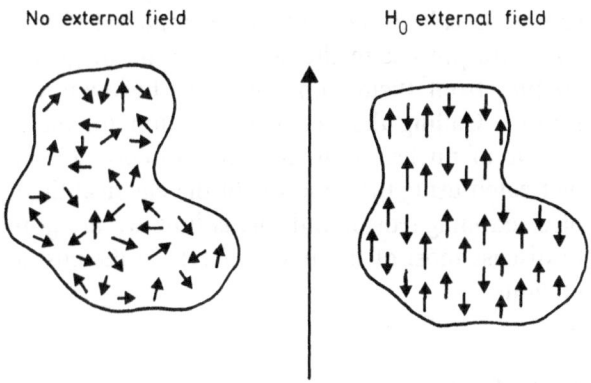

No external field H_0 external field

Fig. 1.1. The protons in a sample outside a magnetic field are oriented randomly. When an external magnetic field H_o is applied, there are two possible orientations for the component along the external field: either parallel or antiparallel. There are slightly more spins pointing along the energetically more favorable direction

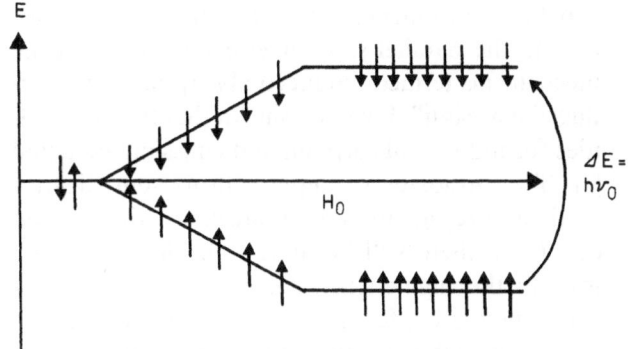

Fig. 1.2. The difference between the two energy levels ΔE increases in proportion to the strength of the external field H_o and is zero without external field. If an electromagnetic wave with the proper frequency v impinges on the sample, some spins will change from the energetically more favorable state into the less favorable state and vice versa

ture. Nevertheless, NMR can be understood using simple physical models from classical physics. We like to think of a spin as something like a compass needle, which will orient itself along an external magnetic field if it is placed in it. Being governed by the laws of quantum mechanics, spins can align not only parallel, but also antiparallel to an external field. Thus, a system of spins pointing in all spatial directions outside a magnetic field, will end up with some spins aligned parallel and some antiparallel to an external magnetic field, once such a field is applied (Fig. 1.1).

The state in which the spin is aligned parallel to the magnetic field is energetically more favorable than the one in which the spin is antiparallel, and the difference between the energies ΔE of the parallel and the antiparallel state is a linear function of the magnitude of the external magnetic field H_o and the magnetic moment of a proton $\mu = \gamma_p h/4\pi$. For a proton this energy difference is

$$\Delta E = -2\mu H_o = -\gamma_p h H_o/2\pi \qquad (1.1)$$

where γ_p is the magnetogyric ratio of the proton ($\gamma_p = 2.6752 \times 10^8$ rad s^{-1} Tesla^{-1} = 2.6752×10^4 rad s^{-1} Gauss^{-1}, h is Planck's constant (6.6262×10^{-34} Joule s = 6.6262×10^{-27} erg s, and $\pi = 3.1415$. Hence, the energy needed to lift a spin from the low- into the high-energy state (Fig. 1.2) grows in proportion with the external magnetic field.

1.1.1 Boltzmann Distribution

If the spins can align parallel and antiparallel to the field, the question arises as to how they are distributed between the two states, as the difference in number between parallel and antiparallel spins determines the net magnetization of a sample. A system of independent nuclear spins, being in thermal equilibrium with its environment, obeys the Boltzmann distribution law. If we call the number of proton spins per unit volume in the lower energy state N_o, then the number of proton spins N per unit volume in the higher energy state is given by [1]

$$N = N_o exp(-\Delta E/k_B T)$$

$$= N_o exp(-\gamma_p h H_o/2\pi k_B T), \qquad (1.2a)$$

where T (degrees Kelvin) is the absolute temperature and k_B is Boltzmann's constant ($k_B = 1.3807 \times 10^{-23}$ Joule Kelvin^{-1} = 1.3807×10^{-16} erg Kelvin^{-1}). Thus, at room temperature with T = 300° and a field strength of 1 Tesla, the ratio $N/N_o = 1-7 \times 10^{-6}$, that is, there are roughly only 7 spins in two million in the lower than in the higher engery state. In this limit Eq. 1.2a can be written as (Appendix A)

$$N = N_o(1 - \gamma_p h H_o/2\pi k_B T) \qquad (1.2b)$$

The fact that the ratio $\gamma_p h H_o/2\pi k_B T$ is only on the order of 10^{-5}-10^{-6} tells us that the NMR phenomenon is a low-energy phenomenon. The thermal energy in the environment $k_B T$ is much higher, and the energy needed to disrupt molecular bounds is even another factor of 10^2 higher, hence the safety of MRI in living systems. It is the slight difference in the population of the two energy levels which is responsible for the net magnetization of a sample containing spins when placed into a magnetic field.

1.1.2 Magnetic Susceptibility

The magnetization M ist the volume density of magnetic dipole moments or the magnetic moment per unit volume of the sample. Its component in the direction of the magnetic field M_z is readily computed using Eq. 1.2b:

$$M_z = (N_o - N)\mu = (N_o - N)\gamma_p h/4\pi$$

$$= N_o\gamma_p h/4\pi \{1 - (1 - \gamma_p h H_o/2\pi k_B T)\}$$

$$= N_o\gamma_p^2 h^2 H_o/8\pi^2 k_B T$$

$$= N\gamma_p^2 h^2 H_o/4\pi^2 k_B T \qquad (1.3)$$

The factor $\chi_C = N\gamma_p^2 h^2/4\pi^2 k_B T$ is called the Curie susceptibility for a system of protons, with N being the number of spins per unit volume. i.e., $N \approx 2N_o \approx 2N$. Equation 1.3 shows that is the very simple case of protons the magnetization of a sample is proportional to the applied magnetic field, and in

fact many substances behave in this way. In classical electromagnetism the proportionality factor between magnetization M_z and the magnetic field H_o for isotropic substances is the magnetic susceptibility χ:

$$M = \chi H_o \qquad (1.4)$$

The susceptibility is a measure of how strongly a given sample can be magnetized, that is, how many spins of what strength are present in a unit volume of the sample under study. When a sample contains unpaired proton (or neutron) spins or unpaired electrons which can align in an external magnetic field, the susceptibility is positive and the sample is called paramagnetic. However, if spins are paired, canceling the magnetic moments of each other to first order, the electrons tend to screen off and hence reduce the external magnetic field inside a sample. Then the susceptibility is negative and the sample is called diamagnetic. If unpaired electron spins are present in the substance, the magnetism coming from them dominates the behavior of a sample. Calling the net magnetization for an ensemble of nuclear spins M, such an ensemble can be treated using the concepts of the classical theory of electromagnetism, and this is how we are going to discuss most of the NMR effects in the ensuing sections.

1.1.3 The Resonance Phenomenon

The NMR phenomenon is based on the fact that in a system of nuclear spins transitions between low- and high-energy states present in the external magnetic field can be achieved by irradiating the sample with electromagnetic waves. These waves are capable of producing a transition from the antiparallel to the parallel state or vice versa through the mechanisms termed "induced absorption" and "induced emission". It can be shown that the probabilities for induced absorption and emission are equal [2]. If we irradiate a sample with its spins distributed according to the Boltzmann distribution (Eq. 1.2a), there will be more transitions from the low- to the high-energy state than vice versa because there are a few more spins in the low-energy state. Eventually, the numbers will be equalized and the system is what is termed "saturated". After irradiation, the spin system is no longer in thermal equilibrium. The relaxation mechanism back to equilibrium occurs through interactions of the spins with the surrounding molecules of the "lattice" (hence the term "spin-lattice" relaxation discussed below), which by their motion generate small electromagnetic fields and can absorb electromagnetic waves, and thus come into resonance with the spin system. It is important to note that in induced emission the emitted wave has a fixed relation of its phase to the initially absorbed wave (Fig. 1.3). The result is that NMR is sensitive to intrinsic or extrinsic effects producing phase changes, hence as an example of an external phase change forced upon the system - the possibility to use phase encoding in 2DFT imaging, or - as an example of an intrinsic phase change - to detect motion by its effect on phase (Chapter 3). This is a fundamental difference to nuclear medicine, where the emission of γ-rays through radioactive decay occurs spontaneously and the phase of this electromagnetic wave contains no useful information.

Assume now a system of spins which has been saturated by irradiation with a pulse of electromagnetic waves and thus has as many spins in the parallel as in the antiparallel state. This system relaxes back to a state where the difference in the spin populations is governed by the thermal equilibrium condition of Eq. 1.2a. However, it can relax back only by exchanging energy with the surrounding molecules, as will be discussed in Sect. 1.3. In the equilibrium state the probability W_+ for a spin to absorb energy from the surroundings and to change from the low- into the high-energy state, times the number of spins N_0 in the low-energy state, has to equal the probability W_+ for a spin to give off energy to the surroundings and thus to change from the high- to the low-energy state, times the number of spins N in the high-energy state:

$$W_+ N_0 =$$
$$W_- N = W_- N_0 \exp(-\gamma_p h H_o / 2\pi k_B T)$$
or
$$W_+ / W_- = \exp(-\gamma_p h H_o / 2\pi k_B T) \qquad (1.5)$$

In the saturated state away from equilibrium the numbers of spins in the lower and higher energy states are both $(N + N_0)/2$ or $N_0 - n_0$ and $N + n_0$, respectively, where $n_0 = (N_0 - N)/2$ (Fig. 1.4). The population of the lower state is n_0 away from its final state and so is the population of the upper state (Fig. 1.4).

The rate of change of n back to the equilibrium dn/dt can again be expressed in terms of the transition probability W_+ and W_- and the populations of the spins at the two levels:

$$dn/dt = W_+(N_0 - n) - W_-(N + n)$$

$$= W_+ N_0 - W_- N + (W_+ + W_-)n$$

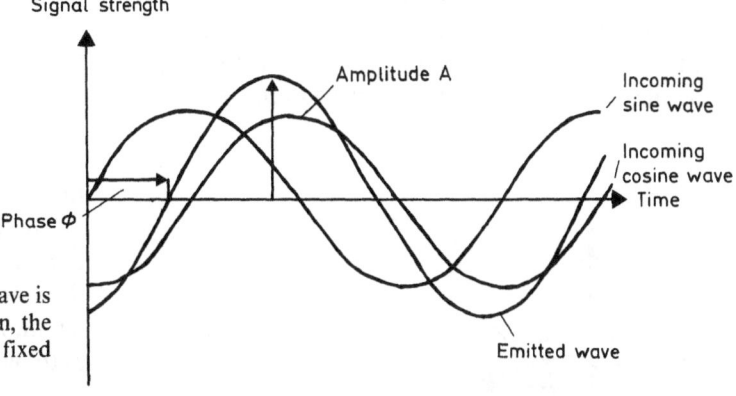

Fig. 1.3. In a simple NMR experiment, the incoming wave is a sine or cosine wave. In the process of induced emission, the electromagnetic wave emitted from the sample has a fixed phase Φ relative to the incoming wave

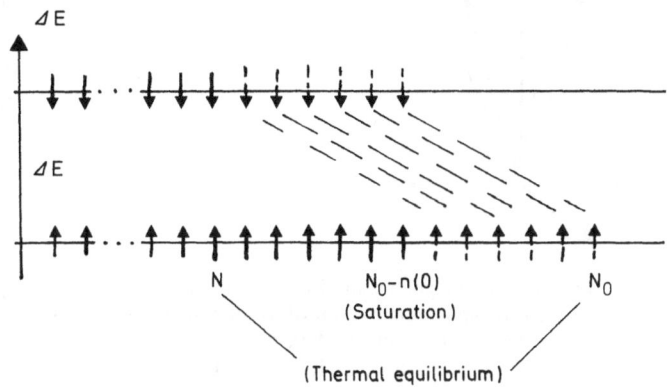

Fig. 1.4. In thermal equilibrium, there are $2n(0) = N_0 - N$ more spins in the lower than in the higher energy state. The difference between populations is very small, on the order of 1–10 spins per million. Upon irradiation of the sample with a saturation pulse, this equilibrium will be disturbed and one finds equal numbers of spins in the high- and the low-energy state

With $1/T1 = W_+ + W_-$ and $W_+N_o - W_-N = 0$ (Eq. 1.5) this equation takes the form

$$dn/dt = -n/T1 \qquad (1.6)$$

where T1 is the "spin-lattice" relaxation time. The inverse of the spin-lattice relaxation time is thus the sum of the probabilities of the spin system to gain or lose some energy respectively. Upon integration of Eq. 1.6 we find the solution

$$n = n_o[1 - \exp(-t/T1)]$$

Since the magnetization M_z in the direction of the main magnetic field H_o, which henceforth will be assumed to lie along the z-axis, is proportional to the number difference of parallel and antiparallel spins (Eq. 1.3), we obtain by analogy to Eq. 1.6 an expression for the rate of change of magnetization

$$dM_z/dt = (M_{zo} - M_z)/T1 \qquad (1.7)$$

where M_{zo} is the thermal equilibrium magnetization. In general, in an NMR experiment a sample is irradiated with a pulse of an electromagnetic wave. As a result, the magnetization, initially aligned along the axis of the main field, tips away from this direction and starts to precess, describing a circle in the plane perpendicular to the main field (Fig. 1.5). This precession is the result of the equations of motion for a system of magnets subject to a torque by an external field and is quite analogous to the precession of a top. If the magnetization vector has

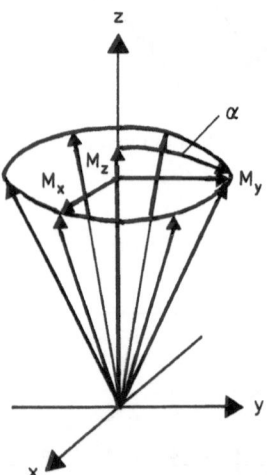

Fig. 1.5. The net magnetization M_z along the main magnetic field is tilted by some angle α out of its alignment parallel to the z-axis. The component of M in the xy-plane, M_{xy}, precesses, that is, it rotates on a circle around the z-axis

been tipped by an external field pulse (an electromagnetic wave pulse), thus altering the magnitude of M_z, Eq. 1.7 describes how M_z grows back after the pulse has been turned off. On the other hand, if such a pulse has generated a magnetization in the xy-plane perpendicular to the main magnetic field, the M_x and M_y components of the magnetization will disappear after the pulse because the magnetic moment tends to line up with the main field H_z. If we assume that the disappearance of these magnetizations happens with a characteristic time T2, we have

$$dM_x/dt = M_x/T2$$
$$dM_y/dt = -M_y/T2 \qquad (1.8)$$

These equations represent the simplest form of the so-called Bloch equations, which describe the behavior of the temporal evolution of the magnetization of a spin system subject to external magnetic fields [3], and their solutions are

$$M_z = M_{zo}[1 - \exp(-t/T1)]$$
$$M_{xy} = M_{xyo}\exp(-t/T2) \qquad (1.9)$$

T1, as well as T2, depends on the interaction of the spin system with its environment and contains much of the information which we are interested in obtaining in MRI. T1 and T2 are strongly influenced by the texture of biologic tissues, by paramagnetic substances in these tissues, and by motion. Thus, it will be a central task in the following sections to obtain some understanding of how the biologic environment influences these relaxation times.

The precession of the magnetic moment around the z-axis occurs at the resonance frequency, called the Larmor frequency, that is in phase with the oscillations of the pulse of the incoming electromagnetic wave. The relation between the resonance frequency and the magnetic field strength is obtained from Eq. 1.1 by noting that the energy of an electromagnetic wave is proportional to its frequency v_o and that the angular velocity ω_o is related to v_o by $v_o = 2\pi\omega_o$

$$\Delta E = hv_o = h\omega_o/2\pi = \gamma_p hH_o/2\pi$$
or
$$\omega_o = \gamma_p H_o \qquad (1.10)$$

With the values given above and a magnetic field strength of 1 Tesla we find that $v_o = 42.5 \times 10^7$ Hz = 42.6 MHz. Thus, for the typical field strengths used in MRI, the resonance frequencies are in the radiofrequency (RF) range, and an NMR experiment requires an RF wave generator and an RF amplifier.

For the sake of convenience, the theoretical analysis of the precessional motion in NMR is carried out in a so-called rotating frame; that is, we imagine analyzing events by looking from a reference frame which rotates about the main magnetic field H_{zo} with the frequency ν_o. In such a frame, only magnetization vectors precessing somewhat faster or slower than with a frequency ν_o will be seen to move away from their initial position. In our further discussions we shall take our vantage point on the rotating coordinate frame.

1.2 Diffusion

NMR in liquid samples is strongly influenced by diffusion processes, as was already recognized by Carr and Purcell [4], and it does not have to be emphasized that diffusion processes are extremely important in living systems. Since diffusion strongly influences the speed of the relaxation processes in NMR and thus the values of the relaxation times T1 and T2, it is necessary to make a short digression into the physics of diffusion. Diffusion occurs in all systems where molecules randomly jiggle around by bumping into the molecules surrounding them. Molecules in a liquid environment show not only translational but also rotational diffusive motion. As will be seen, the distance over which a diffusing molecule travels (or the angle through which it rotates) in a given time span depends on the size of the molecule, the characteristics of the medium (viscosity), and the temperature. This latter is the case because the higher the temperature, the more thermal energy a molecule possesses, which makes it jiggle around faster and thus bump into other molecules more often. In addition, the viscosity itself is a function of temperature.

To get a quantitative understanding of the diffusion process we want to analyze the simplest possible "diffusion" problem. A molecule, let us say a water molecule, is bumped into by another water molecule (Fig. 1.6). We assume that by such a bump it is moved equally likely to the left or the right by a distance a. We are interested in finding out where this molecule is after i bumps. If the molecule has arrived at an average position $<X_{i-1}>$ after $i-1$ bumps, the next bump will either push it to $<X_{i-1}> + a$ or $<X_{1-1}> - a$, on the average the molecule will end up at

$$<X_i> = (<X_{i-1}> + a + <X_{i-1}> - a)/2$$
$$= <X_{i-1}> \qquad (1.11)$$

Since the molecule was at a position $X_o = 0$ before the first bump, on the average it will still be at position 0 after the first bump according to Eq. 1.11, and the same is true for X_2, X_3, etc., as is clear from the iterative relation of Eq. 1.11. As expected, on the average the position of the molecule remains at zero, independent of the number of bumps, as it is equally likely to move towards the left or the right in each step. However, this position is only the most probable but not the only position the molecule could be at after i bumps (Fig. 1.6). In fact, a statistical analysis can provide the probability of finding a molecule a given distance away from its intitial position after i bumps. A measure of the width of such a probability distribution function can be obtained by computing the mean square distance $<X_i^2>$. Proceeding the same way as we did to obtain Eq. 1.11, we find that, given $<X_{i-1}^2>$, the expected value of X_i^2, $<X_i^2>$ is the average of the two expressions

$$<(X_{i-1} - a)^2> = <X_{i-1}^2> - 2a<X_i> + a^2$$

$$<(X_{i-1} + a)^2> = <X_{i-1}^2> + 2a<X_i> + a^2$$

$$\begin{aligned}<X_i^2> &= \{<(X_{i-1} - a)^2> + \\ &\quad <X_{i-1} + a>^2\}/2 \\ &= <X_{i-1}^2> + a^2 \qquad (1.12)\end{aligned}$$

Since for $i = 1$, $<X_{i-1}^2> = 0$, $<X_1^2> = a^2$, $<X_2^2> = a^2 + a^2 = 2a^2$ etc., we obtain

$$<X_i^2> = ia^2 \text{ or } \sqrt{<X_i^2>} = a\sqrt{i} \qquad (1.13)$$

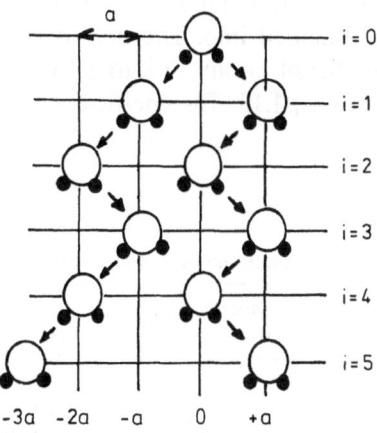

Fig. 1.6. A water molecule engaged in a one-dimensional random walk gets hit by other molecules and takes a step *a* to the right or the left with each bump i

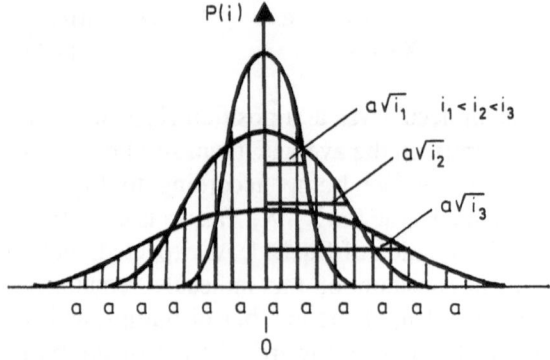

Fig. 1.7. The probability distribution function P(i) of finding a molecule at a position $\pm a$, $\pm 2a$, $\pm 3a$, etc. gets flatter, the more bumps the molecule has undergone since its start. The standard deviation, which is a measure of the width of the probability distribution function, is proportional to the square root of the number of bumps $\sqrt{i}$

Hence, the width or standard deviation of the probability function (Fig. 1.7) of finding a molecule sitting initially at zero is proportional to the square root of the number of bumps i, and if we assume a fixed number of bumps per unit of time, it is also proportional to the time elapsed: the propability distribution function becomes wider and flatter with increasing time (Fig. 1.7). The simple model yields similar results if expanded to a three-dimensional random walk of molecules. For molecules in solution if can be shown that

$$<x^2> \ = \ 2(k_B T/6\pi r\eta)t \ = \ 2Dt \qquad (1.14)$$

where k_B is again the Boltzmann constant, T the absolute temperature, $\pi = 3.1415$, r the radius of the molecule and η the coefficient of viscosity. The term in parentheses is called the diffusion constant D, and the above expression is called the Stokes-Einstein relation. In a sence, D is a measure of the distance over which a molecule moves more or less straight after being bumped into. The time is proportional to the number of bumps or i, thus the analogy of Eq. 1.14 with Eq. 1.13. The coefficient D is

for translational diffusion. In similar ways, a rotational diffusion constant D_{rot} can be defined, which relates the angle of rotation Φ to time t.

$$<\Phi^2> \ = \ 2(k_B T/8\pi r\eta)t/r^2 \ = \ 2D_{rot}t/r^2 \qquad (1.15)$$

Values for the translational coefficients are shown in Table 1.1. As will be seen in the next section, these relations between mean square distance or mean square angle and the time are extremely important for the understanding of relaxation mechanisms.

1.3 Relaxation Mechanisms

1.3.1 T1 and T2 Relaxation

The relaxation processes determining the temporal changes of the magnetization in an NMR experiment (Eqs. 1.7 and 1.9) are intimately linked to diffusion in the sample under investigation, because the jiggling molecules can set up oscillating magnetic fields at the place of a nuclear spin (Fig. 1.8). These oscillating fields are precondition that transitions from the high- to the low-energy state in the nuclear spin system occur. It is by such mechanisms that the spin system gives up energy to the surrounding molecules, i.e., the lattice, hence the term "spin-lattice" relaxation. It will be recalled that when writing the equation for the relaxation of the magnetization in the z-direction along the main magnetic field (Eq. 1.6), we defined 1/T1 as the sum of the probabilities per unit time of a transition from the high- to the low-energy and the low- to the high-energy state. It is the aim of this section to provide insight into the nature of these relaxation processes in biologic systems.

Since the oscillating fields set up by the molecules have to have the proper frequency at which they can be in resonance with the nuclear spin system, we have to know what kind of oscillating field

Table 1.1. Translational and rotational diffusion coefficients

Molecule	Molecular weight	Radius ($m \times 10^{-10}$)	Translatinal diffusion coefficient (m^2/s)
Water	18	≈ 1.5	2.0×10^{-9}
Glucose	180	≈ 5	6.7×10^{-10}
Hemoglobin	68 000	≈ 31.0	6.9×10^{-11}
Catalase	250 000	≈ 52.2	4.1×10^{-11}
Tobacco mosaic virus	50 000 000		3.9×10^{-12}

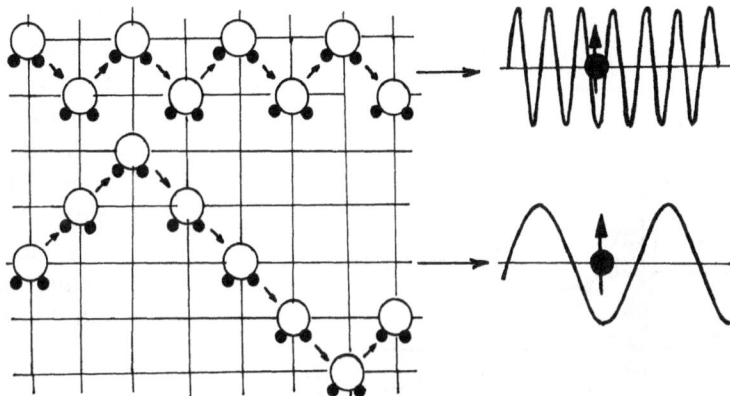

Fig. 1.8. Molecules undergoing their zigzag random walk give rise to small oscillating magnetic fields. The frequency range of these fields is from very low (molecules being pushed in the same direction with each bump) up to high frequencies (molecules being pushed forward and then backward with each random walk jump)

frequencies molecules can generate when they tumble and jiggle around in their diffusive random walk. Obviously, the highest frequencies occurring are the ones where a molecule is bumped into alternately from, let's say, above and below like the top molecule in Fig. 1.8, but, as shown with the bottom molecule in this figure, lower frequencies of oscillation are also possible. If we can estimate the average distance or angle over which a molecule in solution moves before it changes its direction or orientation, we can figure out from the Stokes-Einstein relation (Eqs. 1.14 and 1.15) over what typical time scale τ_c a molecule keeps its direction of motion or rotation. τ_c is called the correlation time (time over which the motion is typically correlated to the previous state of motion). A water molecule, for example, will move approximately a distance its own size before it turns around. From Table 1.1 and Eq. 1.14 we can compute τ_c to be on the order of 10^{-12} s. For a larger molecule like hemoglobin, which will also travel approximately its size before it turns around, τ_c is more on the order of 10^{-8} s. Knowing the time τ_c, we can estimate the frequencies up to which the jiggling and tumbling molecules produce oscillating fields. This is done as follows: Assume that we freeze all molecules in place and then let them go at time zero. It is reasonable to suppose that the number of molecules $-dN$ which undergo a collision and therefore lose correlation to their initial state of motion during a time interval dt is proportional to the number of molecules and the probability P per unit time that the molecule undergoes a collision changing its state of motion. Thus

$$-dN = PNdt \qquad (1.16)$$

This probability is just the average number of colli-

sions which occur per second, that is, $1/\tau_c$ because τ_c is the average time between collisions. Integration of Eq. 1.16 yields

$$N/No = \exp(-t/\tau_c) \qquad (1.17)$$

This function is called correlation function, as it tells us the fraction of molecules that are still moving the same way a time t after time zero, thus whose motion is still correlated to their initial state of motion. The distribution of frequencies generated by molecules characterized by a correlation time τ_c is obtained by obtaining the Fourier transform of Eq. 1.17. A Fourier transformation is a mathematical method used, for example, to extract information on the frequency components contained in time varying signals (see Sect. 1.2.4 and Appendix C). The distribution function of these frequencies generated by an exponential correlation function like the one of Eq. 1.17, called spectral density function $J(\omega)$, has typically the form

$$J(\omega) = \tau_c/(1 + \omega^2\tau_c^2) \qquad (1.18)$$

This distribution function of frequencies is plotted in Fig. 1.9 for different values of τ_c, with our water molecule being represented by the curve labeled τ_{c4}, whereas a hemoglobin molecule would be characterized more typically by the curve with τ_{c2}. This function tells us what fraction of molecular jiggling or tumbling motions will produce oscillating fields in a given frequency range $\Delta\omega$, e.g., around the Larmor frequency ω_o. The more such oscillations occur around ω_o, the more effective is the relaxation or the higher is the relaxation rate $1/T1$. Since in MRI we are using Larmor frequencies ω_o on the

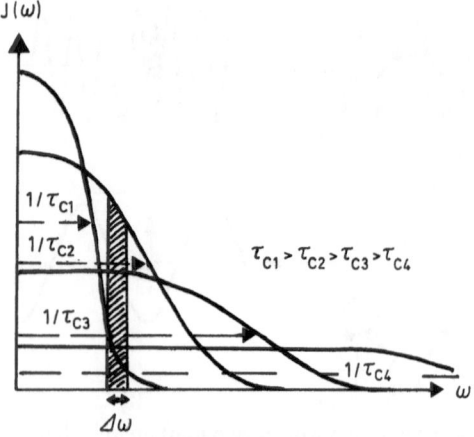

Fig. 1.9. The spectral density function J(ω) tells us how many electromagnetic wavelets per unit volume within a given frequency range Δω are induced by the jiggling motions of molecules in a sample. The shorter the correlation time τ_c, the wider the function J(ω)

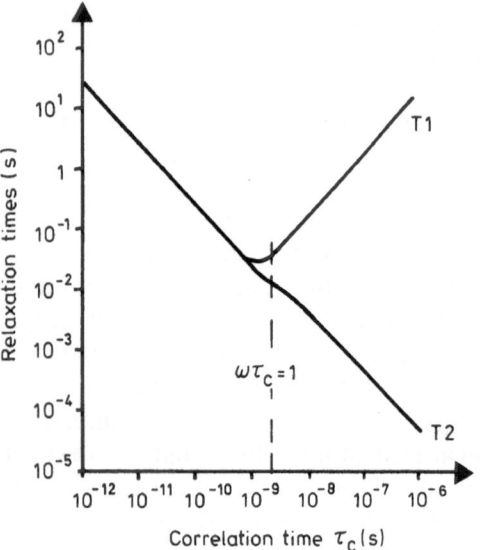

Fig. 1.10. The T1 and T2 relaxation times are functions of the molecular correlation time τ_c. Whereas T2 relaxation is increasingly more efficient with increasing correlation times, T1 relaxation efficiency is maximal when $\omega\tau_c \approx 1$. (With permission from Gadian et al. [9])

order of 10^7–10^8 Hz, a jiggling or tumbling macromolecule like hemoglobin will produce more field oscillations with suitable frequencies than a water molecule (Fig. 1.9).

In addition, it can be expected that the relaxation is the more effective, the stronger the oscillating molecular field. Since the power of the electromagnetic field is proportional to the square of the molecular magnetic field H_m, we expect the relaxation rate 1/T1 to have the following form:

1/T1 proportional to $H_{mxy}^2 J(\omega)$

$$H_{mxy}^2 J(\omega) = H_{mxy}^2 \tau_c / (1 + \omega^2 \tau_c^2) \tag{1.19}$$

The indices xy denote that only magnetic fields in the xy-plane, i.e., perpendicular to the direction of the magnetization M_z, can alter its value. In Fig. 1.10, T1 is plotted for H_2O as a function of the correlation time and a resonance frequency $\nu = 2\pi\omega = 100$ MHz. Here we assume that by some magic mechanism we can vary the correlation time. It is seen that it is shortest for values of $\omega\tau_c = 1$ corresponding to the case τ_{c2} in the spectral density function of Fig. 1.9. Thus, molecules having a correlation time on the order of 10^{-9}–10^{-8} s will produce the shortest T1 relaxation times.

Let us now consider T2 relaxation. T2 is the time constant which describes the decrease of the magnetization in the xy-plane M_{xy}, which is generated by tilting M_z out of its orientation parallel to the z-axis (Fig. 1.5) and the main magnetic field H_0. If the only field present is H_0, there is a single resonance frequency ω_0, and there will be no decay of M_{xy}. However, if there are local variations in the main magnetic field H_0 for some reason, there will be a range $\Delta\omega_0$ of precession frequencies around ω_0. In the rotating coordinate frame (Sect. 1.1.3), only the spins precessing with ω_0 will remain fixed; the oth-

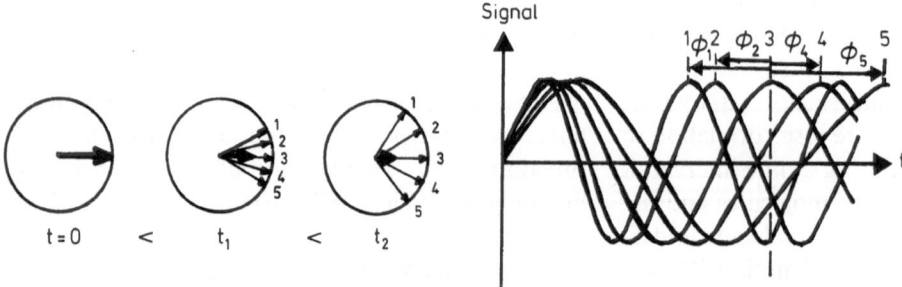

Fig. 1.11. If there are local variations in the main magnetic field, spins at various locations precess at different Larmor frequencies. Thus, some spins precess faster, others slower, and the wavelets emitted by them quickly lose coherence; that is, their relative phase differences quickly increase with time

ers will start to move ahead or lag behind (Fig. 1.11). The net magnetization, which is the vector sum (Appendix B) of all components, will thus start to decrease, and the greater the range of frequency spread, the quicker the decrease of M_{xy}; that is: $1/T2 \approx \Delta\omega_o$, because $\Delta\omega_o$ measures how many more (fewer) times per second the fastest (slowest) spins go around on the circle relative to the ones with ω_o. Once the fastest (slowest) are ahead (lag) by one revolution, M_{xy} has decreased considerably. Spin-spin relaxation therefore occurs due to all processes that produce a spread of the resonance line width. Such a spread comes about through the H-field fluctuations producing the T1 relaxation process. In fact, the finite lifetime of a spin in a given energy state is determined by the Heisenberg uncertainty principle [5]: $\Delta E T1 = T1h\Delta\omega_o/2 \approx h$ or $\Delta\omega_o \approx 1/T1$. Thus, all processes that cause spin-lattice relaxation also produce spin-spin relaxation, and T2 cannot be longer than T1. However, for spin-spin relaxation, the local field does not have to oscillate in synchrony with the spins to produce relaxation. Even a local field variation not oscillating in time will be able to produce a spreading of spins as shown in Fig. 1.11. Thus, the frequencies around zero ($\omega = 0$) in the spectral density function will also contribute to spin-spin relaxation and can dominate T2 relaxation, so that it is usually much shorter than T1 in biologic systems. As with T1 relaxation, the power of the magnetic field will also determine the relaxation efficiency; thus

$$1/T2 \text{ proportional to } H_{mz}{}^2\tau_c \qquad (1.20)$$

where H_{mz} designates the component of the local molecular field perpendicular to the magnetization M_{xy}. In Fig. 1.10, T2 is also plotted as a function of the correlation time for a frequency of 100 MHz. The small irregularity in the steadily decreasing curve is the result of a somewhat more detailed calculation of the T2 dependence on τ_c. Note that for correlation times smaller than 10^{-9}–10^{-8} s, T1 and T2 differ strongly. This corresponds to a situation where the molecules rotate and translate so slowly that they cannot produce oscillating fields with frequencies around ω_o, corresponding to the case of τ_{c1} in Fig. 1.9.

After this general discussion we are going to take a closer look at the different relaxation mechanisms effective in biologic systems.

1.3.2 Interactions Producing Relaxation

There are a number of relaxation mechanisms which have been recognized to influence T1 and T2. In biologic systems in most instances the dominant mechanism seems to be the so-called dipole-dipole relaxation process. In this mechanism, it is the interaction of a dipole on one molecule which interacts with another dipole on the same molecule (Fig. 1.12). The local magnetic field H_m of one dipole S sensed by the other dipole I is given by

$$H_m = \mu_s f(\Theta)/r_{IS}{}^3 \qquad (1.21)$$

where f is a function of the angle Θ between the main magnetic field and the distance r_{IS} between the two dipoles and μ_s is the magnetic moment of dipole S. As the molecule goes through its random tumbling motions, the angle Θ varies, and dipole S thereby sets up an oscillating field at the position of dipole I. For dipole-dipole interactions the relaxation rates 1/T1 and 1/T2 thus vary with $1/r_{IS}{}^6$ (Eqs. 1.19 and 1.20), and the strength of this interaction is strongly dependent on the separation of the two dipoles because it decreases with the inverse distance to the sixth power! As discussed in the section on diffusion, the correlation time τ_{cR} for the tumbling motion of a water molecule is on the order of 10^{-12} s. However, in body tissues, a large fraction of the water molecules (up to 10%) are protein bound and diffuse, with characteristics of the protein to which they are bound rather than those of free water. For proteins the tumbling correlation time τ_{cR} is much longer than that of a free water molecule, on the order of 10^{-9}–10^{-8} s. According to Fig. 1.10, relaxation is much more effective for

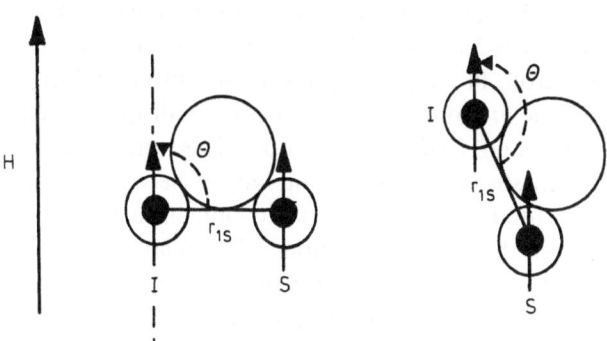

Fig. 1.12. The two protons of a water molecule aligned along an external field change the spatial orientation of their respective spins as the water molecule tumbles. This change in spatial orientation gives rise to small, fluctuating electromagnetic fields

the bound than for the free water molecules. If the correlation time τ_{ce} characterizing the exchange between free and bound molecules is substantially shorter than T1 (fast-exchange regime), the relaxation rate 1/T1, i.e., the probability per unit time of relaxation for such a system, is the sum of the probabilities that a bound or a free molecule of water relaxes. The relaxation process is then simply an average of the relaxation of the free and bound water relaxations. Since τ_{ce} is in the range of 10^{-6}-10^{-5} s, the fast-exchange limit applies. If we denote the fraction of bound water molecules F_b and the relaxation rates of bound and free molecules $(1/T1)_b$ and $(1/T1)_f$, respectively, we have [6]

$$(1/T1) = (1/T1)_b F_b + (1/T1)_f(1 - F_b)$$
$$\quad\quad\quad\quad\text{bound}\quad\quad\quad\quad\text{free}$$

$$= (1/T1)_f + F_b\{(1/T1)_b - (1/T1)_f\} \quad (1.22)$$

Provided that the relaxation rate of the bound water molecules does not depend on the concentration of the water in the sample, the overall relaxation rate 1/T1 is proportional to the fraction of bound water F_b. This has been found to be true experimentally. T2 relaxation of the bound water molecules is much faster than T1 relaxation, because for tumbling macromolecules we are in the regime with $\omega\tau_c \approx 1$ rather than in the regime $\omega\tau_c \ll 1$ (Fig. 1.10).

1.3.3 Paramagnetic Relaxation

Relaxation enhancement due to the paramagnetic substances in biological tissues is extremely important because such substances are abundantly present in vivo. Also, paramagnetic agents can be introduced into the body to alter tissue contrast. Paramagnetic ions are typically transition metals (Mn, Fe) or lanthanides (Gd, Eu, Dy), which have unpaired 3d and 4f electrons, respectively. Since an electron, like a proton, has a spin and therefore a magnetic moment, it can interact with the nuclear spins and produce relaxation. This interaction is much stronger than the interaction between nuclei because the electron magnetic moment is 658 times larger than that of protons. The relaxation rates 1/T1 and 1/T2 are again determined by relaxation mechanisms similar to spin-lattice relaxation for nuclear spins, and in fact, in paramagnetic relaxation the electrons are part of the lattice. Theoretical expressions for the relaxation rates of a system of nuclear spins in the presence of paramagnetic substances were found in the early days of NMR in

the form of the Solomon-Bloembergen equations [7, 8]. These equations contain terms like the ones in Eqs. 1.19 and 1.20:

$$\tau_c/(1 + \omega_I^2\tau_c^2) \text{ and } \tau_c/(1 + \omega_S^2\tau_c^2)$$

where ω_I and ω_S are the proton and electron Larmor frequency, respectively, the latter being higher by a factor of 658. Thus, the paramagnetic relaxation mechanisms are also dependent on the correlation times, which determine the time scales of the interactions between nuclear and electron spins sitting on various types of molecules. For small paramagnetic ions or metal complexes such as Gd^{3+} and Gd-DTPA, dipole-dipole coupling seems again to be the dominant relaxation mechanism [9]. The correlation time τ_c governing the dipolar relaxation mechanism of protons in paramagnetic solutions depends on three processes:

$$1/\tau_c = /\tau_{cR} + 1/\tau_{ce} + 1/\tau_{cs} \quad (1.23)$$

where τ_{cR} is the correlation time of rotational tumbling of the molecule carrying of the paramagnetic ion, τ_{ce} is the correlation time of exchange between bound and free water, and τ_{cs} is the electron spin relaxation time. Typical values for these different correlation times are shown in Fig. 1.13. For Gd^{3+} and small Gd complexes, it can be computed from Eq. 1.15 that the tumbling correlation time τ_{cR} is less than 10^{-10} s, and hence from Eq. 1.21 $\tau_c < \approx 10^{-10}$ s independent of the values of τ_{ce} and τ_{cs}. Within this limit the Solomon-Bloembergen equations predict that T1 and T2 increase as the Larmor frequency increases, so that small paramagnetic

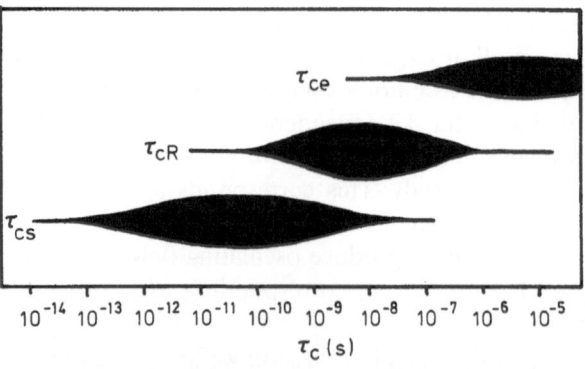

Fig. 1.13. The correlation time τ_c in paramagnetic relaxation depends on three contributions, the electron spin relaxation time τ_{cs}, the rotational correlation time τ_{cR}, and the exchange correlation time τ_{ce}. The typical orders of magnitude of these correlation times are given here. (Reprinted with permission from Bertini and Luchinat [10])

molecules are not as efficient in promoting relaxation at high as at low field strength.

For large paramagnetic complexes, τ_{cR} can be so long (10^{-8}–10^{-9} s) that $1/\tau_{cR}$ and the proton resonance frequency ω_I are comparable. If τ_{ce} and τ_{cs} are also in the same range, which for τ_{ce} is generally true and for τ_{cs} is true with Gd, Mn and in some cases [10] Fe^{3+}, $1/\tau_c$ is comparable to ω_I, according to Eq. 1.23. Within this limit, a behavior of T1 and T2 is found which is similar to the results of Fig. 1.10. Thus, an increase in the size of the molecule to which Gd is bound will result in more efficient relaxation than if Gd is part of a small molecule or free. This has been confirmed with a Gd-immunoglobulin G complex [11]. Bound to large molecules, Gd is a more efficient paramagnetic relaxation agent than when bound to small molecules, particularly at higher field strengths.

For Fe, the situation is much more complicated because, depending on its binding environment, it has an electronic relaxation time which varies considerably. In its $3+$ oxidation state it exists in a high-spin state ($\tau_{cs} = 10^{-10}$–10^{-11} s) or a low-spin state ($\tau_{cs} = 10^{-11}$–10^{-12} s), and in its $2+$ oxidation state only in a high-spin state ($\tau_{cs} = 10^{-12}$ s). Thus, for Fe, even when bound to macromolecules, the overall relaxation rate $1/\tau_c$ will be determined by the electronic relaxation rate in most cases, but the relaxation behavior cannot be analyzed by the Solomon-Bloembergen Equations [10].

For high concentrations of paramagnetic molecules, the field inhomogeneities become so important that dephasing of proton spins on the water molecules occurs quickly, as they diffuse between the paramagnetic centers. T2 relaxation is strongly affected, resulting in the well-known decrease in signal intensity at high concentrations of paramagnetic agents [12]. Very large paramagnetic molecules such as ferrite particles [13, 14], which may be superparamagnetic [15] or ferromagnetic [3] (staying magnetized even after the removal of an external field), tumble very slowly and cannot produce efficient T1 relaxation, but by introducing field inhomogeneities they again promote dephasing and T2 relaxation (qualitatively speaking, they fall on the right of the curve 1 of Fig. 1.10). In addition, the magnetic environment may be altered so strongly that the macroscopic magnetic susceptibility is changed.

While the various correlation times expressing the molecular properties of motion and interaction with the environment are an important determinant of relaxation, the accessibility of the paramagnetic ion by the water molecules is also important in de-

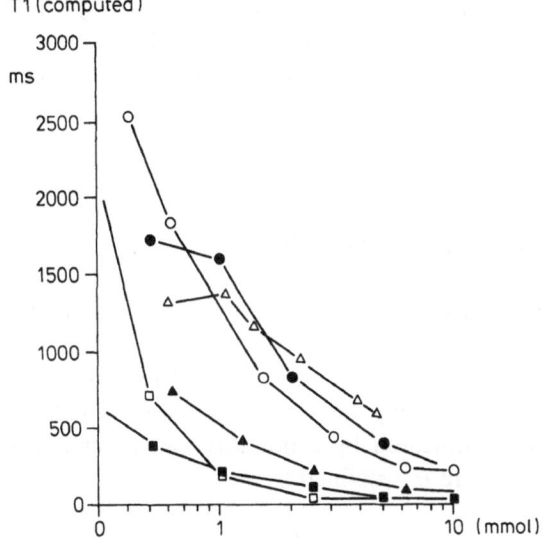

Fig. 1.14. T1 relaxation times as a function of Fe^{3+} concentrations for various compounds. For reference sake, the same curve is also plotted for Gadolinium-DTPA. (-□- FeCl, -▲- Ferrioxamine, -○- Hemin, -●-Meth-Hb, -△- Ferritin, -■- Gd-DTPA). Note that the larger the molecule, the smaller the relaxation-enhancing effect

termining the effectiveness of a paramagnetic molecule in promoting relaxation (remember the $1/r_{IS}^6$ dependence of the relaxation rate in Eqs. 1.19, 1.20 and 1.21). Such steric hindrance probably determines the effectiveness of paramagnetic relaxation in iron-containing molecules, resulting in the decrease in T1 relaxation with increasing molecular size, as shown in Fig. 1.14 [16]. Since the interplay of the various physical effects producing paramagnetic relaxation is difficult to analyze, a prediction of whether a paramagnetic agent is a good or a poor relaxation enhancer cannot be made on theoretical grounds, but has to be made experimentally.

It should be stated here that the relaxation times T1 and T2 depend also on the temperature. However, since MRI of human subjects occurs mostly at 37° Celsius and the temperature dependence of T1 and T2 is not very strong, temperature effects will not be considered further.

1.3.4 Chemical Shift

The electrons surrounding the hydrogen atom protons tend to shield them from the external magnetic field H_o by setting up atomic currents which will counteract this field. How effectively the electrons can shield H_o and reduce it to H_{eff} depends on the molecular structure of the compounds in which the hydrogen atoms are bound. For example, hydrogen atoms bound in fatty-type molecules are screened more effectively than hydrogen atoms bound in water. Introducing a screening constant σ, we can write

$$H_{eff} = H_o(1 - \sigma)$$

or with the help of Eq. 1.10

$$\omega = \gamma_p H_o(1 - \sigma) \tag{1.24}$$

This screening constant is on the order of 10^{-3}–10^{-6}. Usually, the screening in a certain compound is indicated by a quantity called chemical shift δ, where δ is defined as

$$\delta = (\omega_s - \omega_r)/\omega_r \times 10^6 \tag{1.25}$$

a dimensionless quantity given in ppm (parts per million), ω_s is the resonance frequency of the atom of interest and ω_r the resonance frequency of an arbitrary reference atom. The chemical shift of body fat relative to water is approximately -2.75 ppm. In MRI, the chemical shift is responsible for some image degradation, and it can also be used to generate true "water" and "fat" images. In magnetic resonance spectroscopy (MRS), the chemical shift is an extremly important phenomenon, because it contains the information on the molecular environment of protons and other spin-carrying nuclei, and therefore the molecular structure.

1.4 Pulse Sequences

In the foregoing sections the physics of the NMR effect was discussed. We saw that any sample is characterized by relaxation times T1 and T2, which predominantly determine the tissue contrast in MRI and reflect tissue composition. It can be seen in Table 1.2 that T1 and T2 of various tissues vary considerably. Since MRI relies on strong contrast between tissues, imaging should take place in ways which emphasize such differences. Hence, we have to understand the methods by which the influence of T1 and T2 can be manipulated for a given sample. This is done by choosing the proper pulse sequence.

As MRI uses only pulsed NMR methods, whereby the equilibrium magnetization is somehow disturbed in its alignment parallel to the main magnetic field H_o by a radiofrequency (RF) pulse, it is only such pulse sequences that we are going discuss in the ensuing sections. By pulse sequence we mean in

Table 1.2. T1 and T2 values [17] for various body tissues

Tissue	T1 (ms)	Field strength (MHz)	T2 (ms)	Field strength (MHz)
Blood	870	24	90	44
Brain (white)	470	24	110	20
Brain (gray)	640	24	110	20
Heart	630	24	35	15
Kidney (cortex)	410	24	50	15
Kidney (medulla)	800	24	50	15
Liver	310	24	50	15
Muscle	540	24	35	15
Fat	220	15	60	15
Spleen	510	24	60	15

general a sequence of RF and field gradient pulses which is repeated many times with the aim of either improving the signal-to-noise ratio or acquiring an image. The use of gradient pulses to spatially localize a signal will be discussed in the sections on imaging (1.5).

1.4.1 Free Induction Decay

The simplest MR pulse sequence is the free induction decay (FID). The schematics of this pulse sequence are shown in Fig. 1.15. In this pulse sequence an RF pulse is sent into the sample, tilting the magnetization vector by 90° into the xy-plane. The magnetization starts to precess in this plane, but in the rotating reference frame it remains stationary. Due to the spin-spin interactions, some spins precess a little faster and others a little slower, resulting in a spread of the components of M_{xy}' (' denoting the fact that we are looking from the vantage point of the rotating frame of reference). As a result, the MR signal detected in the receiver coil decreases in time. After a repetition time TR, another 90° pulse is sent into the system. The signal decrease does not occur with the rate constant $1/T2$, as we may expect, because this rate constant results from spin-spin relaxation only. However, there are mechanisms other than spin-spin relaxation which affect the local field H_{eff} around the relaxing spins. These mechanisms are extrinsic and intrinsic in nature. Extrinsic mechanisms are field inhomogeneities due to, e.g., a slightly inhomogeneous external magnetic field. Intrinsic mechanisms are related to the presence of paramagnetic substances and are due to diffusive processes of spin diffusion through environments with slightly different field strengths. Let us call ΔH_o the varia-

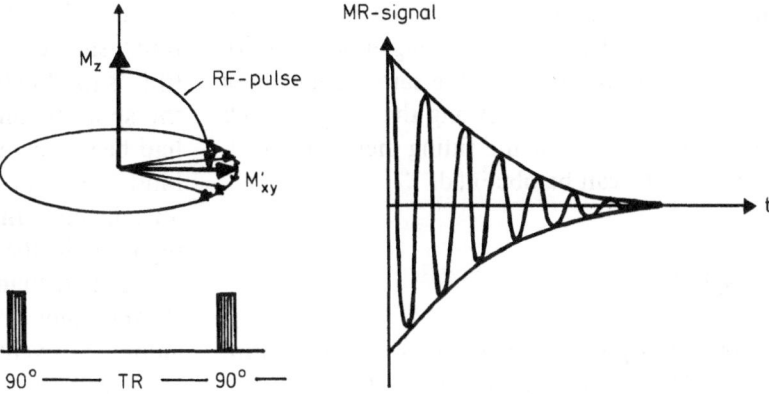

Fig. 1.15. In a free induction decay experiment (FID), the magnetization in the z-direction M_z is first flipped by a 90° pulse. The signal coming from the precessing magnetization $M_{xy'}$ is measured and the whole sequence repeated after a repetition time TR, which can be selected by the operator

tion of the main magnetic field over the sample due to an extrinsic field inhomogeneity; it will produce a faster dephasing of the spins and hence a faster decrease in MR signal intensity. According to Eq. 1.10, ΔH_o will generate a variation in precession frequencies given by

$$\Delta\omega_o = \gamma_p\Delta H_o \qquad (1.26)$$

and lead to a spread of phases (see Fig. 1.11) which occurs faster than by spin-spin interactions alone. Relaxation rates are additive, as they represent the probability that relaxation occurs through spin-spin interaction or due to field inhomogeneities, and the effective T2 relaxation time T2* can be written as

$$1/T2^* = 1/T2 + \gamma_p\Delta H_o/2 \qquad (1.27)$$

where the factor of 2 is included to conform with the definition of a Lorentzian line width (Sect. 1.4.4 and Appendix C). The relaxation time T2* measured is thus an expression of the field inhomogeneity in the sample in addition to the molecular relaxation mechanisms, and FID measurements are not suitable for measuring T2 relaxation times. As will be seen in Sect. 1.4.3, an elegant trick has been devised in the form of the so-called spin echo experiment to overcome this problem. However, the measurement of an FID is useful, when T1 is to be determined (see below).

1.4.2 Inversion Recovery

Inversion recovery pulse sequences are useful in the determination of T1 values. In this pulse sequence, the magnetization M_z is inverted by a 180° at the start of the pulse sequence. With the initial condi-

tion that $M_z = -M_{zo}$, M_z grows back according to Eq. 1.7 and the curve in Fig. 1.16 and obeys the following equation:

$$M_z = M_{zo}[1 - 2\exp(-t/T1)] \qquad (1.28)$$

After a variable time TI – the so-called inversion time – the magnetization is flipped into the xy-

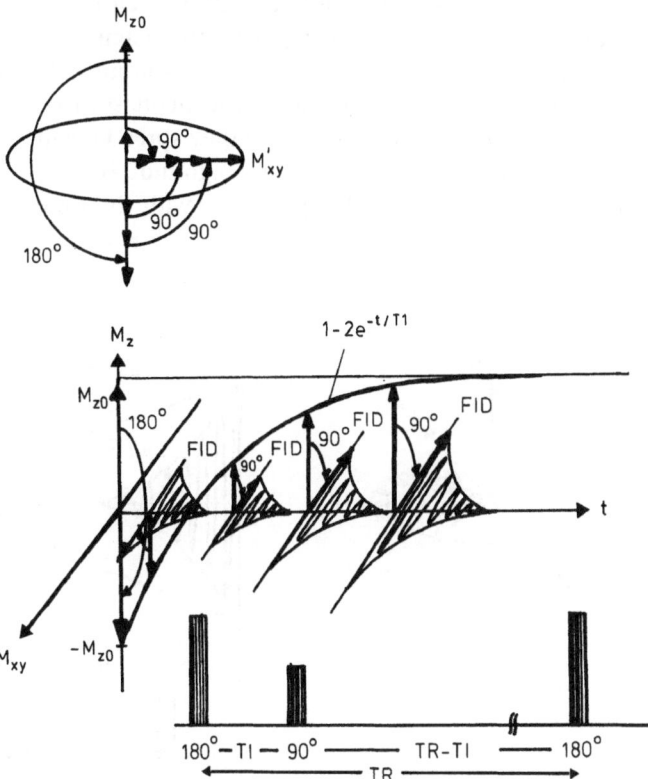

Fig. 1.16. In an inversion recovery experiment (IR), the magnetization M_{zo} is first flipped by a 180° to become $-M_{zo}$. After an operator-dependent waiting period TI, the inversion time, the instant magnetization M_z is flipped into th xy-plane by a 90° pulse and the free induction decay is measured. This sequence is repeated with a repetition time TR

plane and there the signal generated is measured as an FID. Eventually, after a time long enough for M_z to recover (typically $t > 5T1$), the same sequence of pulses is repeated. By measuring the various FIDs on the curve of Fig. 1.16 and fitting them on a logarithmic plot, T1 can be obtained.

1.4.3 Spin Echo

The spin-echo pulse sequence was originally proposed by Hahn [18] as an ingenious trick to overcome the problem associated with measuring T2 in an FID experiment. It is no doubt the most important pulse sequence used in present-day MRI, permitting data collection a few to several hundred milliseconds after the initial 90° pulse and thus permitting also the acquisition of data from the heart in conjunction with ECG triggering (see Chap. 3), and by using multi-echo sequences bringing out the T2 characteristics of the tissues studied. As seen in Sect. 1.4.1, the FID experiment can measure only T2*, which is smaller than T2. The "Hahn" spin echo pulse sequence was modified by Carr and Purcell [4] and later by Meiboom and Gill [19] to reduce effects of self-diffusion, as will be seen in the next section. As shown in Fig. 1.17, the magnetization is initially subject to a 90° pulse as in an FID experiment, and the spins are left to dephase; that is, in the rotating reference frame they spread again around the initial position. The magnitude of M_{xy} decreases, as in an FID experiment, with the time

constant T2*. However, after a time TE/2, a 180° refocusing pulse is applied along the y'-direction (this is the Meiboom-Gill modification), which flips the spins running ahead into a position as if they had been lagging behind, and the spins lagging behind into a position as if they had been running ahead. Since the faster moving spins are still at a higher field than H_o and the slower spins still at a lower field than H_o, the faster spins gain and the slower spins lose on the reference spin staying along x'. Eventually, after an echo time TE, all spins will coincide again along the x'-axis, giving rise to an echo. A picture for this has been drawn in the so-called race track analogy (Fig. 1.18). If the signal is measured when it peaks, a point on the T2 decay curve is obtained. By varying the echo time, various such points can be measured and T2 obtained from a semilogarithmic plot. Alternatively, the spins are again left to defocus and a second refocusing pulse is sent into the sample at 3TE/2, which leads to a second echo at 2TE. In this way a multi-echo sequence can be generated. The magnetization measured in such a sequence, M_{xy}, is given by

$$M_{xy} = FH[1 - \exp(-TR/T1)]\exp(-nTE/T2)$$
(1.29)

where F is a factor containing various dependences such as flow-related signal alterations, H is the proton density, and the factor in brackets represents the amount of M_z magnetization which has been recovered after a repetition time TR, and is thus avail-

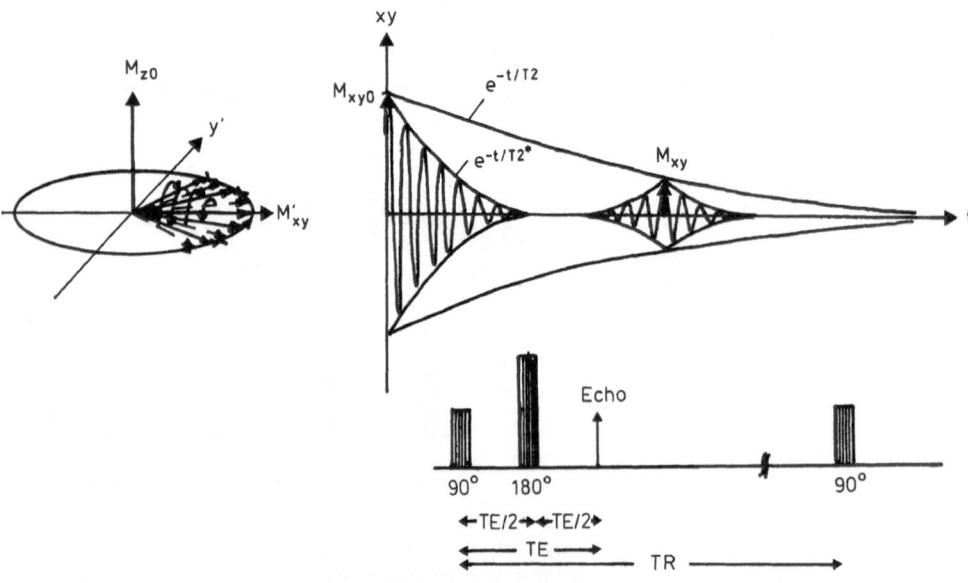

Fig. 1.17. In a spin-echo experient (SE), the magnetization M_z is first flipped into the xy-plane as in an FID experiment and the magnetization M_{xy} decays in this way. However, after a time TE/2, a 180° pulse is sent into the system which refocuses the spins at TE, resulting in a strong signal. This sequence is repeated after a time TR

able to be flipped into the xy-plane with the next 90° pulse. The repetition time TR and the echo time TE are parameters which can be set by the operator. It is often convenient to emphasize either the T1 or the T2 character and suppress the influence of the other of the image, producing so-called T1-weighted or T2-weighted images. If TR and TE are chosen such that $TR \ll T1$ and $TE \ll T2$, a Taylor series expansion of the exponential expressions in Eq. 1.29 (Appendix A) yields

$$M_{xy} \approx FH\, TR/T1 \qquad (1.30)$$

thus, the conditions $TR \ll T1$ and $TE \ll T2$ produce T1-weighting. Alternatively, if TR and TE are chosen such that $TR \gg T1$ and $TE \gg T2$, the exponentials in Eq. 1.29 become small and $1 - \exp(-TR/T1) \approx 1$, thus

$$M_{xy} \approx FH\, \exp(nTE/T2) \qquad (1.31)$$

The conditions $TR \gg T1$ and $TE \gg T2$ produce T2-weighting.

The spin-echo method can also be used to measure the signal after an IR experiment. A 180° refocusing pulse has then to be added to the pulse sequence in Fig. 1.16 after the 90° pulse.

Experimentally, it was found in liquids that the decrease of the magnetization M_{xy} was exponential for relatively short TEs yielding T2 rather than T2* values, but much more rapid than exponential for longer TEs. Analysis of this problem led to the conclusion that the self-diffusion of spins in an environment where H changes slightly due to extrinsic or intrinsic factors (field inhomogeneities, paramagnetic ions) could not be ignored.

1.4.4 Diffusion-Sensitive Pulse Sequences

The effects of diffusion on MR experiments were first analyzed by Carr and Purcell [4]. They assumed that the variations of the magnetic field due to inhomogeneities linear over the distances over which water molecules diffuse in a typical time TE, i.e., the field they experience, could be approximated by

$$H_{eff} = H_0 + (G.r) \qquad (1.32)$$

Using this type of magnetic field they solved the equation of motion for the spins in the xy-plane (Eq. 1.18) under inclusion of diffusion effects. Here G is the gradient field vector of the magnetic field

$(G = G_x, G_x, G_z)$, r is the positional coordinate vector $(r = x, y, z)$ and $(G.r)$ the inner product: $(G.r) = (G_x x + G_y y + G_z z)$ (Appendix B). With the help of Eq. 1.14 and Table 1.1, we find that a water molecule moves approximately 10 μm in a typical echo time of $TE = 30$ ms. It can be safely assumed that over such distances the external field inhomogeneity does not oscillate and thus, higher order terms than the linear one can be ignored (Appendix A). Inclusion of diffusion effects in the equation of motion of the precessing spins (Eq. 1.8) leads to the following result:

$$M_{xy} = M_{xyo}\exp(-TE/T2 - \gamma_p^2 G^2 DTE^3/12) \qquad (1.33)$$

Hence, diffusion enhances the rate of T2 decay, particularly if $\gamma_p^2 G^2 DTE^2/12 > 1$ when the second term in Eq. 1.33 starts to dominate the decay of M_{xy}.

It is intuitively clear that such enhanced relaxation occurs when diffusion effects are included,

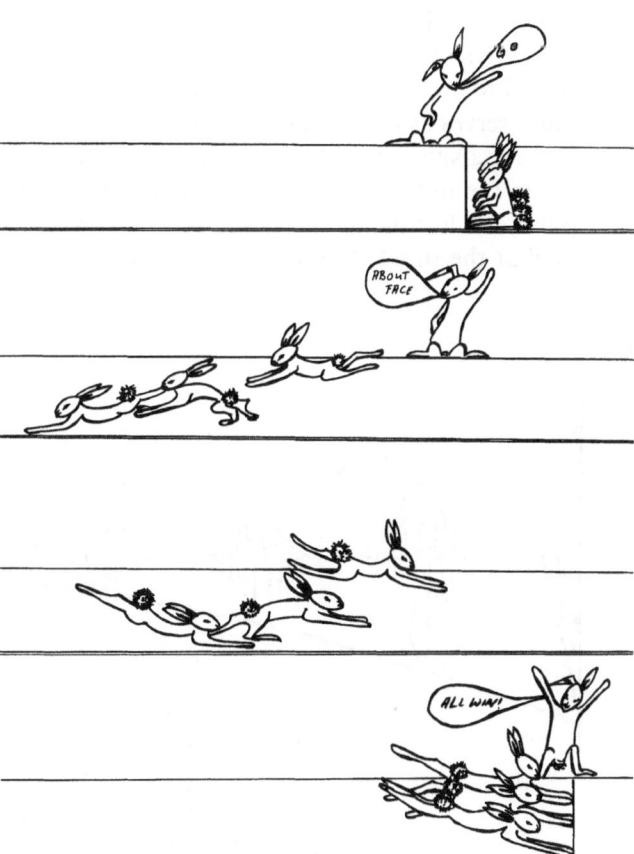

Fig. 1.18. The refocusing effect of an SE experiment was likened to a race track by Hahn. Spins in a somewhat higher magnetic field precess faster. Thus, at the command "go," these spins (rabbits) will run ahead. If the starter orders "about face," the fastest runners have a distance handicap but still run (precess) faster, so that all of them cross the starting line simultaneously

because the 180° refocusing pulse can refocus only spins which experience the same deviation ΔH_o from the main magnetic field over the entire time TE from the 90° pulse to the echo. In the case of diffusion, however, the spins are wandering at random from one field strength to another during this time. Thus, if a spin is precessing a bit too fast from t=0 to TE/2 because it is experiencing a slightly higher field strength, this puts it at a disadvantage on the race rack (Fig. 1.18) after the 180° refocusing pulse. If between TE/2 and TE the spin has wandered to a site of lower field strength, it will not be able to catch up and get back to the starting line when the echo occurs and thus will not contribute to it.

To reduce diffusion effects in spin echo experiments, Carr and Purcell proposed their multi echo sequence (Fig. 1.19). In this sequence, the spins are left to dephase after forming the first echo at TE. A second 180° refocusing pulse is sent into the sample after 3TE/2, which gives rise to a second echo at 2TE. In the same way, a refocusing pulse after a time $(2n + 1)$TE/2 will generate the n-th echo at the time nTE. For this pulse sequence diffusion effects are reduced, because each 180° refocusing pulse serves as a new starting point for diffusive effects: if a spin happened to be at a higher field between the n-th echo and $(n+1)$-th 180° refocusing pulse, the likelihood that it will still be at a higher field at the $(n+1)$-th echo and thus properly refo-

cus is the higher, the shorter the echo time TE. The expression for the magnetization for the CPMG (Carr-Purcell-Meiboom-Gill) pulse sequence including diffusion is

$$M_{xy}(nTE) = M_{xyo}\exp[-nTE/T2 \\ - nTE(\gamma_p^2 G^2 DTE^2/12)] \qquad (1.34)$$

where $\gamma_p^2 G^2 DTE^2/12$ can be viewed as a diffusive T2 relaxation rate. Compared with the Hahn spin echo sequence, the CPMG pulse sequence is less sensitive to diffusion, and, in principle, this sensitivity can be arbitrarily reduced by reducing TE (Eq. 1.34). For technical reasons this is not possible below a few ms, particularly in MRI.

The notion that a (natural) magnetic gradient field applied during an MR experiment is responsible for alterations in the observed T2 relaxation is an interesting one, and the question arises immediately whether, by intentional application of external gradients, diffusive effects could be amplified and thus measured. This is indeed the case.

If we want to measure diffusion, we obviously want the externally applied magnetic field gradient to be larger than the field gradients resulting from field inhomogeneities present in the system. The basic diffusion- and motion-sensitive sequence was designed by Stejskal and Tanner [20] and is shown in Fig. 1.20. In fact, in MRI, field gradients like the ones used in the Stejskal-Tanner experiment are

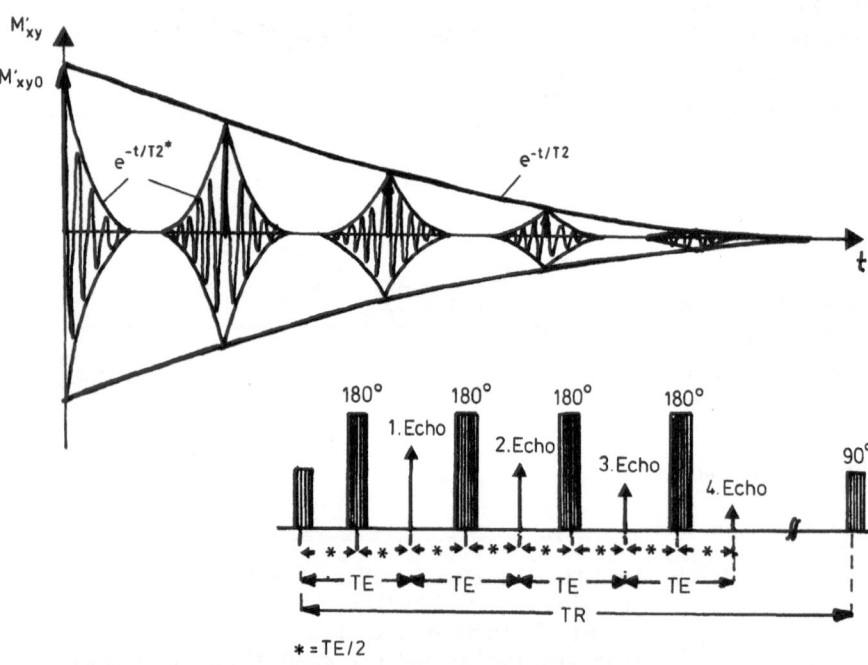

Fig. 1.19. The SE experiment can actually be extended to obtain multiple echoes. Instead of waiting for the next 90° pulse, a second 180° pulse is sent into the system after 3TE/ 2, which refocuses the spins again at 2TE, and so on. Measuring the peak amplitudes at each echo results in a decaying exponential permitting the measurement of T2

switched on for spatial localization purposes (Fig. 1.20), as will be seen in Sect. 1.5. Hence, all standard MRI sequences "accidentally" sensitize MR images to motion effects. It is by this pulse sequence that information on diffusion may be obtained, and in the case where Δ and δ are the times defined in Fig. 1.20, M_{xy} is given by

$$M_{xy'} = M_{xyo'}\exp[nTE/T2 + n\gamma^2 G^2 D\delta^2(\Delta - \delta/3)] \tag{1.35}$$

for a multiecho sequence. In a cellular environment, diffusion is not free but restricted by the cell walls. For short times Δ, the molecules in a diffusion-sensitive spin echo experiment diffuse over short distances according to Eq. 1.14 and are not restricted by the cell walls. Thus, a constant diffusion coefficient D will be found. However, for longer

times Δ the diffusion coefficient will appear to become smaller, this being a result of the molecules bouncing off the cellular walls and thus of restricted diffusion. From the time Δ_c above which this occurs and the diffusion constant D for short Δ, representing unrestricted diffusion, approximate cellular dimensions can then be computed according to Eq. 1.14: $d = \sqrt{D\Delta_c}$.

As implied above, additional field gradients not only sensitize the MR experiment to diffusion but also to bulk motion, such as flow. Understanding flow phenomena in MRI is extremely important, as such effects occur on almost every MR image. However, in bulk motion the magnetization at the echo time TE is no longer aligned parallel to the x-axis but is turned away from it by a certain angle Φ (Fig. 1.21). MR is capable of measuring this angle Φ, as we shall see below.

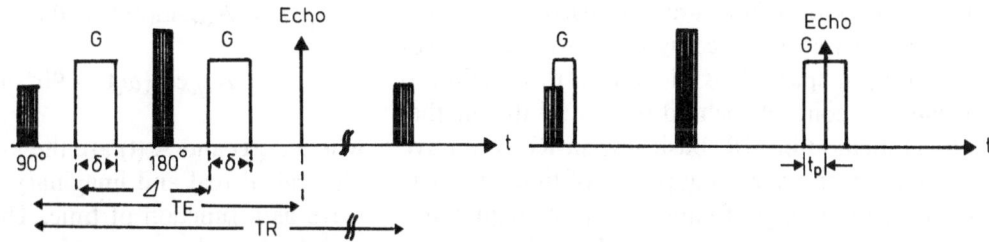

Fig. 1.20. If during an SE experiment symmetric magnetic gradient fields G are switched on during a time δ before and after the 180° refocusing pulse separated by a time Δ, these pulses sensitize moving spins by inducing a change in their precessional phase relative to the stationary spins. In MRI this occurs accidentally, because for spatial localization purposes, gradient fields have to be switched on in any case

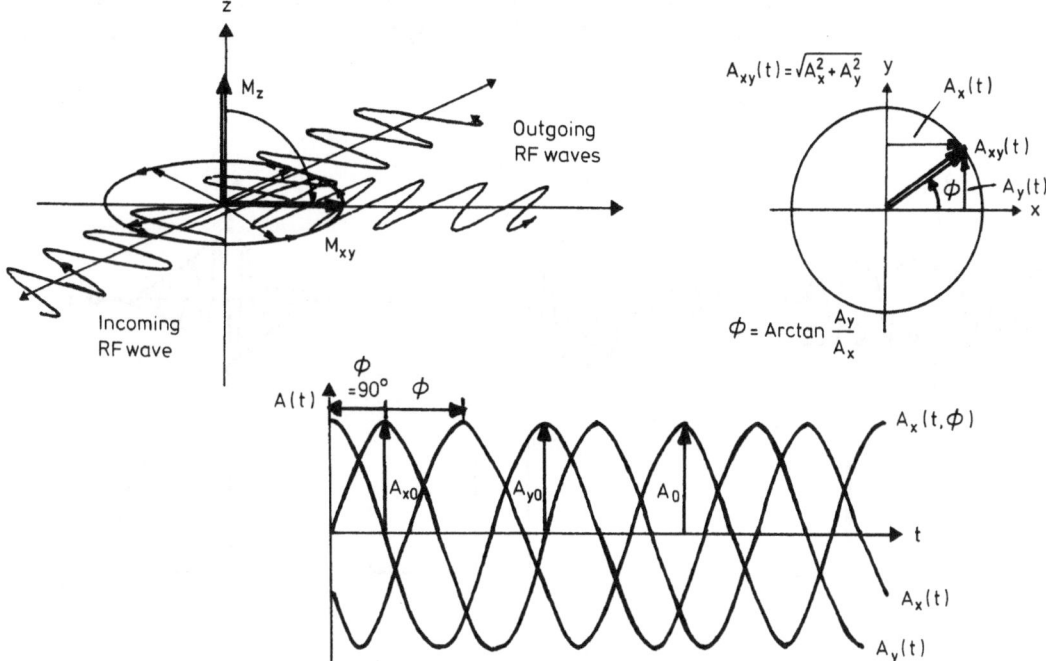

Fig. 1.21. An incoming RF wave gives rise to two RF waves coming from the sample, which are phase shifted by 90° against each other. These two outgoing RF waves are generated by the magnetization vector M_{xy}, precessing in the xy-plane. Thus, an instant amplitude $A_{xy}(t)$ is obtained using the Pythagorean theorem by measuring $A_x(t)$ and $A_y(t)$. The instantaneous phase angle Φ can also be measured and is obtained using standard trigonometric functions

1.4.5 A Mathematical Tool: The Fourier Transformation

So far, we have discussed only situations where the magnetization could be examined by looking at a decaying MR signal. If we want to obtain information on flow or motion, additional information has to be extracted from this decaying MR signal. Furthermore, in the case of MRI the signal measured is a superposition of many distinct sine waves with different frequencies and, again, these have to be extracted from the signal. To extract such information, a wonderful mathematical tool, termed the Fourier transformation, named after its inventor Fourier, has to be used. Fourier transform play an extremely important role in all areas of physics where sinusoidal waves occur. The Fourier transformation is a tool which can decompose, e.g., a time-varying signal into its frequency components. However, Fourier transform are also used to fit functions which vary in space by a series of sine waves oscillating in space. It is the aim in this section to explain the concepts behind the use of this mathematical method in MR. Basically, an RF sine wave extending over a very long period of time t is characterized by a single frequency ν_o or angular frequency ω_o and an amplitude B_o (Fig. 1.21)

$$B(t) = B_o\cos(\omega_o t) \tag{1.36}$$

Such an RF wave impinging on a system of spins gives rise to a circularly polarized RF wave, which has components in the x- and the y-directions with amplitudes A_{xyo}:

$$A_{xo}(t) = A_{xyo}\cos(\omega_o t)$$

$$A_{yo}(t) = A_{xyo}\sin(\omega_o t)$$

$$= A_{xyo}\cos(\omega_o t - 90°) \tag{1.37}$$

but with a phase difference of 90° of the wave in the y-direction relative to the x-direction; i.e., when the wave is maximum (or minimum) in the x-direction it is zero in the y-direction and vice versa. If by some means the spin system has changed the phase Φ of the wave but not the frequency, such a wave can be described by

$$A_x(t) = A_{xyo}\cos(\omega_o t + \Phi)$$

$$A_y(t) = A_{xyo}\sin(\omega_o t + \Phi) =$$

$$= A_{xyo}\cos(\omega_o t - 90° + \Phi) \tag{1.38}$$

where $A_x(t)$ and $A_y(t)$ are the x- and y-components, also called real and imaginary components, of this wave as a function of time. The components $A_x(t)$ and $A_y(t)$ can be measured in an MR experiment as induced currents in coils placed perpendicularly to the x- and y-directions (so-called quadrature detection.). Alternatively, and more commonly, a phase sensitive detector is used, and only the component $A_x(t)$ or $A_y(t)$ along the x- or the y-axis is measured

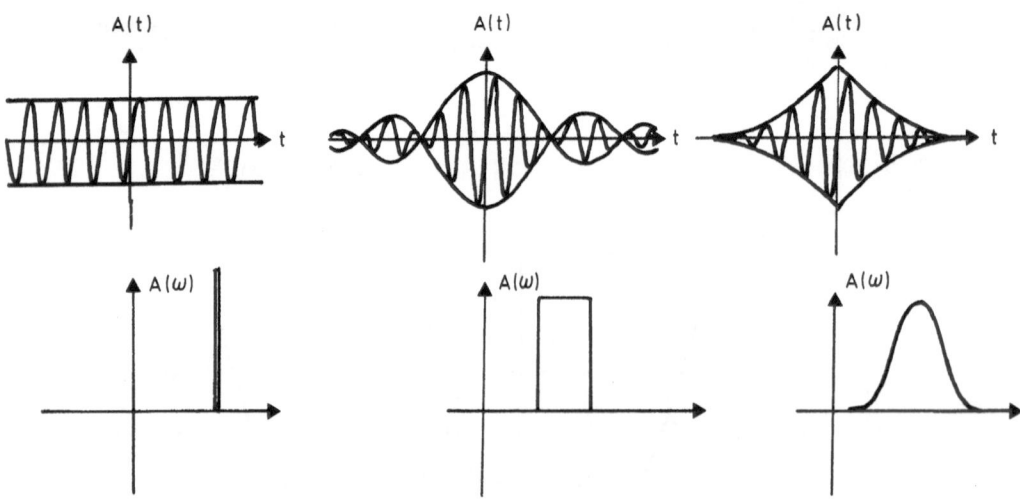

Fig. 1.22. An oscillatory function of time, characterized by an instant amplitude A(t), can be transformed into a function of frequency by means of the Fourier transformation. For example, a sine wave gives rise to a single peak in frequency space, a so-called δ function, a sinc function (sinωt/t) to a square function, and a decaying exponential to a Lorentzian in frequency space. Such functions are called Fourier pairs

and multiplied with the incoming wave B(t). The Fourier transformation of these sine waves extracts the values $A_x(0)$ and $A_y(0)$ from the measured signals, which according to Eq. 1.38 and Fig. 1.21 are $A_{xyo}\cos(\Phi)$ and $A_{xyo}\sin(\Phi) = A_{xyo}\cos(90° + \Phi)$ respectively. The amplitude or modulus and phase are then found by computing

$$A_{xyo} = \sqrt{A_x(0)^2 + A_y(0)^2} \qquad (1.39)$$

$$A_y(0)/A_x(0) = A_{xyo}\sin(\Phi)/A_{xyo}\cos(\Phi)$$
$$= \tan(\Phi)$$

$$\text{or } \Phi = \arctan[A_y(0)/A_x(0)] \qquad (1.40)$$

In MRI, we are usually interested only in the amplitude A_{xyo}, which in standard MR images is represented for each pixel. However, as will be seen, motion information resides in the value of the phase Φ. If we represent Φ on a pixel by pixel basis, this is called a phase image, whereas $A_{xy}\cos(\Phi)$ and $A_{xy}\sin(\Phi)$ are the real and imaginary images respectively.

If a time-varying signal is composed of several frequencies, as in MRI, then a Fourier transformation permits the extraction of the amplitudes and the phases relative to the incoming wave for all these frequency components. In fact, an RF pulse itself contains not only one, but an entire spectrum $J(\omega)$ of frequencies (Fig. 1.22). The narrower the pulse, the wider the spectrum, and vice versa. Only the limit of the pulse actually being not a pulse but a continuous sine wave does the spectrum contain a single frequency component (Fig. 1.22). In Appendix C we give a few Fourier pairs of functions which are often used in MRI.

1.4.6 Flow and Spin Phase Graphing

Pulse sequences identical to the one shown in Fig. 1.20 can be used to detect bulk motion or directed flow with MR. As spins move from one field strength to another within a sample volume over which a magnetic field gradient G is applied, they gain or lose phase Φ relative to nonmoving spins according to Eqs. 1.26 and 1.32:

$$\omega_0 + \omega = d\Phi/dt = \gamma_p H_{eff} = \gamma_p[H_0 + G.r]$$

which in the coordinate frame rotating with $\omega_0 = \gamma_p H_0$ reduces to

$$\omega = d\Phi/dt = \gamma_p(G.r) \qquad (1.41)$$

Here r is the position vector. The field gradient G is linear in MRI, but spins can move with constant velocity, i.e., when moving in small straight veins or undergo complicated accelerated motion as in the arteries, particularly when turbulence occurs or in any curved vessel. To understand the effects of various types of motion on the MR signal, it is useful to write r decomposed into its various motion components (Appendix A) by a Taylor series expansion.

Table 1.3. Phase angles Φ for stationary spins and spins moving at constant velocity and acceleration in a balanced gradient

180° pulses and echoes	Phase angle Φ_s/b for constant position ($b = \gamma G_x x_o$)	Phase angle Φ_v/c for constant velocity ($c = \gamma G_x v_{xo}/2$)	Phase angle Φ_a/d for constant acceleration ($d = \gamma G_x a_{xo}/6$)
TE/2	t_p	t_p^2	t_p^3
TE (1st echo)	0	$2TEt_p - 2t_p^2$	$3TE^2t_p - 3TEt_p^2/2$
3TE/2	t_p	$4TEt_p - ti_p^2$	$6TE^2t_p + t_p^3$
2TE (2nd echo)	0	0	$6TE^2t_p - 3TE^2t_p - 3TEt_p^2$
5TE/2	t_p	$4TEt_p + t_p^2$	$18TE^2t_p + t_p^3$
3TE (3rd echo)	0	$2TEt_p - 2t_p^2$	$9TE^2t_p - 9Tt_p^2/2$
7TE/2	t_p	$8TEt_p - t_p$	$36TE^2t_p + t_p^3$
4TE (4th echo)	0	0	$12TE^2t_p - 6TEt_p^2$
(2n + 1)TE/2 (n-th refocusing pulse)			
n even	t_p	$2nTEt_p + t_p^2$	$3(n^2 + n)TE^2t_p + t_p^3$
n odd	t_p	$2(n + 1)TEt_p - t_p^2$	
2nT (n-th echo)			
n even	0	0	$3n(TE^2t_p - TEt_p^2/2)$
n odd	0	$2TEt_p - t_p^2$	

If we assume that motion occurs only along the x-axis, r can be written as

$$r(t) = x_o + v_{xo}t + a_{xo}t^2/2 +$$

$$+ (\text{higher order motion terms}) \qquad (1.42)$$

with x_o being the position, v_{xo} being the velocity, and a_{xo} being the acceleration of a spin. Equation 1.42 can be inserted into Eq. 1.41 and the latter integrated for a typical MRI spin echo sequence (Fig. 1.19). The results of such an integration for balanced gradients in a spin echo sequence (same height and duration of gradients before and after 180° pulse) are shown in Table 1.3, where the phase angles are given for constant velocity and constant acceleration motion at the echo times and the times where the refocusing pulses occur [21]. The corresponding calculations are carried out in Appendix D.

There are several points worth noting in this table. First, stationary spins in a CPMG sequence always refocus to the zero position at the echoes. Second, the spins undergoing constant velocity motion do not refocus to zero at the odd numbered echoes but rather to a constant value of the phase angle $\Phi = b(2TEt_p - t_p^2)$ away from the zero position; that is, they have non-zero phase at odd-numbered echoes (Fig. 1.23). As this phase can be determined, velocity measurements can be made with MR. Third, for balanced gradients, the phase angle for even-numbered echoes vanishes identically; it is zero independent of the velocity of a spin (Fig. 1.23). This is a special result and is at the base of a well-recognized phenomenon often observed in MRI, termed "even echo refocusing" [22]. Fourth,

for motion with constant acceleration, the phase angle increases linearly with the echo number, hence it is also non-zero on even-numbered echoes. The measurement of the phase angle on even echoes yield motion contributions from acceleration only. A detailed understanding of how the phase angle varies with different types of motion is essential for motion and flow velocity determinations which now come into use in MRI.

When the flow-sensitizing gradient is not strictly balanced, as is typically the case with the slice-selection gradient in MRI, the results of Table 1.3 no longer hold, but similar expressions can be calculated. In general, the refocusing phenomenon no longer occurs. On the other hand, it can be shown that spin echo pulse sequences can be constructed which are not sensitive to motion at all. Such pulse sequences have been called "MAST" sequences [23]. They are very useful because when a bright structure is moving during MR image acquisition, it produces strong motion artifacts which can be suppressed by the MAST technique. MAST sequences appear to be particularly useful in gradient echo imaging of blood vessels, where flowing blood appears very bright (Sect. 1.4.8).

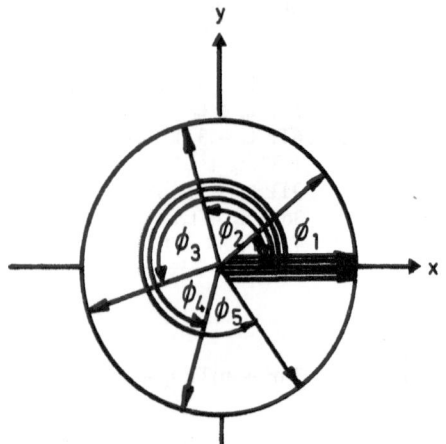

Fig. 1.23. Depending on the velocity, acceleration, or higher order motion terms, the phase angle Φ is turned away from the zero position. For stationary spins, the phase angle should always be zero in an ideal MR system

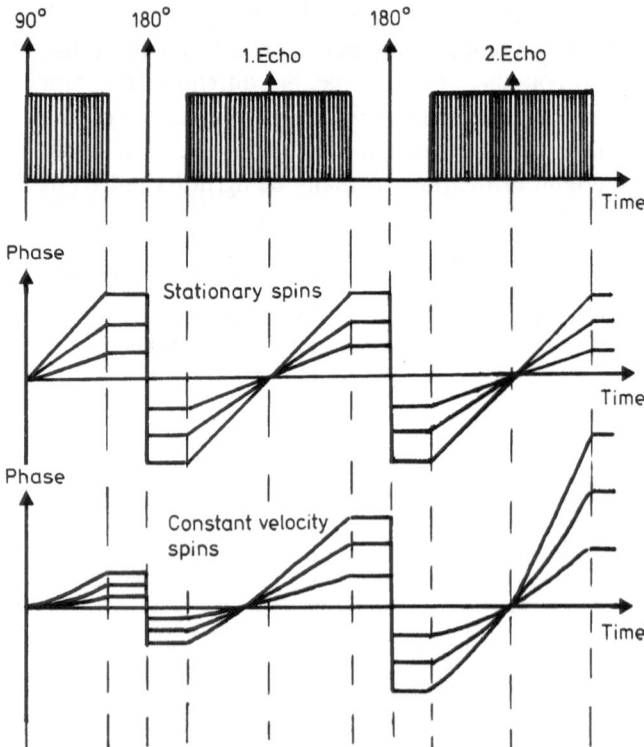

Fig. 1.24. The so-called phase graphs give the instant phase angle during the progress of a sequence. Here, the phase graphs for three spins with slightly different positions and velocities are shown. Note, that spins moving at constant velocity show parabolic changes in phase during the time the gradient is switched on

A convenient method for looking at the behavior of spins under the influence of various gradients has been proposed by Singer [24] with the so-called spin phase graphing method. An example is given in Fig. 1.24. There we represent the phase angle of spins as a function of time under the influence of a balanced gradient, which can be seen to be symmetrical around the 180° refocusing pulses. Whereas phase increases linearly for stationary spins, it increases quadratically for spins moving with constant velocity and does not refocus on the first (or any odd-numbered) echo. This can be easily seen in Fig. 1.24, where the phase graphs do not intersect the zero line at the first echo, but earlier. Using this method, the actual phase of a spin can be found at any time during a pulse sequence. Flow-sensitive pulse sequences are a first example of how the phase information available in an MR experiment can be used to obtain additional information not present if only the amplitude of the MR signals is evaluated. A second example is the so-called chemical shift pulse sequence used to obtain separate water and fat information, initially proposed for imaging by Dixon [25].

1.4.7 Chemical Shift Sequences

In Sect. 1.3.4 we indicated that the different shielding of water and fat protons results in a slightly different precession frequency for a given external field. For body fat this chemical shift is approximately -2.75 ppm relative to water and can be used to separate water and fat images as follows [26]. At the echo time in a spin echo experiment, the water and fat spins both refocus at the zero position, because the spin echo experiment is insensitive to slightly different magnetic fields which do not

vary over the echo time (Sect. 1.4.3). The "field inhomogeneity" present for fat relative to water protons satisfies this condition. Acquisition of such data yields a so-called in-phase signal, as fat and water protons are in phase (Fig. 1.25). However, if we delay our sampling for a few milliseconds until the water spins have moved 180° ahead of the fat spins due to their higher precession frequency, signal acquisition yields a so-called opposed-phase signal (Fig. 1.25). If we call the contributions to the signal from water and fat U and V, we apparently measure the in-phase signal $I = U + V$, and the opposed-phase signal $O = U - V$. These two equations can be solved to obtain pure water and fat contributions:

$$\text{WATER:} \quad U = (I + O)/2$$

$$\text{FAT:} \qquad V = (I + O)/2 \qquad (1.43)$$

There are various clinical situations where the separation of water from fat is desirable, such as in the distinction of dermoids from hemoglobin-containing cysts, or in the identification of avascular necrosis of the femoral head. Furthermore, whenever a sample contains comparable amounts of water and fat, the signal in the opposed-phase image will be small. In imaging, this is found, e.g., at the interface of the kidneys with the perirenal fat. In MR imaging, this results in a dark line interface between the two structures which is very useful for automatic edge detection (see Chap. 6).

1.4.8 Gradient Echo Sequences

As noted in Table 1.2 the typical T1 relaxation times of body tissues are on the order of several hundred milliseconds. After a 90° pulse in a spin

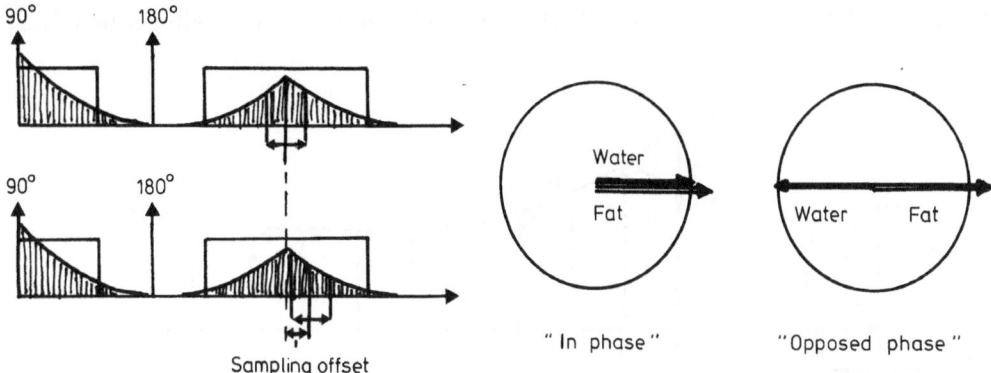

Fig. 1.25. In a water/fat separation experiment two sequences are used. The first in a simple SE sequence. In it, water and fat protons align during the echo. To obtain an op-

posed phase image, the echo is sampled with a slight offset, corresponding to the time needed to just have the water spins move 180° ahead relative to the fat spins

echo experiment, a considerable amount of time, the repetition time TR has to elapse before the magnetization M_z has grown back to such a height that another 90° pulse will produce substantial M_{xy} magnetization. To acquire an image with 256 lines, a similar number of repetitions of the basic pulse sequence have to be carried out. For TR = 1 s, acquisition of an image thus requires several minutes. The use of gradient echoes, first introduced into imaging independently by Haase et al. [27] and by van der Meulen et al. [28], has the great advantage that MR images can be acquired in a matter of seconds rather than minutes.

There are two basic differences between gradient echoes and spin echoes. The first difference is that for gradient echoes an RF pulse is used, which tilts the magnetization typically by a nutation angle α of less than 90°, thus not fully saturating (destroying the M_z magnetization of) the system. In repetitive excitations as used in MRI, some magnetization in the z-direction is left after the first RF pulse. In subsequent excitations, an equilibrium between destruction of magnetization by the RF pulse and magnetization recovery during TR is established (Fig. 1.26) at a relatively large M_z. Thus, there is substantial M_{xy} magnetization to be measured after each nutation pulse, even when TR is below 100 ms. The angle $α_E$, for which the measured signal is maximized in a gradient echo sequence, the so-called Ernst angle, depends on the repetition time TR and the T1 relaxation time in the following way:

$$α_E = \arccos[\exp(-TR/T1)] \tag{1.44}$$

Second, instead of using a 180° pulse to refocus the spins, no such refocusing is done as long as no gradient field is applied for spatial localization, as necessary in imaging (Sect. 1.5). The result is that the M_{xy} magnetization in a gradient echo experiment decays with T2* rather than T2 (see Sect. 1.4.1), and

that a gradient echo sequence corresponds in a sense more to a free induction decay rather than to a spin echo pulse sequence. In order to still measure an appreciable signal in a gradient echo sequence, the requirements for magnetic field homogeneity are much more stringent than these for SE sequences because it is the field inhomogeneities which are responsible for the shortening of T2 (Eq. 1.27). On the other hand, shorter echo times can be achieved, because no 180° refocusing pulse requiring several milliseconds has to be inserted between the initial nutation (90° or α) pulse and the measurement of the signal.

The fact that in gradient echo pulse sequences we measure T2* rather than T2 has important consequences on the information contained in the signal. First, field inhomogeneities due to chemical shift of water versus fat affect the signal. Depending on the time delay between nutation pulse and signal measurement, in-phase or opposed-phase images are obtained. For a field strength of 1.5 Tesla (64 MHz), the time for the water protons to precess half a circle ahead of the fat protons is approximately 2.33 ms. Hence, for all odd multiples of this number an opposed-phase signal is obtained, whereas for even multiples an in-phase signal is measured. Second, if we assume the field of the main magnet to be perfect, field inhomogeneities in a sample are due only to variations in local susceptibility, e.g., to local differences in the presence of paramagnetic substances in one region compared with another. Measurement of the signal phase accumulated in a given region is thus related to the magnetic susceptibility, which enters into Eq. 1.27, because the difference in susceptibility in a region 1, $χ_1$ and a region 2, $χ_2$ corresponds to $ΔH_o$:

$$ΔH_o = (χ_1 - χ_2)H_o \tag{1.45}$$

In MRI, gradient echo imaging can thus be used to produce susceptibility maps [29].

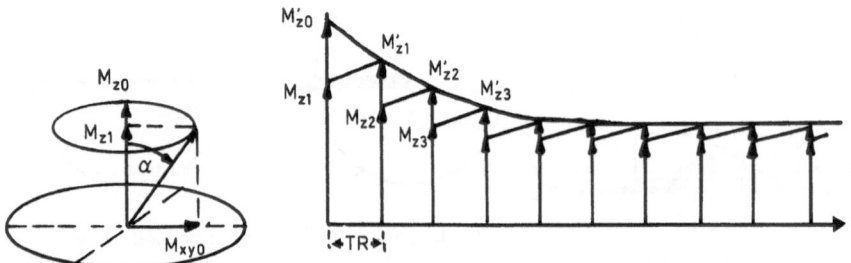

Fig. 1.26. In gradient echo experiments, an FID is measurend, but after an RF pulse generating a flip angle α usually smaller than 90°. As a result, not all longitudinal magneti-zation M_{zo} is destroyed and a short repetition time TR can be used. After several short TR, an equilibrium between destruction and recovery of longitudinal magnetization is established

1.4.9 Gradient Echo Sequences for Measuring Flow

It was shown in Sect. 1.4.6 that switching on a magnetic gradient field after the 90° nutation pulse in a spin echo MR experiment leads to a sensitization of spins to motion. This can also be achieved in gradient echo imaging, by using a so-called bipolar gradient (Fig. 1.27). If a gradient field is applied during a time t_p (as is necessary for imaging) and its sign inverted after a time TE/2, stationary spins which were losing phase coherence due to the influence of the additional localizing gradient field will refocus after TE. However, spins moving at constant velocity will continue to gain or lose phase relative to the stationary spins, as discussed in Sect. 1.4.6. Thus, a bipolar gradient echo pulse sequence is in a sense equivalent to a balanced gradient with two equal gradient pulses around the 180° refocusing pulse in a spin echo experiment (Fig. 1.20). Application of a symmetrical gradient whose sign is inverted twice, such as the bimodal gradients shown in Fig. 1.27, will produce even echo refocusing similar to an SE experiment and thus be velocity insensitive (Sect. 1.4.6). Such bipolar gradients are the base of the so-called FEER sequence (Field Even Echo Refocused) [30]. This results in extra-strong intravascular signals in MRI on second echos. If only these second echoes are studied and a slight time shift is introduced into the bipolar gradient, as shown in Fig. 1.27, the flow-insensitive pulse sequence can be arbitrarily flow sensitized

and used for flow velocity (or motion) measurements. Several schemes have been proposed in which gradient echo refocusing sequences are used for the measurement of blood flow velocities [31].

1.5 Magnetic Resonance Imaging

Formation of an MR image requires three steps. First the appropriate pulse sequence has to be chosen. We discussed a variety of them in the preceeding section. Second, spatial localization of the signal has to be accomplished, and third, the time domain data measured with the RF receiver of the MR imager have to be transformed into an image. We shall discuss only two- or three-dimensional Fourier transformation (2DFT and 3DFT) imaging methods as they are the only ones in clinical use. The initial experiments by Lauterbur [32], the Fourier transformation MR imaging by Kumar et al. [33], and its spin-warp modification proposed by Edelstein et al. [34] all make use of the fact that by applying external magnetic gradient fields in addition to the main magnetic field, the resonant Larmor frequency becomes a function of position. In this way, imaging is accomplished. In 2DFT and 3DFT, furthermore, use is made of the fact that the phase of an MR signal can also be measured (Sect. 1.4.5). As suggested when flow and diffusion were discussed (Sects. 1.4.4, 1.4.6, and 1.4.9), the addition of gradient fields to pulse sequences sensi-

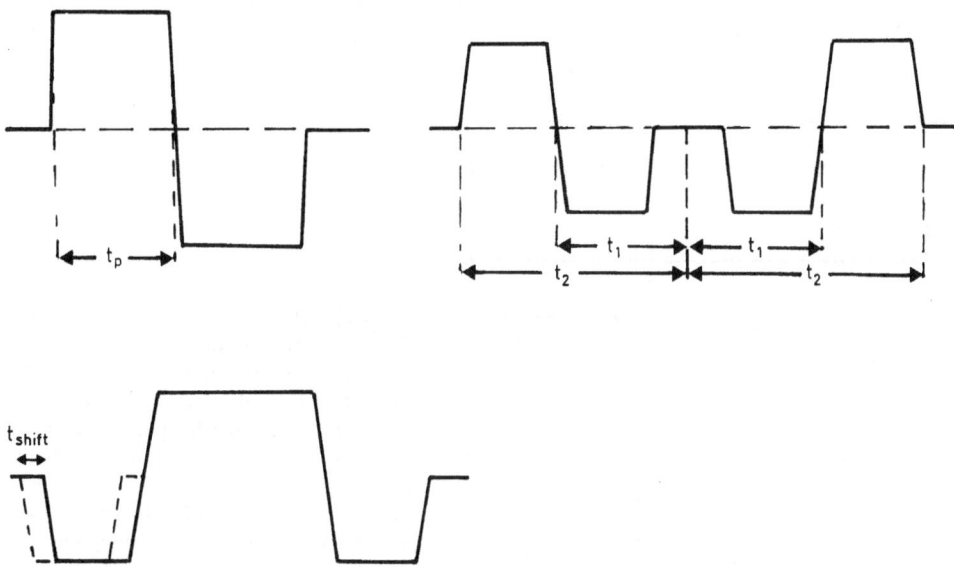

Fig. 1.27. In a gradient echo experiment, the gradient field is inverted after a pulse time t_p (*left*). For stationary spins this results in zero phase shift at the gradient echo time. However, moving spins gain or lose phase relative to the stationary spins according to Table 1.3. A bimodal gradient produces neither a phase shift for stationary spins nor one for spins moving a contant velocity (*middle* and *right*). A slight time shift t_{shift} may be used to produce a controllable velocity sensitization of the sequence (*right*)

tizes MR to motion and flow phenomena. A good understanding of the imaging process thus not only promotes insight into the basics of MRI but also into the reasons for the variety of flow phenomena observed in MRI. In 2DFT an image is built up as follows: a slice of arbitrary orientation in space is selected and then the magnetization values of pixels within this slice are measured.

1.5.1 Slice Selection

For the sake of simplicity we shall discuss MR image acquisition in the ensuing sections only for a slice perpendicular to the main magnetic field, that is, perpendicular to the z-axis of the reference coordinate system at the z = 0 position. Any other slice can be imaged by analogy. The first step in MRI is the selection of the slice to be imaged. This is ac-

complished by superimposing a magnetic field gradient G_z on the main magnetic field. As a result, the Larmor frequency ω varies along the z-direction according to Eqs. 1.10 and 1.29:

$$\omega = \gamma_p(H_o + G_z z) \qquad (1.46)$$

Hence, if an RF pulse of a certain band width (frequency range) is used to irradiate the sample, only spins precessing with frequencies in this range will experience the RF pulse; spins at larger or smaller z will not feel the RF pulse, as they do not satify the Larmor condition (Fig. 1.28). The RF pulse sent into the patient needs to have a temporal shape such that it contains all the frequencies with which it can flip the spins in a slice with thickness s. It turns out that the RF pulse needed for this purpose has the form of a so-called sinc function, that is, $\sin(\omega t)/\omega t$ (Fig. 1.22). Exciting different slices along the z-axis then simply requires shifting the center frequency of the sinc function slightly upward or downward. This temporal encoding of a square frequency profile requires that the RF pulse have a certain duration, which in practice is on the order of several milliseconds. As a result, the minimal echo time which can be achieved in MRI with good slice definition is on the order of 10 ms. In MR SE (spin echo) imaging in the multislice mode, the 180° refocus pulses also have to be slice selective (Sect. 1.5.4), putting further constraints on the minimal echo time. In gradient echo imaging, where no refocusing pulses are necessary, shorter echo times are possible. Typical SE and gradient echo pulse sequences for imaging are depicted in Fig. 1.29. Note that the

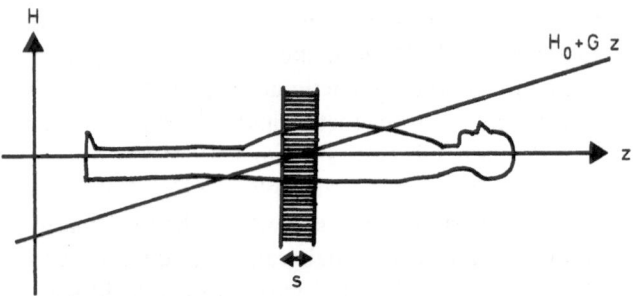

Fig. 1.28. In MRI, a transverse slice is selected by applying, e.g., a gradient field G_z along the axis of the patient. The net magnetic field strength then varies as a function of position along the patient. A sinc function (Fig. 1.22) with its square frequency spectrum will flip the spins in only a narrow range around the center frequency of the sinc function

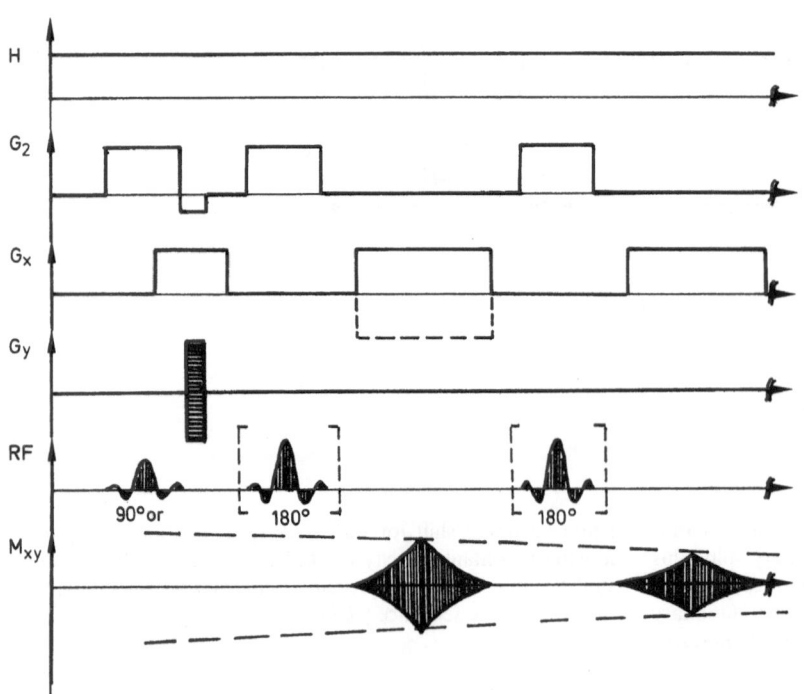

Fig. 1.29. Pulse sequence schematic for an SE (in *brackets* gradient echo) imaging sequence. In addition to the main magnetic field H, a slice-selecting gradient G_z field is turned on during the RF pulses. The read gradient G_x is switched on first shortly after the 90° pulse and then while the echoes are received. The phase-encoding gradient G_y is applied in variable strength along the y-axis. At the echo time TE, a signal M_{xy} is measured. The read and phase-encode gradients can be interchanged, and if other spatial slice orientations are desired, the slice-selecting gradient has to be applied along another direction, which can be arbitrary

gradient G_z becomes negative for a short period just after the 90° pulse. This is done to refocus the spins with a kind of gradient echo after the application of the slice-selection gradient has somewhat refocused them.

Using the process described above, selection of a slice in the object under study is accomplished. The next step is to identify from which pixel within the selected slice the MR signal is coming. This is done by the process of frequency encoding in one dimension and, in the case of 2DFT, by the process of phase encoding in the other dimension.

1.5.2 Frequency Encoding

To spatially localize an object along one in-plane axis, assume the horizontal x-axis, a method called frequency encoding is used. During data acquisition, i.e., when the radio receiver records the signal coming from the patient, a magnetic gradient field is applied across the patient from left to right. This is the so-called read or read-out gradient. This field has the effect that the resonant Larmor frequencies

are lowest on the left and highest on the right of the patient. All the parts of the patient lying in a pixel column (Fig. 1.30) in the imaging plane emit sine waves of identical Larmor frequencies, but the overall signal measured is a superposition of sine waves with many different frequencies: by the process of frequency encoding a spatial position along the x-axis is uniquely represented by a frequency in the MR signal. The signal amplitudes coming from these pixel columns are extracted from the received signal by means of a Fourier transformation (the first in 2DFT). The timing of the read gradient in an SE sequence is shown in Fig. 1.29. It is usually a balanced gradient (Sect. 1.4.6), and it is the read gradient which is responsible for in-plane flow sensitization in MRI (Chap. 3). The reason why the read gradient is turned on for a short time shortly after the 90° nutation pulse in this: Under the influence of an external gradient field the spins defocus as discussed in Sect. 1.4.4. However, switching on the gradient G_x, as shown in Fig. 1.29, leads to a situation where stationary spins all refocus at the echo time TE (Sect. 1.4.6) and a sizable signal is recorded at the echoes.

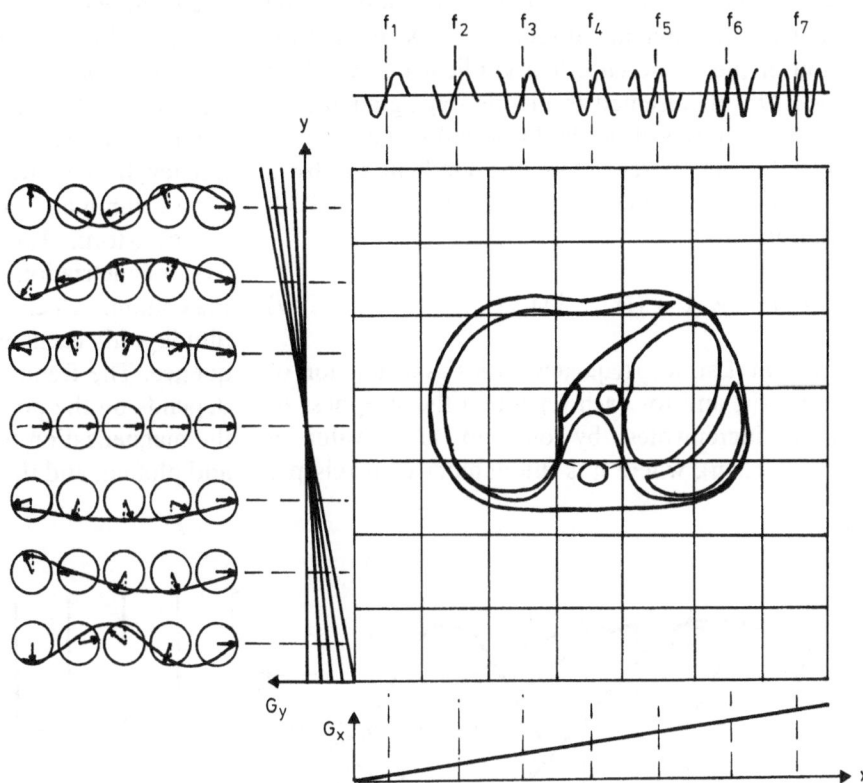

Fig. 1.30. In order to spatially localize a signal in the imaging plane in 2DFT, a gradient G_x is applied across the patient. The resonant Larmor frequency thus varies in space, and the wavelets coming from the various columns of the pixel grid have different frequencies f (here f_1-f_7). Identifying the signal as coming from a particular pixel requires an additional localization process, which in 2DFT is phase encoding.

By systematically increasing the gradient G_y with each repitition of the basic pulse sequence, spins at the top and the bottom of the image run ahead and lag behind the spins on the horizontal center line, respectively, giving rise to another set of oscillating functions, whose frequencies encode for position

In gradient echo imaging, the same scheme is used for spatial localization. The only difference is that now no 180° refocusing pulse is used, but rather the read gradient is inverted (dashed lines in Fig. 1.29), which makes the spins precess backwards and in that way leads to refocusing. Note, however, that in gradient echo imaging it is only the phase dispersion induced during the read process which can be refocused by switching on the read gradient after the 90° nutation pulse. Quasi static field inhomogeneities due to system imperfections are not refocusable in gradient echo imaging as they are in SE imaging (Sect. 1.4.8).

By the process of frequency encoding we can thus localize from where along the x-axis a certain signal is coming. This is done in one SE or gradient echo sequence shown in Fig. 1.29 in a time on the order of tens to hundreds of milliseconds.

1.5.3 Phase Encoding

The localization of the signal into individual pixels within a column is accomplished by a process called phase encoding in both conventional and gradient echo imaging. It requires a systematic variation of the phase encoding gradient G_y, which in Fig. 1.29 is represented as a ladder-type gradient. G_y is varied by repeating the basic pulse sequence of Fig. 1.29, but incrementing the gradient G_y by a constant amount yG_y for each repetition (Fig. 1.30) according to

$$\omega(y) = \gamma_p H = (H_o + kyG_y) \qquad (1.47)$$

Thus, the Larmor frequency varies as a function of the y-axis, and for each repetition the steepness of G_y is incremented by one up to a value n $(k = 1,2,...,n)$, where n is the number of pixels per column. In order to assign a signal equivocally to one pixel in a column, n measurements at different gradient settings are required, hence the basic need to repeat a pulse sequence n times with different G_y settings, and the repetition time of the basic pulse sequence is TR. In conventional SE imaging TR is usually taken to be anywhere between 300 and 2500 ms.

Let us consider a signal coming from a single pixel in a column. When G_y is switched on, the precessing spins gain or lose phase relative to the spins in the reference pixel in the center of the column, where the gradient field G_y is always zero (Fig. 1.30). After switching off the phase-encode gradient G_y, all the spins precess again with the Larmor frequency of the reference spins, but with some defined (encoded) phase gain or lag. With each phase-encode step, the phase gain (lag) increases (decreases) by a constant for a given pixel. Hence, when measuring the magnetization M_{xy}, the phase for this pixel is found to be turned, e. g., first by 30°, then by 60°, then by 90°, etc., as indicated on the left of Fig. 1.30. If we measure the projection of the magnetization M_{xy}, let us say along the y-axis for each phase-encoding gradient setting, a sinusoidal curve is obtained, and this sinusoidal curve is seen to vary according to the pixel position along the y-axis (Figs. 1.30, 1.31). The further away the pixel is from the center, the higher is the oscillation frequency. In MRI we measure the magnetization M_{xy} for a column and know its value after the first Fourier transform. This value is a superposition of the M_{xy} magnetizations of the individual pixels within the column, which in turn vary sinusoidally in magnitude with each repetition of the basic pulse sequence. The frequency of this sinusoidal variation depends on the position along the y-axis. Hence, if the magnetization in a column is measured n times and plotted, and then subjected to a second Fourier

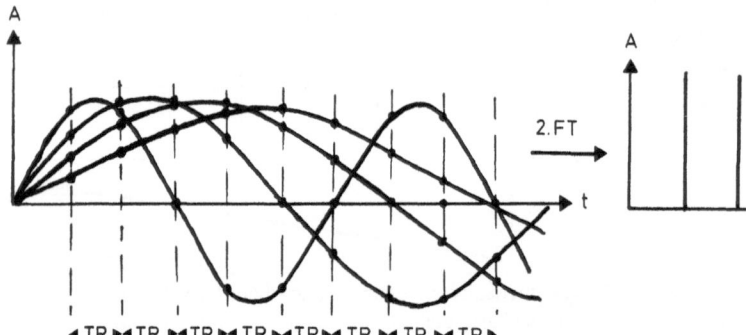

Fig. 1.31. Measurement of the amplitude along the x- or y-axis results in an oscillating signal for each pixel. The further the row is away from the center row in the phase-encode direction, the higher is the frequency of the oscillations. Thus,

the frequency obtained in a second Fourier transformation yields a frequency which encondes for the vertical position of the measured signal

transform, the pixel magnetization is obtained (Fig. 1.31).

Frequency and phase encoding and a two dimensional Fourier transform yield the real and imaginary or amplitude and phase values for the magnetization vector of each pixel. Using the concepts of Sect. 1.4.5, we may thus represent amplitude or modulus images, as the usual MR images are called, or produce phase images, which contain information on motion and susceptibility. In principle, real images and imaginary images can also be obtained, but the information content of such images is not readily extracted. The frequency- and phase-encoding directions can be chosen arbitrarily at right angles to each other. So it is not necessary that frequency encoding be done along the horizontal and phase encoding along the vertical axis. By limiting the range of frequencies measured in the frequency-encoding direction, the size of the field of view is determined. In the phase-encoding direction the field of view is not limited, because phase encoding is not a unique process: whether a spin is not phase-shifted at all or is phase-shifted by 360° with each phase-encode gradient increment cannot be distinguished. The result of this is the so-called backfolding phenomenon, by which structures above the upper border of the field of view appear again at the bottom of the image (Fig. 1.32). This apparent drawback can be used to good advantage

in many situations, particularly if high-resolution surface coil images of structures in a noncentral location have to be acquired.

The process of three-dimensional Fourier transformation imaging (3DFT) is analogous to that of 2DFT except that instead of a slice-select gradient, a second phase-encode gradient is applied. Image reconstruction can also be done as in computed tomography with back-projection reconstruction [35, 36], but this method is not widely used.

1.5.4 Multislice Imaging

We have seen that in imaging pulse sequences such as an SE sequence the read process for an echo occurs after 10–30 ms, but in order for the magnetization M_z to grow back to a sizable magnitude, a repetition time TR of several hundreds of milliseconds has to elapse. During this time, the MR imager is idle and can be used for further data acquisition. For this reason, all present-day imagers have the capacity of multislice imaging: several slices are examined "quasi simultaneously." The process of multislice imaging is as follows: The first pulse sequence es applied to a first slice with not only the 90° pulse but not also the 180° refocusing pulse(s) being slice selective so as not to disturb spins in adjacent slices. Note that for single-slice imaging, the 180° refocusing pulses do not have to be slice selective. This first slice is then left to recover its magnetization M_z for a time TR. However, after the echo has been received from the first slice, a second slice is subjected to a pulse sequence starting with the 90° pulse, then a third, and so on. The number of slices which can be examined simultaneously in this way depends on TE and TR. The longer the TR, the more SE sequences can be applied to the subject under investigation, and thus slices examined, before the first slice will have to be reexamined using the second setting of the phase-encode gradient. The read process is repeated for all slices with the second phase-encode gradient value, and this process is repeated until the n-th phase-encode value has been used on all examined slices (Fig. 1.33). The result is an interleaved data acquisition of many slices simultaneously. The sequence in which the slices in a stack are read is arbitrary and can be chosen in many imagers. To minimize "cross-talk" between slices, a sequence 1,3,5,7,...2,4,6,8,... is advantageous. When imaging the cardiovascular system a sequence of acquisition of, e.g., 1,2,3,4,5,6,7,8,... may be preferable, as will be seen in Chap. 3.

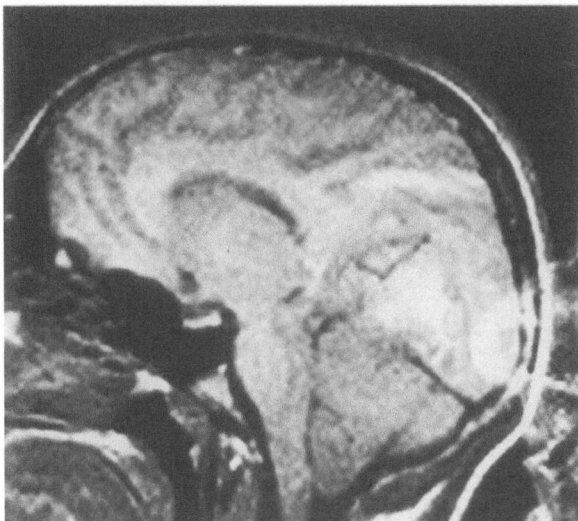

Fig. 1.32. The position of the signal along the phase-encode direction is not unique. If an object is beyond the border of the image, the phase-encoding gradient will turn the phase at each step such that it appears again at the other end of the image. In this direction, the image wraps around

Slice

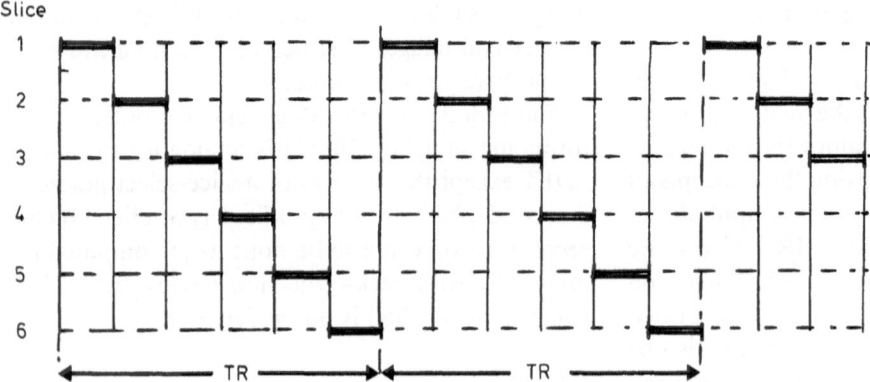

Fig. 1.33. The first slice is read and then the machine is idle, waiting for TR to elapse, before it is read again. However, in multislice imaging the machine is used during this idle time to look at a second, third, etc. slice, until the first slice has to be looked at again. In this figure at total of six slices are examined, one after the other. In principle, the sequence in which the slices are looked at is arbitrary

1.5.5 Chemical Shift Artifacts and Chemical Shift Imaging

In Sect. 1.3.4 we discussed the chemical shift phenomenon, which, due to the different screening of water and fat protons by the surrounding electrons, leads to slight differences in their precession frequencies. Since in imaging, slice selection is accomplished by exciting spins precessing in a given frequency range, the different precession frequencies of water and fat protons translate into a situation whereby the actual image is a sum of a water and a fat image taken at slightly different anatomic levels. The difference between these two levels is determined by the steepness of the applied slice-select gradient field: the steeper it is, the more exact is the superposition of the water and fat images. The same is true for the read gradient, where again the precessional frequency encodes for position. The fat spins, precessing at slightly slower frequencies, are placed in the image slightly to the right of the water spins in the same anatomical position. This phenomenon is more pronounced in high-field imagers because of the higher precession frequencies and the higher absolute value of the chemical shift in terms of frequency. It is readily noted in many MR images (Fig. 1.34).

In gradient echo imaging, the chemical shift has an additional effect on the images. Since the water spins are precessing somewhat faster than the fat spins, there will be in-phase and opposed-phase echoes, as discussed in Sects. 1.4.7 and 1.4.8, depending on the echo time chosen. In the opposed-phase images with pixels containing comparable amounts of water and fat spins, the total signal will cancel approximately, thus leaving a black pixel.

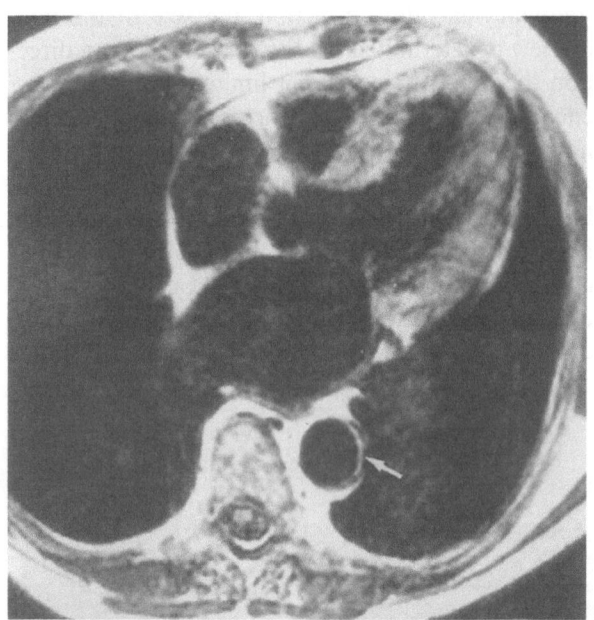

a

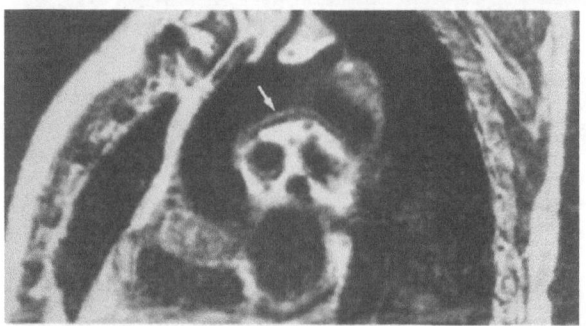

b

Fig. 1.34. a Chemical shift artifact appearing as a fine line on the left side of the descending aorta *(arrow)*. In this transverse image, the read-gradient direction is left-right and it is in this direction that the chemical shift occurs. **b** On a sagittal image in an other patient, a duplication of the caudal outline of the aortic arch *(arrow)* is due to a chemical shift artifact, which, because the read gradient is cranio-caudal in this image, now occurs along this direction

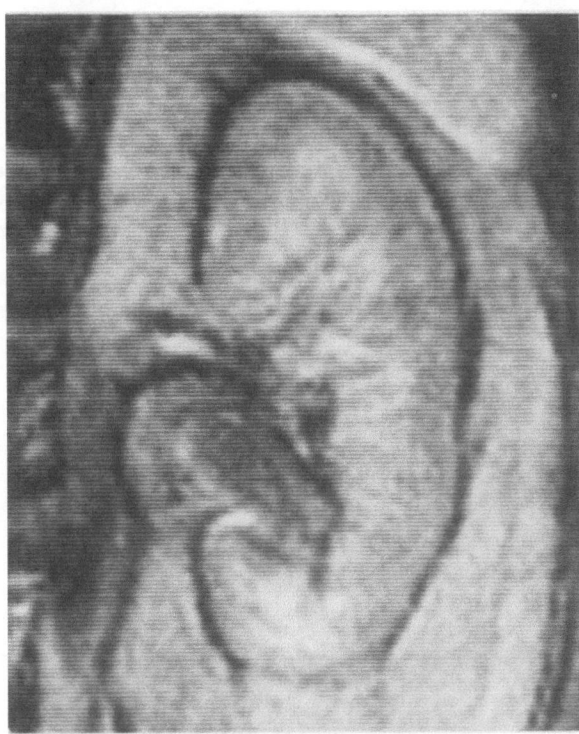

Fig. 1.35. Gradient echo image of a kidney taken with an echo time of approximately 16.1 ms, for which at 1.5 Tesla an opposed-phase image is obtained (phase shift between water and fat protons = 180° after 2.3 ms: 7 × 2.3 = 16.1 ms). Note the dark rim around the edges of the kidney marking the pixels which contain similar amounts of renal tissues (mainly water) and perirenal fat

This effect is noted whenever a fat-containing and a water-containing structure are adjacent to each other. As an example, this is the case with the kidneys and the perirenal fat. In opposed-phase images, the kidneys are nicely outlined by a dark rim (Fig. 1.35). This facilitates automated edge detection in region-of-interest (ROI) analysis, as will be seen in Chap. 6.

References

1. Pake GE (1950) Fundamentals of nuclear magnetic resonance absorption, part 1. Am J Phys 18: 438–452
2. Schiff LI (1968) Quantum mechanics (3rd edition). McGraw-Hill, New York
3. Slichter CP (1963) Principles of magnetic resonance. Harper and Row
4. Carr HY, Purcell EM (1954) Effects of diffusion on free precession in nuclear magnetic resonance experiments. Phys Rev 94: 630–635
5. The Heisenberg uncertainty principle states that certain pairs of variables, such as the energy or frequency of the quantum mechanical state and the life time of the system in such a state, cannot be known more exactly than given by the relation $\Delta E \Delta t \approx h$, where h is Planck's constant
6. Mansfield P, Morris PG (1982) NMR imaging in biomedicine. Acadamic Press, New York 1982
7. Solomon I (1955) Relaxation processes in a system of two spins. Phys Rev 99: 559–565
8. Bloembergen N (1957) Proton relaxation times in paramagnetic solutions. J Chem Phys 27: 572–573
9. Gadian DG, Payne JA, Bryant DJ, Young IR, Carr DH, Bydder GM (1985) Gadolinium-DTPA as a contrast agent in MR imaging - theoretical projections and practical observations. J Comp Ass Tomogr 9: 242–251
10. Bertini I, Luchinat C (1986) NMR of paramagnetic molecules in biological systems. Benjamin/Cummings Publishing Co, Menlo Park, Ca
11. Burton DR, Forsen S, Karlstrom G, Dwek RA, McLaughlin AC, Wain-Hobson S (1976) Difficulties in determining accurate molecular motion parameters from proton relaxation enhancement measurements as illustrated by the immunoglobulin G-Gd(III) system. Eur J Biochem 71: 519–528
12. Grodd W, Brasch RC (1986) Magnetopharmazeutische Kontrastveränderungen in der Kernspintomographie. Fortschr Röntgenstr 145: 130–139
13. Saini S, Stark DD, Hahn PF, Wittenberg J, Brady TJ, Ferrucci JT (1987) Ferrite particles: a superparamagnetic agent for the reticuloendothelial system. Radiology 162: 211–216
14. Widder DJ, Greif WL, Widder KJ, Edelman RR, Brady TJ (1987) Magnetite albumin microspheres: a new MR contrast material. Am J Roentgenol 148: 399–404
15. Bean CP, Livingston JD (1968) Superparamagnetism. J Appl Physiol 30: 1205–1298
16. Duewell S, Wüthrich R, Buck A, von Schulthess GK (1988) Signal loss in intravoxel incoherent motion: evaluation of different perfusion types and pulse sequences. SHRM book of abstracts 221
17. Beall PT, Amtey SR, Katsturi SR (1984) NMR data handbook for biochemical applications. Pergamon Press, New York
18. Hahn EL (1950) Spin echoes. Phys Rev 80: 580–585
19. Meiboom S, Gill D (1959) Modified spin echo methods for measuring nuclear relaxation times. Rev Sci Instr 29: 688–692
20. Stejskal EE, Tanner JE (1965) Spin diffusion measurements: spin echoes in the presence of a time-dependent field gradient. Chem Phys 42: 288–293
21. von Schulthess GK, Higgins CB (1985) Blood flow imaging with MR: spin-phase phenomena. Radiology 157: 687–695
22. Waluch V, Bradley WG (1984) NMR even echo rephasing in slow laminar flow. J Comput Ass Tomogr 8: 594–598
23. Pattany PM, Phillips JC, Chiu LC, et al (1987) Motion artifact suppression technique (MAST) for MR imaging. J Comput Ass Tomogr 11: 369–377
24. Singer JR (1978) NMR diffusion and flow measurements and an introduction to spin phase graphing. J Phys E Sci Instrum 11: 281–291
25. Dixon WT (1984) Simple proton spectroscopic imaging. Radiology 153: 189–194
26. Brateman L (1986) Chemical shift imaging: a review. AJR 146: 971–980
27. Haase A, Mattaei D, Hänicke W, Merboldt KD (1986) Flash imaging: rapid NMR imaging using low flip-angle pulses. J Magnetic Resonance 67: 258–266
28. van der Meulen P, Groen JP, Cuppen JJ (1985) Very fast MR imaging by field echoes and small-angle excitation. Mag Res Imag 3: 297–299

29. Young IR, Khenia S, Thomas DGT et al (1987) Clinical magnetic susceptibility mapping of the brain. J Comput Ass Tomogr 11: 2-6

30. Nayler GL, Firmin DN, Longmore DB (1986) Blood flow imaging by cine magnetic resonance. J Comput Ass Tomogr 10: 715-722

31. Wehrli FW, Shimakawa A, Gullberg GT, MacFall JR (1986) Time-off-flight MR flow imaging: selective saturation recovery with gradient refocussing. Radiology 160: 781-785

32. Lauterbur PC (1973) Image formation by induced local interactions: examples employing NMR. Nature 242: 190-196

33. Kumar A, Welti D, Ernst RR (1975) NMR Fourier zeugmatography. J Mag Resonance 18: 63-89

34. Edelstein WA, Hutchinson JMS, Johnson G et al (1980) Spin warp NMR imaging and applications to human whole-body imaging. Phys Med Biol 25: 751-756

35. Hounsfield GN (1973) Computerised transverse axial scanning (tomography). 1. Description of system. Br J Radiol 46: 1016-1022

36. Gordon R, Herman GT, Johnson SA (1975) Image reconstruction from projections. Scientific American 233: 56-68

Chapter 2   Functional Aspects of the Cardiovascular System

The purpose of the cardiovascular system ist to oxygenate body tissues by pumping blood through vessels. Thus, any imaging method which permits accurate assessment of the movements associated with the cardiovascular system may have a major impact on cardiovascular diagnosis. Since MRI is very sensitive to motion and flow and also to perfusion (Chap. 3), in addition to its ability to depict morphology in great detail, MRI has many excellent advantages as a tool for studying the cardiovascular system. In this chapter we discuss the basics of motion and flow in the cardiovascular system, keeping in mind existing and potential applications of MRI to the study of cardiovascular function. Hence, this chapter will not review cardiovascular physiology in general but rather will highlight areas of cardiovascular physiology amenable to study by MRI.

The basic components of the cardiovascular system are simple: a pump and a network of pipes. The pumping action is by contraction and expansion of the cardiac walls. In addition, the large arteries, particularly the aorta, are elastic in young people and thus can provide some "passive" pumping action during diastole. Due to the cardiac valves, this pumping action results in directed flow in large and small blood vessels: the tubes and pipes. We shall discuss first motion, then flow.

2.1 Motion in the Cardiovascular System

2.1.1 Motion of Cardiac Walls and Valves

The combination of anatomic and functional data is very important in the evaluation of the cardiac patient, because only functional data are able to indicate the severity of cardiac disease. In congenital heart disease, identification of the morphological abnormality is the most important task, but in patients with left-right shunts and consequent pulmonary hypertension, it is the pulmonary vascular resistance, a function parameter, which determines,

whether correction of the lesion can still be accomplished. A rise in pulmonary vascular resistance eventually leads to a right-left shunt with cyanosis, termed "Eisenmenger's syndrome" [1]. In acquired heart disease, the diagnosis of ventricular hypertrophy, dilatation, and ventricular aneurysms is made using morphological criteria, but in coronary artery disease, the earliest indicators of disease are regional wall motion abnormalities, and cardiac arrhythmias are functional derangements which may or may not have morphological correlates recognizable on anatomic images. In cardiac valvular abnormalities, the gradient across the diseased valve, another function parameter, is an important determinant of severity of the disease.

Cardiac walls and valves move as the cardiac cycle evolves. The events of the cardiac cycle will be discussed here in their relation to the ECG, as is the ECG which is readily available for study and is used in MRI to provide ECG-synchronous data acquisition. In Fig. 2.1 we depict an ECG cycle together with a ventricular volume curve, showing the hypothetical variation of the blood volume in the left ventricle. With the onset of the QRS complex in the ECG, the ventricular walls start to contract. This contraction is first isovolumetric and involves little change in cardiac geometry, because the pressure inside the left ventricular chamber has to rise from left atrial pressure, being around 0 mm Hg, to the aoritc pressure of around 100 mm Hg in a normal person. The time during which this happens is called the preejection period (PEP) and lasts for 80–100 ms. Since SE data acquisition in MRI takes only several to 50 ms, starting a pulse sequence with the onset of the QRS complex will produce at least one end-diastolic image during the preejection period. The mitral valve closes during this time, and the aortic valve opens at the end of the preejection period and systole begins. During systole there is first slow but accelerating, then constant high, and finally decelerating motion of the cardiac walls, pushing the blood into the aorta. During this time, the cardiac walls thicken, typically by 50%. End-systole (ES)

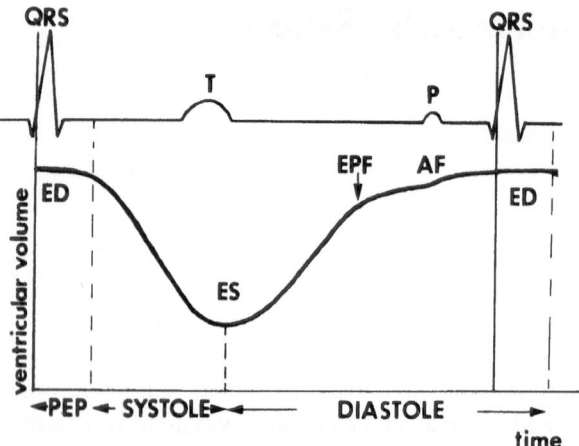

Fig. 2.1. Temporal relations of events in the cardiac cycle showing an ECG and a hypothetical ventricular volume curve. End-diastole *(ED)* lasts approximately 50–100 ms after the onset of the ECG-QRS complex and corresponds to the time of isovolumetric contraction *(PEP)*. Systole starts, and its end *(ES)* coincides more or less with the T wave of the ECG. The ventricle then relaxes and blood flows into it until the end of passive ventricular filling *(EPF)*, marked by a inflection on the volume curve. With the onset of atrial contraction, marked by the ECG-P wave, there is a short additional inflow of blood *(AF)*. The diastolic time interval between EPF and AF is the most variable part of the cardiac cycle, and it is mainly this interval which changes with variations in heart rate

coincides essentially with the T wave in the ECG, which is a good marker for this event, and it has been shown that for heart rates between 50 and 80 beats per minute (BPM), there is very little variation in the occurrence of these initial events after the QRS complex. In fact, PEP decreases from 110 to 80 ms and ES from 410 to 360 ms after the onset of the QRS complex [2]. ES proper is marked by the onset of relaxation of the ventricular walls with a consecutive intraventricular pressure drop, the closure of the aortic valve, and the passive inflow of blood through the now open mitral valve. Passive inflow subsides towards the end of diastole because the ventricle is filled (EPF). This diastolic phase of the cardiac cycle is most variable in length, lasting from approximately 400 to 700 ms with a decrease of the cardiac frequency from 80 to 50 BPM, and it is also in this phase that the normally existing sinus arrhythmia affects the timing of the cardiac events relative to the preceding QRS complex the most. A last injection of blood is brought about by the onset of atrial contraction (AF), which is marked by the P wave in the ECG. The right ventricle behaves essentially like the left one, except that the opening of the tricuspid valve is somewhat earlier than that of the aortic valve due to the lower pressure in the pulmonary vascular system. The atria are essentially

passive chambers which have the function of collecting the blood before it enters the cardiac ventricles. Their pumping action is minor, and in fact, the active filling phase contributes only about 10% to the total blood volume in the cardiac chambers at end-diastole (ED).

Many quantities describing global ventricular function have been studied with the aim of obtaining information on the function state of the myocardium. Among these are ventricular wall thickness (WT) and percent of ventricular wall thickening, defined as

$$\% \text{ wall thickening} = (WT_{ED}WT_{ES})/WT_{ED} \qquad (2.1)$$

This quantitiy is useful in the assessment of the remaining contractile myocardium after infarction. Other functional data obtainable through anatomic measurements are the left ventricular mass, which yields information on the extent of cardiac hypertrophy, and the venticular volumes in the end-diastolic (EDV) and endsystolic (ESV) states.

These volumes can be calculated from cine ventriculography or echocardiography. For this calculation the following hypothesis is made, which was originally developed by Dodge et al. [3]. The left ventricular cavity is approximated by a prolate ellipsoid [4] with one major and two minor diameters. These diameters are obtained by the so-called area-length method. For this method, the longest length of the ventricle L obtained is measured, as is the area of the ventricle A. The diameter C of the ventricle is then obtained by computing $C = 4A/\pi L$. This calculation is ordinarily made for both an anteroposterior (ap) and a lateral (lat) projection. With this, the left ventricular volume V is then computed as

$$V = 4/3\pi (L/2) (D_{ap}/2) (D_{lat}/2) \qquad (2.2)$$

Corrections have to be made for the volume occupied by the papillary muscle. This calculation can be performed to obtain the EDV as well as the ESV.

The difference etween EDV and ESV is called the stroke volume (SV). An important quantity derived from these volumes is the so-called ejection fraction (EF), defined as

$$EF = (EDV - ESV)/EDV \qquad (2.3)$$

which is a good global indicator of ventricular function and a quantity independent of the patients size. EDV, ESV, and SV are usually obtained from cine ventriculograms or echocardiograms using the area-

Table 2.1. Normal values of some cardiac volumetric quantities

End-diastolic volume[a] (ml/m²)	Stroke volume[a] (ml/m²)	Left ventricular mass[a] (g/m²)	LV ejection fraction (%)	End-diastolic wall thickness (mm)
70 ± 20	45 ± 13	92 ± 16	0.67 ± 0.08	10.9 ± 2.0

[a] Normalized to body surface area (normal man: body surface area 1.72 m²)

length method. With this method, the left ventricular cavity is assumed to be an ellipsoid. Measurement of the LV chamber dimensions in an image cutting through the long axis of the heart and an image cutting perpendicularly to it yields the three axes of the ellipsoid. The volume of the ellipsoid is then determined according to the geometric formula.

Alternatively, if volume rather than planar information is available, as is the case in gated blood pool scanning or a tomographic method, direct volume determinations or determinations of the volume from a stack of sections through the cardiac chambers can be used to determine quantities such as EDV, ESV, and SV, as well as the EF.

A quantity less often used is the percentage of fiber shortening (%FS), which is computed from the end-diastolic length (EDL) and the end-systolic length (ESL) of the heart as %FS = 100 (EDL-ESL)/EDL. A further quantity derived from measurements of the cardiac volumes is the cardiac index (CI), which is given by

$$CI = (EDV - ESV) \, HR/BSA = SV \, HR/BSA \quad (2.4)$$

where HR is the heart rate in beats per minute and BSA is the body surface area. Normal values for these quantities are given in Table 2.1 [5, 6].

It has been shown that with coronary artery disease, which is most often focal, global function parameters such as the ones described above are not the earliest indicators of disease. Regional function parameters are more sensitive [7]. For this purpose many of the above variables such as EF have also been defined to yield regional information, for example, by computing regional EFs on ventricular sectors.

When imaging methods are used which produce ventricular volume curves with high temporal resolution [8] rather than just ventricular parameters in end-diastole and end-systole, function parameters such as parameters related to the speed of ventricular wall contraction and relaxation can be obtained, as in cine angiography or nuclear cardiology. Quantities measured are peak ejection and filling rates [9, 10], and such measurements have been advocated by some people [11] as early indicators of myocardial disease, again particularly when measured on a regional basis. One such quantity, peak circumferential fiber shortening (PCFS), is defined as [12]

$$PCFS = [(V)^{-2/3}/3(dV/dt)]max \quad (2.5)$$

where V is the end-diastolic volume.

If the ventricular volume data are obtained from the right as well as from the left ventricular chamber, shunt volumes can be calculated. Determinations of shunt volumes require relatively accurate measurements of ventricular volumetric data. This has been accomplished with nuclear medicine, but in general, cardiac shunts have been quantified by indicator dilution techniques and, more recently, they have been measured and visualized by Doppler echocardiography.

2.1.2 Motion of the Great Vessels

Whereas the veins, except for the vena cava, do not change their dimensions much with the events of the cardiac cycle, the large arteries, particularly the aorta and the pulmonary arteries, show considerable size variations over the cardiac cycle due to

Table 2.2. Percentage diameter change of large arteries from end-systole to end-diastole (after McDonald [17])

	Ascending aorta (%)	Descending aorta (%)	Left pulmonary artery (%)	Right pulmonary artery (%)
$\Delta R/R \times 100\%$	12.0	9.1	60.9	67.5

their natural elasticity, which serves as a means of minimizing the differences between diastolic and systolic blood pressure. The percentage of change in vessel radius 100 $\Delta R/R$, where R is the radius and ΔR the change in vessel radius, is given in Table 2.2 [13, 14]. The elasticity of the aorta, and thus the quantitiy $\Delta R/R$, diminishes with age and the onset of atherosclerosis. This causes the well-known increase in the difference between systolic and diastolic blood pressures [15].

2.2 Flow

The blood vessels conduct blood to the end organs and back to the heart; thus, the contents of the lumina of the cardiovascular system are in almost constant motion. The essentials of the physics of flow in vessels are necessary to understand circulatory phenomena. As we have seen in Chap. 1, MRI is exquisitely sensitive to blood flow, and it is blood flow which is responsible for the fact, that many blood vessels appear dark on MR images. In this section we discuss these basics of flow and present some data on the human circulation.

2.2.1 Shear Forces

The simplest model of a blood vessel is a cylindrical straight tube of length L. The viscosity of any substance flowing through such a tube results in some friction between the fluid and the tube wall. The tangential shear stress σ, or shear force exerted on the vessel wall, is given by

$$\sigma = \mu (dv/dr) \qquad (2.6)$$

with μ being the viscosity coefficient and dv/dr the radial variation of the velocity at the vessel wall. These shear forces are of interest in medicine because abnormal shear stress is thought to be one of the key determinants in the onset of atherosclerosis [16].

2.2.2 Laminar and Turbulent Flow, the Reynolds Number

As long as the layers of fluid within a tube glide along each other withouth actually mixing, so-called laminar flow prevails. For laminar flow in a tube it can be shown that the flow Q is given by

$$Q = (P_1 - P_2) \, \pi R^4 / (8\mu L) \qquad (2.7)$$

where P_1 and P_2 are the pressures at the entry and the exit of the tube respectively, R is the radius, and L is the length of the tube. Equation 2.7 is the famous Hagen-Poiseuille law. It is important to recognize that the flow varies with the fourth power of the vessel radius. The consequence is that the vascular surface area at different levels of branching in the vascular tree has to increase strongly with decreasing vessel diameter so that peripheral resistance is not exceedingly high. Some pertinent data are summarized in Table 2.3 (after McDonald [17]).

For laminar flow the velocity profile, i. e., the distribution of velocities across the tube lumen, is parabolic (Fig. 2.2), and for parabolic flow the average velocity $<v>$ is given by $<v> = v_{max}/2$. For increasing velocities, laminar flow breaks down and fluid layers no longer glide past each other, but vortices are formed along the course of flow; this is called turbulent flow. The velocity profile in a cylindrical tube then takes a more pluglike shape (Fig. 2.2) with a very rapid increase of velocity from the wall into the lumen and little velocity variation across most of the lumen. Under what conditions this change to turbulence occurs is determined by a quantity called the Reynolds number, Re, which is defined as

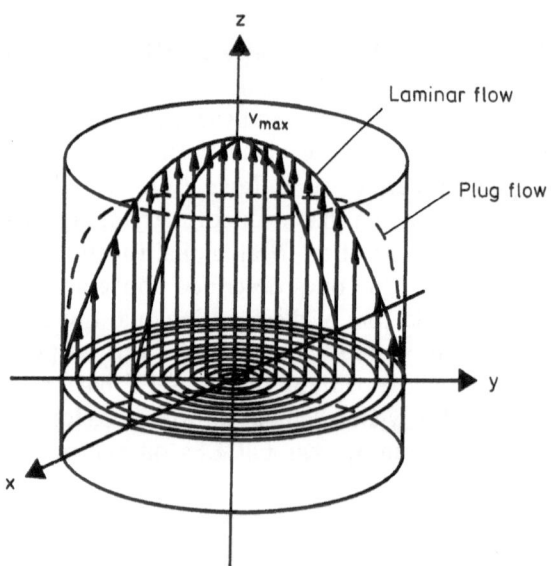

Fig. 2.2 Cylindrical vessel showing a parabolic flow profile. Note that the increase in velocity, when moving from the vessel wall inward is very steep close to the wall, but approaches zero towards the center of the vessel. In plug flow, which occurs under flow conditions approaching turbulence, this change in velocity close to the vessel wall is even more marked, and in the remainder of the vessel there is practically no velocity change as one moves across the lumen

Table 2.3. Estimated dimensions of the arterial tree (after McDonald [17])

Vessel	Length (cm)	No. of tubes	Diameter (mm)			Total area (cm^2)
			Entrance	Exit	Average entrance	
Aorta	40	1	20	7	20	3.2
Large arteries	20	20	10 -1.8	1.8	3.2	3.4
Main branches	10	260	4.0 -1.0	1	3.4	3.4
Secondary branches	4	800	2.0 -0.4	0.4	0.8	4.0
Secondary branches	4	7×10^3	0.8 -0.2	0.2	0.31	5
Tertiary branches	1.4	3×10^4	0.4 -0.1	0.1	0.16	6
Terminal arteries	0.1	2×10^5	0.2 -0.04	0.04	0.08	10
Terminal branches	0.15	2×10^6	0.1 -0.025	0.025	0.032	16
Arterioles	0.2	8×10^6	0.06 -0.015	0.015	0.02	25
Arterioles	0.2	3×10^7	0.03 -0.008	0.008	0.008	80
Capillaries	0.1	2×10^8	0.015-0.008	0.008	0.008	80

$$Re = <v> D\rho/\mu \qquad (2.8)$$

where D is the vessel diameter and ρ the density of the fluid. A lower limit for which fluid flow becomes turbulent is $Re \approx 2300$; however, by careful preparation of the samples, much higher values of Re and thus $<v>$ have been observed.

If the flow in a vessel is no longer constant, but time dependent as in the arterial blood vessels, the definition of laminar and turbulent flow no longer is valid. McDonald coined the term "disturbed" flow for this situation [17]. Nevertheless, in oscillating flow, a Reynolds number can be defined in analogy to constant flow conditions. Theoretical analyses and experimental data show, that for oscillatory flow the change to turbulence occurs for much higher values of the Reynolds number of approximately 7000 or more [18]. The transition from "laminar" to "turbulent" flow occurs the earliest in the deceleration phase of flow shortly after peak ve-

locity conditions. Bends in a tube also result in considerably higher Reynolds numbers, and the increase depends on the ratio of the radius of curvature to the radius proper of the vessel [19].

2.3 Hemodynamics

2.3.1 Flow in Veins and Arteries

In humans conditions resembling laminar flow are found only in veins and capillaries. The great veins of the thorax experience variations in intrathoracic pressure and the active contractions of the atria; thus, blood flow in them is oscillatory, like in arteries, rather than steady. Typical flow velocities in the large veins are between 10 and 20 cm/s (Table 2.4), and conditions leading to turbulent flow are never met in the venous system. Since the venous system is a low-pressure system with little pathology, ather-

Table 2.4. Flow velocities, Reynolds numbers, and shear rates in the human circulation (after McDonald [17] and Fung [20])

Vessel	Diameter (cm)	Velocity (cm/s)	Reynolds number	Shear rate $\partial v/\partial r$ (s^{-1})
Ascending aorta	2.30–4.35	21.3–87.4 (mean systolic)	5,000–12,000	80 (mean)
Main pulmonary artery	2.32–3.50	33.1–63.5 (mean systolic)	5,000–12,000	
Thoracic inferior vena cava	2.0	10.7–16.0 (mean)	1320 –1980	12
Small arteriole	0.01	1.0 (mean)	0.3	400
Capillary	0.0005	0.02–0.17	0.001	400

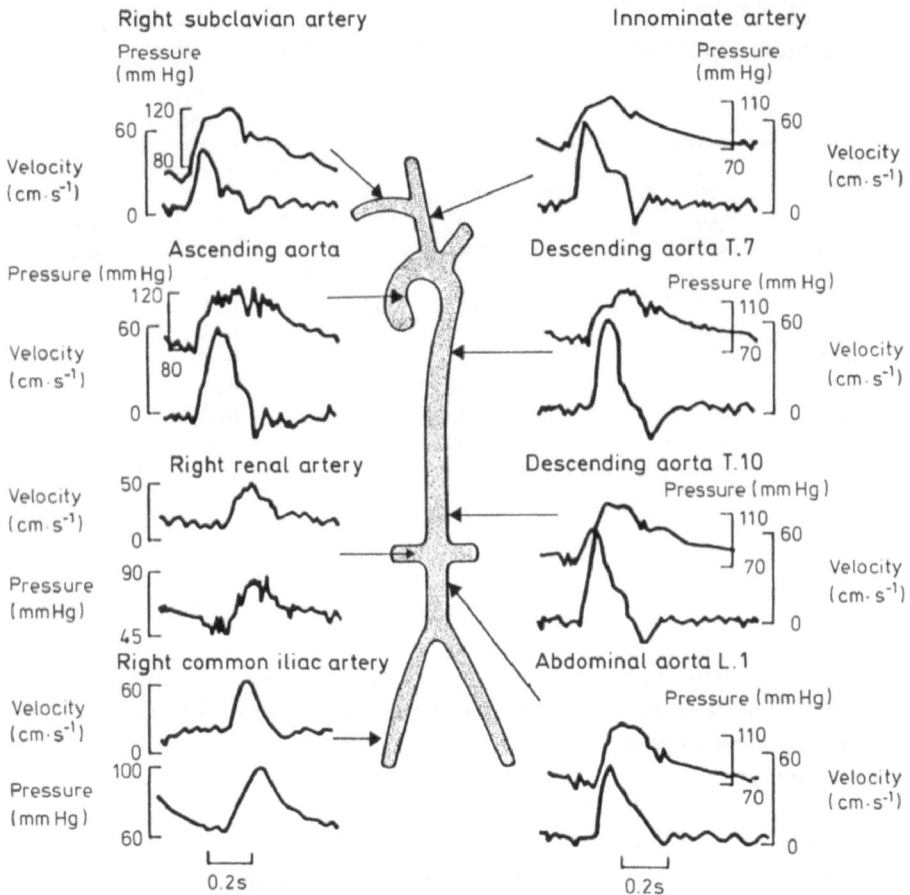

Fig. 2.3. Flow velocities and pressures as a function of the cardiac cycle measured in the aorta and its large branches. Note that the velocity variations are greatest in the aorta, which serves as an expansile reservoir of blood, damping the swings in flow velocity and blood pressure in the branching arteries. (Reprinted with permission from Milnor [21] and Mills et al. [22])

osclerotic changes are not seen. The major problems in the venous bed are caused by intrinsic or extrinsic obstruction, leading to venous stasis in parts of the body and formation of collateral circulations.

In the arterial part of the circulation, blood flow is pulsatile, and, as stated above, the terms "laminar" and "turbulent flow" should be used only in the sense that a Reynolds number can be defined, above which pulsatile flow exhibits "turbulent" characteristics. As can be seen from Table 2.4, the Reynolds number is practically always smaller than 7000: the human blood vessels seem to be "engineered" such that virtually no "turbulent" flow occurs. If it occurs, then only in the largest arteries and only during part of systole [17, 21]. Typical velocity and pressure measurements are given in Fig. 2.3 [22] and are seen to vary from practically zero to even negative velocity around the closure of the aortic valve, to 50–100 cm/s during mid-systole. Only patients with ventricular septal defects and aortic stenosis may show higher velocity jets close to the defect. The result of such defects is a prolongation of the systolic "turbulent" flow phase. Turbulence also can occur in aneurysms, because in aneurysms the "vessel" diameter is enlarged, resulting in a large Reynolds number (Eq. 2.8).

In arteries, blood flows through a system of curving [23] and branching vessels [24] and branching points. As can be seen in Fig. 2.4, complicated flow patterns are established with so-called recirculation zones. Wall stress due to the flowing blood is perpendicular rather than tangential at the sites where recirculation zones and zones of normal flow meet. There, areas of increased shear rates alter with areas of decreased shear rate, and it is in these zones of complicated wall stress patterns where atherosclerotic changes occur with predilection [25]. In the presence of atherosclerotic plaques, stenosed vessels, a stenosis of the aortic valve, or and coarctation of the aorta, "turbulent" flow downstream of the obstacle occurs thereby with shedding of vor-

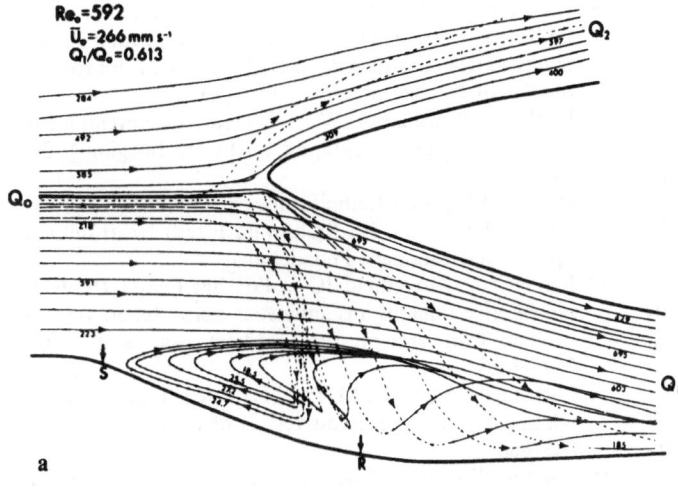

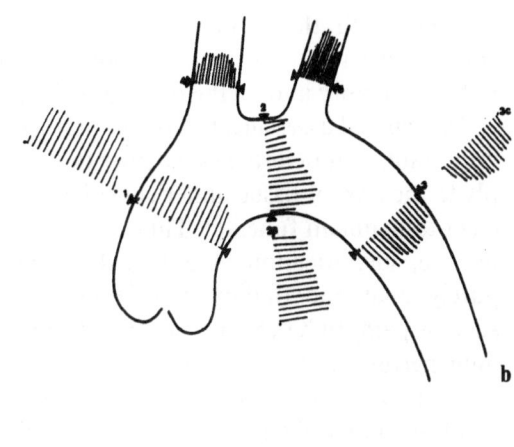

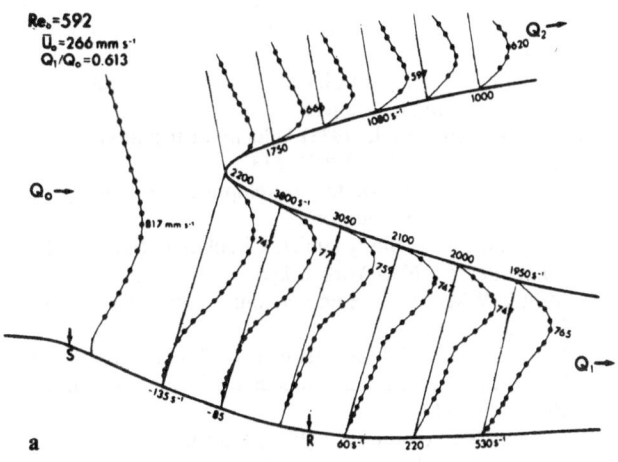

Fig. 2.4. **a** Flow patterns *(stream lines) (above)* and velocity profiles *(below)* in the human carotid artery in the region of the bifurcation. Note complicated flow pattern and high spatial variation of velocities near the flow divider. Shear stress is high along the divider but low opposite to the divider (Reprinted with permission from Motomyia and Karino [24]). **b** Velocity profiles in the aortic arch again show marked asymmetry (velocity profiles shown outside the arch are taken perpendicular to plane of arch). (Reprinted with permission from Farthing and Peronneau [23])

tices, further altering vessel wall stress, which can lead to poststenotic dilatation.

2.3.2 Flow in the Cardiac Chambers

As in the arteries, blood flow in the cardiac chambers is cyclical. Since the ventricular cavities are relatively large open spaces, vortex formation occurs, which results in a thorough mixing of the blood. This fact is well known from cine ventriculography [26]. The vortices die down very quickly in the endphase of diastole in people with low cardiac frequency such as athletes, in whom the ventricular walls do not move for quite some time during the late diastolic phases. At frequencies above 70 BPM, systole and diastole last about equally long, and blood is kept constantly in motion by the cardiac action. However, because of the trabeculations and the papillary muscles there exist pockets of stagnating flow. Proper mixing does not occur in these

areas [27]. In dilated or aneurysmatic ventricles there are also zones of poor mixing [28], as neither inflow nor ejection of blood occurs as quickly as in the healthy ventricle. In the atria, where the velocities generated are slower than those in the ventricles, little vortex formation occurs and "laminar" flow conditions prevail: mixing of blood in the atria is poorer.

2.3.3 Microcirculation

The microcirculation represents the last "directed flow-stage" in the distribution of blood to the end organs. From capillary vessels to cells, nutrients and oxygen are no longer transported by directed motion but by diffusion (see Sect. 1.2). The microcirculatory vasculature represents a branching network of very narrow channels which take more or less random orientations in space, depending on the organ they are perfusing. Flow velocities in the capillaries, with their dimensions of 5–20 μm, are small, and have been found by Bollinger et al. [29] to be oscillatory and on the order of 0.4–0.7 mm/s.

The clinical assessment of organ perfusion is very important, as it determines whether the oxygen supply to the area of tissue under consideration is sufficient to maintain function. Thus, in coronary artery disease, identification of a vascular stenosis is a purely anatomic finding and "function" criteria, such as pain, ECG changes in stress testing, or thallium perfusion abnormalities under stress must be found to warrant coronary surgery or coronary angioplasty. Not only is it important to decide when a preventive procedure such as coronary bypass surgery is indicated; by assessing the regional perfusion state therapeutic success can be evaluated. In cardiac imaging, the most sensitive noninvasive method for assessing perfusion has been found to be thallium scintigraphy stress testing [30], and rapid progress is being made with positron emission tomographic examinations (PET). For the brain, perfusion and function agents for "conventional" and single photon emission computed tomographic studies (SPECT) have been developed recently [31, 32] and tested clinically on a larger number of patients [33, 34]. PET imaging seems to be particularly useful for the study of cerebral and cardiac perfusion and metabolism [35]. Furthermore, CT enhancement using xenon inhalation has been advocated for the study of brain perfusion.

References

1. Perloff JK (1978) The clinical recognition of congenital heart disease. WB Saunders Co, Philadelphia
2. Weissler AM, Harris WS, Schönfeld CD (1969) Bedside techniques for the evaluation of ventricular function in man. Am J Cardiol 23: 577–583
3. Dodge HT, Sandler H, Ballew DW, Lord JD jr (1960) The use of biplane angiocardiography for the measurement of left ventricular volume in man. Am Heart J 60: 762–770
4. Bronstein A, Semendiajev B (1967) Taschenbuch der Mathematik. Verlag Harry Deutsch, Zürich
5. Mackley CE (1976) Quantitative evaluation of left ventricular function by radiographic techniques. Circulation 54: 862–868
6. Kennedy JW et al. (1966) Quantitative angiocardiography. The normal left ventricle in man. Circulation 34: 272–279
7. Rackley CE, Russell RO, Mantle JA jr, Rogers WJ (1977) Modern approach to the patient with acute myocardial infarction. Curr Probl Cardiol, Vol 1, 10: 49 pp
8. Berger HJ, Zaret BL (1981) Nuclear cardiology (second of two parts). New Engl J Med 305: 855–865
9. Green MV, Ostrow HG, Douglas MA et al. (1974) High temporal resolution ECG-gated scintigraphic angiocardiography. J Nuc Med 16: 95–98
10. von Schulthess GK, Pfeiffer A (1983) Global left ventricular function parameters: a systematic investigation of their ability to detect cardiac disease. Conf Proc 21. Int Conf of the Soc of Nuclear Medicine (Europe)
11. Ratib O, Rutishauser W (1985) Recent developments of cardiac digital radiography. Int J Card Imaging 1: 29–40
12. Holman BL (1980) Radioisotope examination of the cardiovascular system. In: Braunwald E (ed) Heart disease, pp 376. WB Saunders, Philadelphia
13. Barnett GO, Greenfield JC jr, Fox SM (1961) The techniques of estimating instantaneous aortic blood velocity in man from the pressure gradient. Am heart J 62: 359–366
14. Luchsinger PC, Sachs M, Patel DJ (1962) Pressure-radius relationship in large blood vessels of man. Circ Res 11: 885–888
15. Kaplan NM (1980) Systemic hypertension: therapy. In: Braunwald E (ed) Heart disease. p 944. WB Saunders, Philadelphia
16. Schettler G, Nerem RM, Schmid-Schönbein H, Mörl H, Diehm C (eds) (1983) Fluid dynamics as a localizing factor for atherosclerosis. Springer, Berlin Heidelberg New York
17. McDonald MA (1974) Blood flow in arteries. Edward Arnold Publishing Co, London
18. Clark C, Schultz DL (1973) Velocity distribution in aortic flow. Cardiovasc Res 7: 601–613
19. Goldstein S (1938) Modern developments in fluid dynamics. Oxford: Clarendon press
20. Fung YC (1984) Biodynamics, Circulation. Springer, Berlin Heidelberg New York Tokyo
21. Milnor WM (1982) Hemodynamics. Williams and Wilkins, Baltimore
22. Mills CJ, Gabe IT, Gault JH et al. (1970) Pressure-flow relationships and vascular impedance in man. Cardiovasc Res 4: 405–417
23. Farthing SP, Peronneau P (1979) Flow in the thoracic aorta. Cardiovasc Res 13: 607–620
24. Motomyia M, Karino T (1984) Flow patterns in the human carotid bifurcation. Stroke 15: 50–55
25. Naumann A, Schmid-Schönbein H (1983) A fluid-dynamicist's and a physiologist's look at arterial flow and arteriosclerosis. In: Schettler G, Nerem RM, Schmid-Schönbein H, Mörl H, Diehm C (eds) Fluid dynamics as a localizing factor for atherosclerosis. Springer, Berlin Heidelberg New York
26. Dodge HT, Hay RE, Sandler H (1962) An angiocardiographic method for directly determining left ventricular stroke volume in man. Circulat Res 11: 739–745
27. Lynch PR, Bove AA (1968) Patterns of blood flow through the intact heart and its valves. In: prosthetic heart valves. Brewer LA (ed). Thomas, Springfield Illinois
28. Wiederhelm CA, Bruce RA, John GG (1957) Continuous recording of oxygen saturation during cardiac catheterization. Amer J Med Sci 233: 542–545
29. Bollinger A, Butti JP, Barras H, Trachsler H, Siegenthaler W: Red blood cell velocity in nailfold capillaries of man, measured by a television microscopy technique
30. Berger HJ, Zaret BL (1981) Nuclear cardiology (first of two parts). New Engl J Med 305: 795–805
31. Kuhl DE, Barrio J-L, Huang SC et al. (1982) Quantifying cerebral blood flow by N-isopropyl-p-(I-123) iodoamphetamine (IMP) tomography. J Nucl Med 23: 196–203
32. Sharp PF, Smith FW, Gemmell HG et al. (1986) 99m-Tc HM-PAO stereoisomers as potential agents for imaging

regional cerebral blood flow: normal volunteer studies. J Nuc Med 27: 135-142

33. Lee RGL, Hill TC, Holman BL, Clouse ME (1982) N-isopropyl-p-(I-123) iodoamphetamine brain scans with single photon emission tomography: discordance with transmission tomography. Radiology 145: 795-799

34. von Schulthess GK, Ketz E, Schubiger PA, Bekier A (1985) Regional quantitative noninvasive assessment of cerebral perfusion and function with N-isopropyl-p-(I-123) idioamphetamine. J Nucl Med 26: 9-16

35. Schelbert HR (1987) Current status of new radiopharmaceuticals for cardiovascular nuclear medicine. Seminars Nucl Med 17: 145-181

Chapter 3   The Effects of Motion and Flow on Magnetic Resonance Imaging

Throughout the human body, motion and flow effects occur due to the cardiovascular system. However, respiration, peristalsis and swallowing are other physiological phenomena associated with motion. This first chapter on cardiovascular imaging is designed to familiarize the reader with flow phenomena as they are observed in routine MR images. Recognition of such phenomena is important in daily clinical practice because blood vessels are present in almost any MR image examined. Blood vessels in MRI exhibit various amounts of intravascular signal, which may make their identification difficult. Being aware of how intravascular signal can appear helps with the proper identification of blood vessels. Two broad classes of flow phenomena can be identified and will be discussed below. They are the spin phase and the time-of-flight or slice transition phemomena.

3.1 Spin-Phase Phenomena

It was pointed out in Sects. 1.4.4 and 1.4.6 that MR is very sensitive to motion and that the magnetic gradient fields used to spatially localize the signal "accidentally" sensitize MR images to motion. In fact, motion affects the precessional phase of the spins and thus the magnetization vector. For constant velocity motion it was found (Table 1.3) that the phase shift is proportional to the velocity for all odd echoes and that it is zero for even echoes. The ensuing sections explore the ways in which spin-phase phenomena affect the appearance of MR images and how they can be used to obtain information on the cardiovascular system. Spin-phase phenomena have different effects on MR images depending on whether the moving structures move uniformly over the entire volume element (voxel) imaged, or whether there are variations in the motional characteristics of the spins within a voxel. An example of the latter situation is the blood flow close to a vessel wall where, due to the steep spatial variation in velocity, the velocities of individual spins (isochromats) contained within a voxel vary substantially. Examples of uniform motion within an entire voxel are the cardiac wall and blood flow in the central area of a vessel. Spin-phase phenomena associated with bulk motion are discussed first.

3.1.1 Spin-Phase Phenomena in Coherent Intravoxel Motion

In conventional SE as well as gradient echo imaging, the read gradient produces phase changes of spins having a motion component along the read direction, and the slice select gradient produces phase changes for spins with a motion component perpendicular to the slice. When all spins[1] within a voxel move identically, the changes in phase angle due to applied external gradient fields are the same for all the spins in the voxel. Thus, the magnetization vectors of all spins in the voxel are characterized by the same magnitude and the same phase. Total signal intensity is not altered, because all magnetization vectors within the voxel add (Fig. 3.1), but the phase angle differs from zero in contradistinction to a voxel containing only stationary spins. The computation of phase images or other images containing phase information thus yields function images coded for motion. In phase images the phase angle is usually represented on a gray scale extending from $-180°$ to $+180°$, black representing $-180°$, gray around $0°$, and white $+180°$

---

[1] We use the term spins in this text somewhat loosely in that we actually mean ensembles of spins, also termed isochromats. These ensembles of spins are so small that the spatial variations in magnetic field strength due to imperfections in the system occur over much larger dimensions than the isochromat dimension. Thus all proton spins within an isochromat precess at the same Larmor frequency. An isochromat is also much smaller than a voxel. On the other hand, an isochromat is so large that a magnetization vector in the classical physical sense can be assigned to it. Thus the laws of classical physics apply to an isochromat.

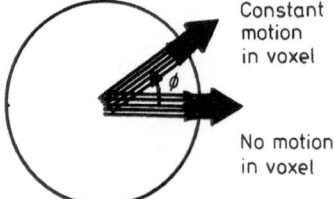
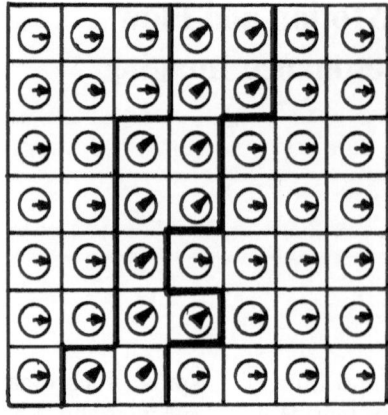

Fig. 3.1. For stationary spins all magnetization vectors point in the 0° direction at the echo time TE, resulting in large signal. If all spins within a voxel move identically, their magnetization vectors are no longer zero, but are all turned by the same phase angle Φ. This still yields the same signal strength, because all magnetization vectors within the voxel point in the same direction. Whether the signal comes from stationary or moving spins can be determined only on a phase image. The pixel grid represented here shows areas of altered phase in a hypothetical vessel

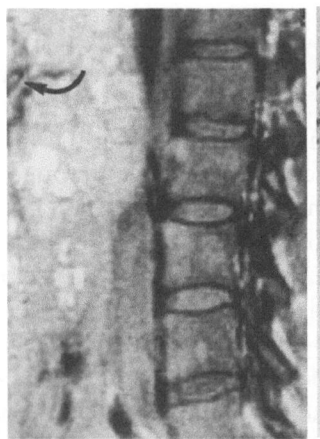
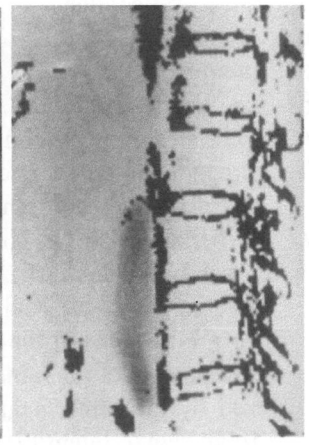
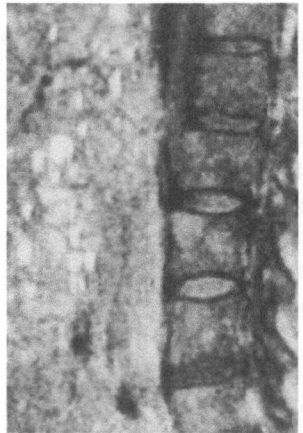
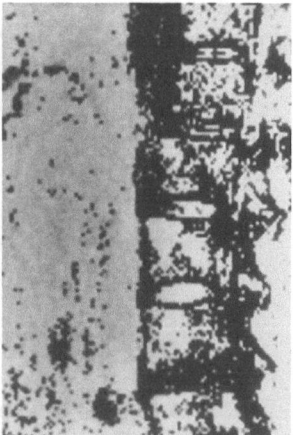

a–d

Fig. 3.2 a–d. Slow constant velocity blood flow in an obstructed inferior vena cava of a patient with a liver tumor (SE 1100/30 ms and SE 1100/60 ms). Note that on the first echo magnitude image (**a**) it is difficult to indentify the vessel (*arrow*), but on the phase image (**b**) this is easy. On second-echo images it is possible to identify the vessel neither on a magnitude (**c**) nor on a phase image (**d**), because of the even echo rephasing effect, occurring for constant velocity motion. Flow is also identified in a branch of the portal vein (*curved arrow*[a]). (Reprinted with permission from von Schulthess and Augustiny [1])

(Fig. 3.2). It is possible that the phase shift induced is larger or smaller than +180° or −180° respectively. Thus, a given gray scale value does not uniquely represent a velocity, but for example a velocity resulting in a phase shift of 42° is indistinguishable from a velocity producing a 360° +42° = 402° phase shift. If the signal intensity of a structure is (close to) zero, the phase angle is not defined. Hence, dark areas on a magnitude image would produce arbitrary phases and a speckled appearance of the phase image. To prevent this, a threshold amplitude value, typically 5% of the maximum amplitude in the image, is often chosen as a cutoff: the phases of pixels with smaller amplitudes are all set to −180° and thus appear black (Fig. 3.2). Gradual changes in the gray scale across the phase image occur and are an expression of imager imperfections. They are much more prominent on phase images obtained with gradient echo pulse sequences.

In practice, the nonuniqueness of the relation between phase and velocity and the phase shifts due to system imperfections are of no concern, if merely moving from nonmoving structures have to be distinguished, such as when distinguishing slow flow from intravascular thrombus [1] or identifying ventricular akinesia [2], because in these cases only a qualitative assessment of the phase is necessary:

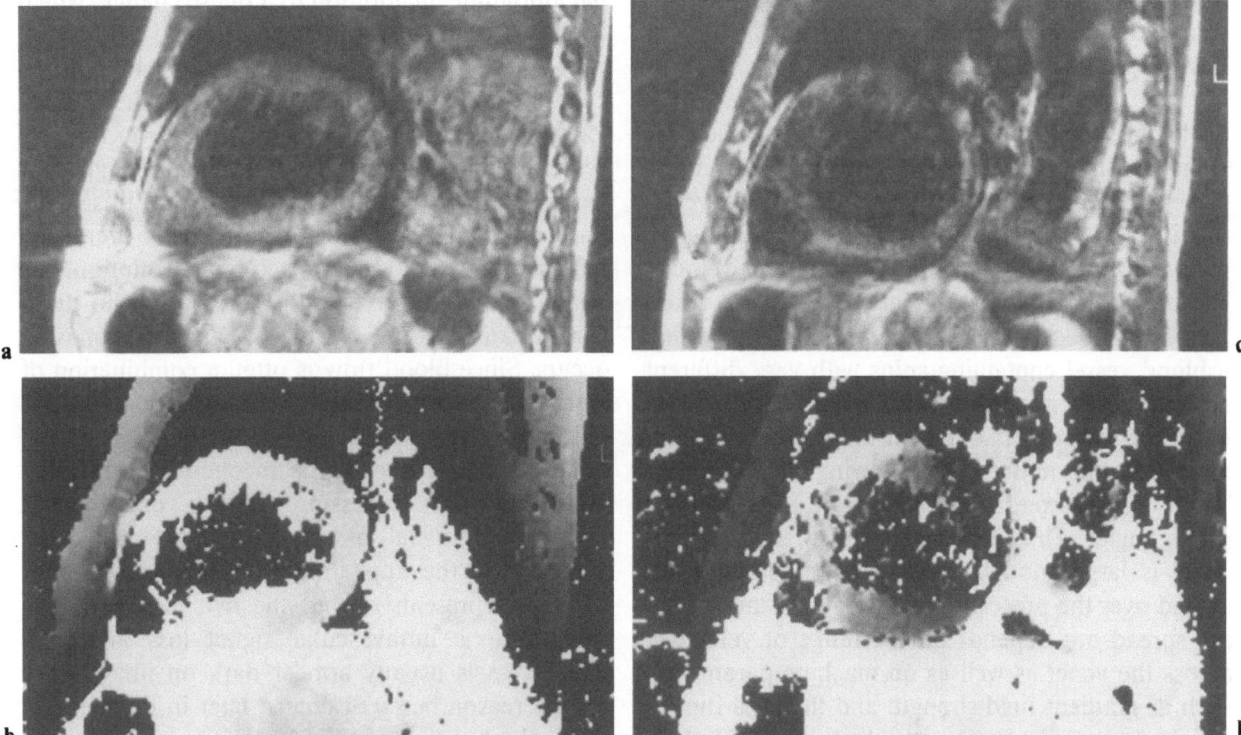

Fig. 3.3. Sagittal amplitude (**a**) and phase images (**b**) through the heart. **a** and **c** magnitude images, **b** and **d** phase images. Few phase changes are noted on the end-diastolic phase image **b**, where the heart is not yet contracting. However, the mid-systole phase image (**d**) shows phases in the region of the heart which are different from the surrounding tissues due to cardiac motion

one has to know whether the phase in the region of interest is different from the phase of the surrounding stationary tissues or not. For a qualitative assessment it is necessary only that the motion sensitizing gradients be sufficiently strong to produce a distinct phase change even for slow velocities. In fact, read- and slice-select gradients typically result in phase shifts of some 10° for velocities down to 0.5 cm/s. Figures 3.2 and 3.3 show examples of such qualitative phase maps, which are true function images representing motion. The moving structures are simply identified by an abrupt jump in phase relative to surrounding stationary tissues [1]. An alternative method using similar concepts is the so-called Zebra Stripe method [3, 4]. Note that for the relatively constant flow velocity in the obstructed inferior vena cava of Fig. 3.2, rephasing of the flowing spins back to a phase angle of 0° occurs on the second (which is an even) echo: no phase difference exists between stationary and moving spins on the second echo phase image, as predicted by Table 1.3.

When quantitative flow measurements are made, system imperfections have to be suppressed and a well-defined relation between phase angle and ve-locity has to be established. This is possible, e. g., with the FEER sequence [5] described in Sect. 1.4.9. In this sequence, the motion sensitization due to the spatial localizing gradients is compensated using the "MAST" technique and additional motion sensitizing gradients are used along the direction of flow, whose strength can be controlled such that for the velocity range of interest a unique relation exists between velocity and phase shift, permitting quantitation. This technique has been used to produce flow profiles across the aortic root, demonstrating the spatial and temporal variations occurring in flow velocities over the cardiac cycle [6]. Flow in coronary artery bypass grafts has also been quantified [7]. Images showing acceleration rather than velocity have also been generated [8], and it is likely that it is this type of MR sequence which will be further developed and used for quantitation of blood flow in the future. The FEER and other similar flow-sensitive pulse sequences draw on the enormous versatility of MR pulse sequence programming, permitting arbitrary selection of the spatial direction in which motion is measured and providing sensitization specifically to the motion component of interest, such as velocity or acceleration.

3.1.2 Spin-Phase Phenomena in Incoherent Intravoxel Motion: Flow in Large Vessels and Intravascular Signal Loss

So far, we have considered only motion where all spins within a voxel move at the same speed in the same direction. However, in a lager blood vessel this is hardly the case, since there exists a flow velocity profile and the spatial variations in velocity can be considerable, particularly close to the vessel wall. In this section we consider the situation where a blood vessel containing spins with very different velocities (and accelerations) is larger than the voxels of the image (Fig.3.4). Considering just constant velocities, one notices the following. According to Table 1.3, different velocities produce different phase angles. Thus, if the velocity spread within a voxel is large enough, the spins are found to be spread over the precessional circle. How much they are spread out depends on the range of velocities across the voxel as well as on machine parameters such as gradient field strength and the time during which the gradients are switched on (Table 1.3). Since in MRI we are able to measure only the net magnetization of a voxel, that is, the vector sum (Appendix B) of all the contributing spins, the signal measured becomes greatly reduced, particularly if the phase difference between slowest and fastest spins in the voxel is more than 360°. Thus, intravoxel velocity differences produce a decrease in sig-

nal amplitude, in addition to a phase change, which itself is determined by the mean velocity in the voxel. This is shown on the right of Fig.3.4. On even echoes the phase angle is zero independent of velocity; hence, the spins are not spread over the precession circle and the signal remains as high as it would be if the spins were not moving: this is the proper explanation for the occurrence of even echo refocusing [9, 10, 11]. For accelerated motion, the phase spread increases with increasing echo number, as can be seen in Table 1.3, and no rephasing occurs. Since blood flow is often a combination of constant velocity and accelerated motion, the rephasing effect is usually not complete.

The fact that due to the incoherence (different phases) of spins precessing within a voxel there is intravascular signal loss has very important consequences for the appearance of flowing blood in MRI. It represents one of the two major reasons why there is intravascular signal loss and why blood vessels usually appear dark on images, the second reason being discussed later in this chapter under the heading of Slice Transition or "Time-of-Flight" Phenomena. When intravascular signal appears, and this is the case for slow blood flow on the order of 5 cm/s or less for conventional SE images, it is usually brighter on second echo images due to refocusing (Fig.3.5). Furthermore, dark rims along the edges of a perfused vessel are common on first echo. This is a qualitative reflection of the vari-

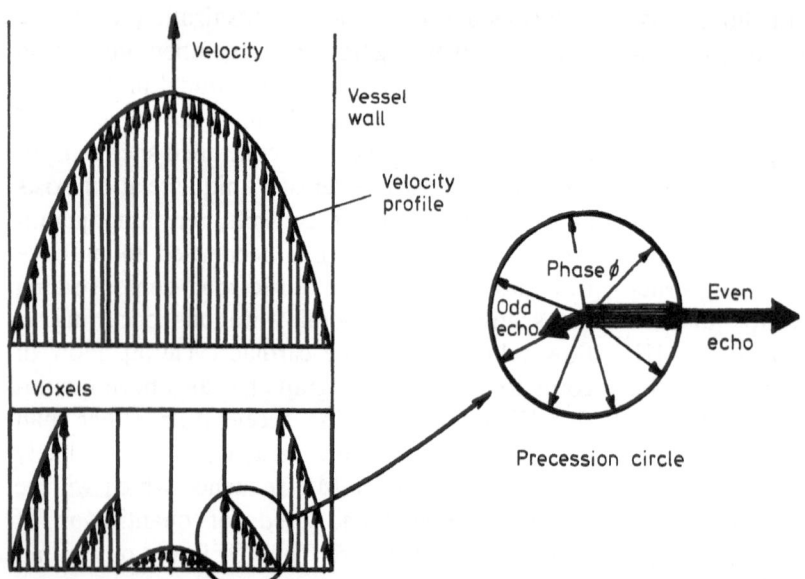

Fig.3.4. Flow velocity profile in a blood vessel. Note that the spatial variation in velocity is much more marked along the walls of the vessel than in its center. MRI divides this vessel into voxels, the ones close to the walls containing a larger range of velocities. As different velocities result in different phase angles in SE or gradient echo experiments, spin mag-

netization vectors are spread over the precession circle. If the intravoxel variation in velocity is such that phase spreading approaches or exceeds 360°, signal loss occurs. However, for constant velocity motion the phase angle is zero on even echoes independent of velocity. In this case, the intravoxel phase spread (incoherence) is refocused

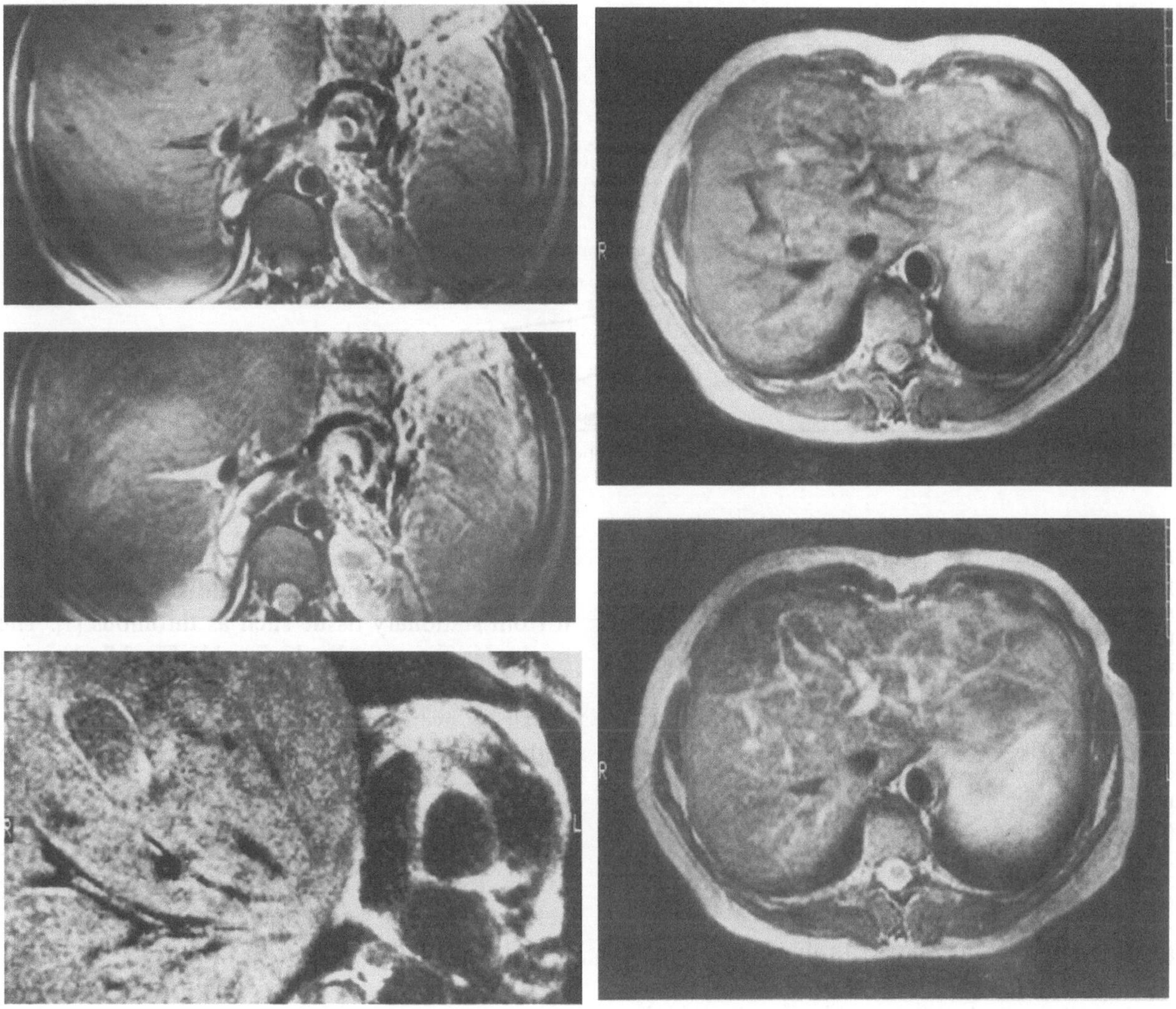

Fig. 3.5. First (**a**) and second (**b**) echo image through the liver at the level of the portal vein in a patient with Budd-Chiari syndrome, showing a dim line of central signal on first echo (**a** SE 2000/30 ms). On second echo, an increase in intravascular signal intensity and reappearance of signal along the vessel wall is observed, which is an expression of rephasing (**b** SE 2000/60 ms). **c** First echo oblique image showing dephasing in a hepatic vein along the vessel wall (SE 750/30 ms). Small hepatic vessels show lack of signal on first echo (**d** 2000/30 ms) and strong signal due to rephasing on second echo (**e** 2000/60 ms)

Fig. 3.6. End-diastolic gradient echo image (first echo) show- ▶ ing very bright intravascular signal in parts of the ventricles, the atria, and the descending aorta. The signal dropout in parts of the left ventricle is a result of inflow turbulence due to aortic insufficiency, which induces dephasing of spins. This image was obtained with a velocity-compensated sequence (Sect. 4.6); thus, spin phase-induced signal loss is due entirely to acceleration and higher order motion terms (Eq. 1.42)

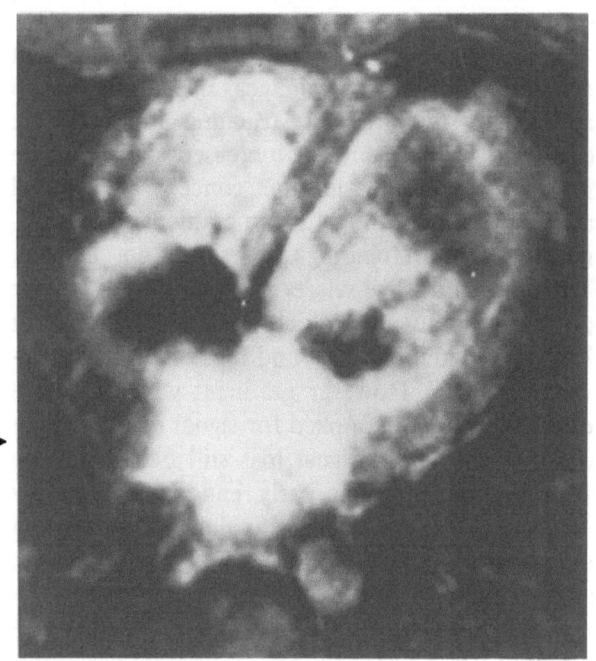

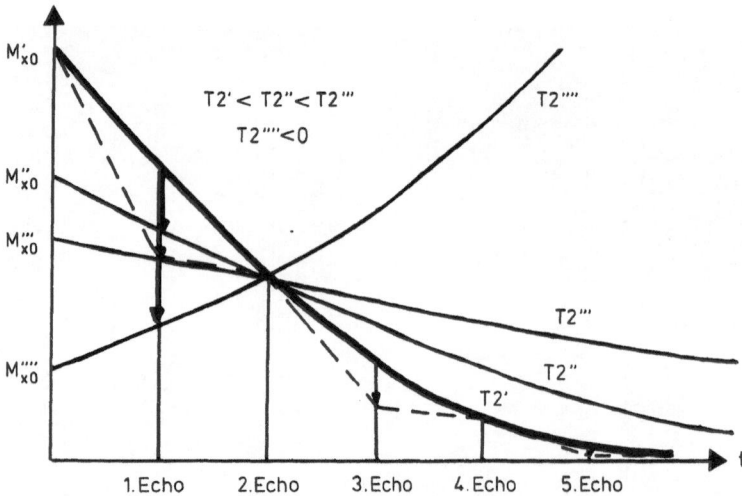

Fig. 3.7. For stationary spins the magnetization in the xy-plane M_{xyo}' decays exponentially, characterized by a spin-spin relaxation time T2'. With flow, there is a gradual reduction in first (and all odd) echo signal, but not on second (and all even) echo. If T2 is calculated from the first and second echo signal, the T2 values appear to increase. When the absolute signal intensity of the first echo drops below that of the second, such a calculation results in negative T2 values. This can only occur due to flow, thus positively identifying it. If many echoes are measured, they fall onto a zigzag line *(dashed line)*

able steepness of the velocity profile across a vessel. As is clear from Fig. 3.5, the velocity profile is steeper along the vessel walls, resulting in more dephasing and signal loss (Fig. 3.4), but for constant velocity flow, the dark rim disappears due to rephasing [11].

Intravascular signal is much stronger in gradient echo images than in SE images, and in fact vessels are usually the brightest structures in the image (Fig. 3.6). The presence of increased signal can be partly understood with the concepts developed above. As noted in Fig. 1.29, in gradient echo imaging the 180° refocusing pulses are not needed. Therefore, no slice-selection gradient has to be turned on, reducing the defocusing influence in at least one spatial direction and thus increasing intravascular signal. However, gradients which produce defocusing are still applied for signal readout. That defocusing-induced signal loss still occurs can be seen in Fig. 3.6, where early end-diastolic inflow turbulence produces almost total signal dropout in part of the left ventricle. The intense intravascular signal cannot be accounted for by spin-phase phenomena alone; entry slice phenomena are also important (Sect. 3.2.2).

Like phase imaging, the refocusing phenomenon can be used to identify blood flow and distinguish it from stationary tissue such as thrombus [1]. The method is chematically depicted in Fig. 3.7, showing dephasing-induced signal loss on odd and normal signal on even echoes. If the T2 value in a region with flow is determined from the measurement of a first and a second echo, artifically long or even negative T2 values may be obtained. The latter result is consistent only with flow, and thus identifies it positively. If multiple echoes are measured, a zigzag behavior of the signal intensity is observed [12] (Fig. 3.7, *dashed line*).

3.1.3 Spin-Phase Phenomena in Intravoxel Incoherent Motion: Flow in Small Vessels, Tissue Perfusion and Diffusion

In the previous section we considered the situation where the vessel under consideration was large compared with a voxel. However, in the case of the microcirculation, a voxel is much larger than the vessel dimension. In this section, we will analyze the effect of perfusion in small vessels and of diffusion on the MR signal.

We have seen that for spins moving with different velocities within a voxel there is signal loss due to loss of phase coherence of the spins. If a voxel contains a network of perfused channels, there are a variety of mechanisms which can bring about such coherence loss. First, the channels contained in a voxel have different diameters, which in general produce quite variable flow velocities according to Poiseuille's law (Eq. 2.7), which predicts the flow to vary with the 4th power of the diameter of the channel! Second, as in large vessels, there is a flow velocity profile in small vessels which results in dephasing even if the vessels course parallel within the voxel, as shown in the first cube of Fig. 3.8. Third, if the vessels are straight but their orientation is random, this will result in an additional coherence loss, because the velocity component parallel to the flow-sensitizing gradient varies, even if the flow velocity is the same for all channels (middle cube in Fig. 8). Fourth, if the channels bend inside the voxel, this produces acceleration and deceleration of spins along the flow-sensitizing gradient, and hence additional coherence loss (right cube in Fig. 3.8). Whether such bends actually produce acceleration and deceleration effects depends on whether the typical curvature of these bends is large or comparable to the distance traveled by the spins within an echo time TE. For capillaries, the randomly oriented straight tube example (Fig. 3.8b) is probably appropriate, because they show flow velocities of <1 mm/s (Table 2.4) and thus move just about 30–50 μm if a TE = 30 ms is chosen. However, for arterioles and venules with their flow velocity approximately ten times higher, the curved-vessel model of Fig. 3.8c is likely to be more appropriate.

There is an additional source of coherence loss due to intravoxel incoherent motion, i.e., diffusion. The random Brownian motion of spins also results in a decrease in the magnetization vector measured in a voxel, as discussed in Sect. 1.4.4. Since diffusion is a random process, no refocusing of the spins is possible, and this effect is always present. However, we stated in Chap. 1 that the CPMG spin echo sequence was specifically designed to minimize this effect. Therefore, if a sequence is to be made particularly sensitive to intravoxel incoherent motions, it is necessary to increase the echo time. Furthermore, additional dephasing gradients should be introduced into the pulse sequence, as was illustrated in Fig. 1.20.

There are clear indications from phantom studies that signal loss due to intravoxel incoherent motion can be observed and quantified [13, 14], and that flow and diffusive contributions to signal loss can be separated [13]. Figure 3.9 shows the signal intensity in a multiecho SE sequence plotted as a function of the echo for two types of perfused phantoms [15]. In the phantom containing small straight capillaries (dialysis filter), the expected zigzag behavior of the signal due to even echo rephasing is noted. There is no signal loss in addition to the normal T2 decay, which was removed from the curve by dividing through the signal obtained on the unperfused control phantom. However, in a phantom made of

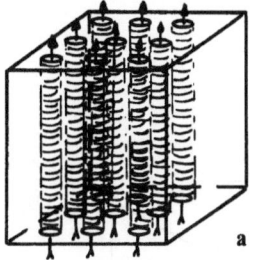
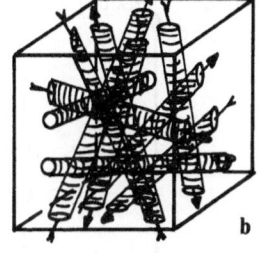

Straight parallel   Straight "random"

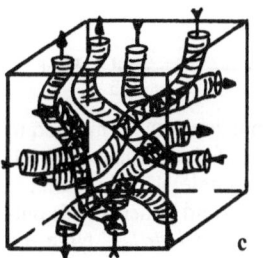

"Randomly" curved

Fig. 3.8 a–c. Three different arrangements of vessels inside a voxel are possible in principle. Either the vessels are **a** parallel inside the voxel, or they are **b** straight but course randomly through the voxel, or **c** they curve in a more or less arbitrary fashion within the voxel

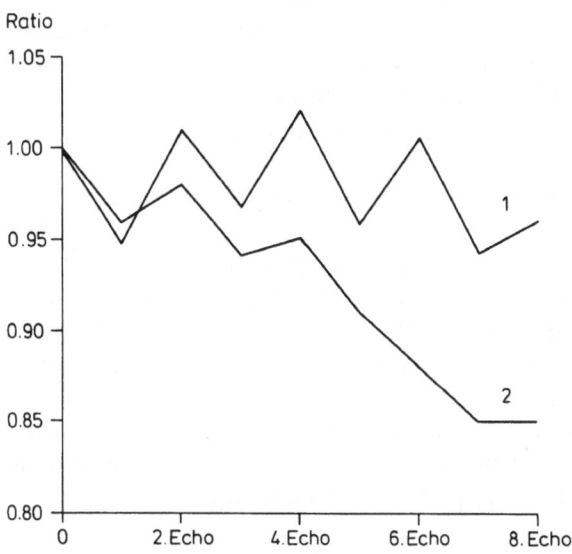

Fig. 3.9. Signal intensity as a function of the echo in a multiecho SE sequence (TR = 1000 ms, TE = 30 ms) obtained in two perfusion phantoms. The values measured were divided by the signal of the nonperfused phantoms. Note the zigzag behavior in both curves as expression of the rephasing phenomenon occurring due to spins flowing with constant velocity. In a phantom containing straight capillaries (1, dialysis filter) almost perfect rephasing occurs, indicating near-constant velocity flow for all spins. In a phantom of densely packed beads (2, ion exchange resin), the flow is around the beads. Some spins undergo acceleration and hence produce additional signal loss, which increases with increasing echo number

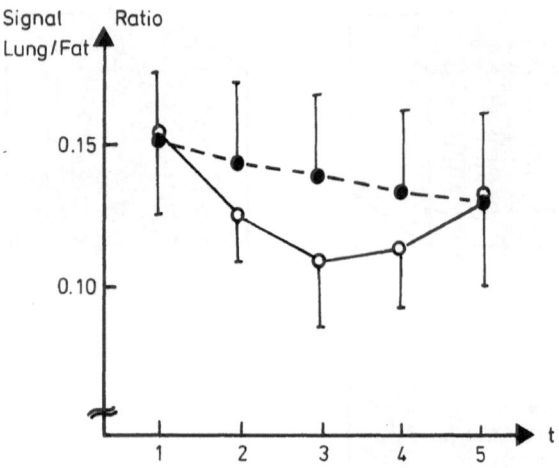

Fig. 3.10. Peripheral lung field signal intensity normalized to axillary fat measured as a function of the cardiac cycle (1, end-diastole; 2, early systole; 3, mid-systole; 4, end-systole; 5, early diastole) in normals *(open circles)* and patients with pulmonary arterial hypertension (PAH) *(solid circles)*. Note the signal decrease during systole in normals, when pulmonary blood flow is faster than in diastole. In patients with PAH, with their increased pulmonary vascular resistance and pulmonary parenchymal abnormalities, this effect is not seen. (Reprinted with permission from von Schulthess et al. [16])

beads (ion exchange resin beads, average bead size 500 μm), additional and progressive signal loss occurs with increasing echo number due to the directional randomization of the flowing spins, diverted in all directions by the beads.

Signal variations which are probably due to tissue perfusion also have been observed using conventional [16] and perfusion/diffusion-sensitive sequences [13]. Figure 3.10 is an illustration of this. The data shown were obtained for normals and patients with primary arterial hypertension (PAH) by ROI analysis in the lung periphery [16]. During systole, when the arterial blood moves fastest, the lung signal intensity is seen to decrease significantly in normals but not in PAH patients, who have an increased pulmonary vascular resistance and thus a pulmonary perfusion abnormalitiy.

3.1.4 Flow Measurements Using Spin-Phase Phenomena

The foundation for MR flow imaging using spin-phase phenomena was laid by Moran [17], who suggested designing pulse sequences which, in addition to signal localization in three dimensions, would also measure the velocity in three dimensions. The problem with this is that six-dimensional data acquisition has to be used, making imaging time pro-

hibitive. For this reason, variations and simplifications of Moran's scheme have been implemented and tested in vitro and in vivo. They all make use of the fact that once the direction of a blood vessel is known, the flow component of interest in this vessel is usually along its axis [18–20]. Using standard SE imaging together with phase imaging, a plane can be imaged and the velocity component perpendicular to it measured [21, 22]. The clinically most advanced flow imaging scheme of this kind is the FEER sequence described by Nayler et al. [23], which has been described in Sect. 1.4.9.

One-dimensional flow profiles across vessels can also be obtained using phase mapping. In such schemes, the 180° pulse is applied in a slice perpendicular to the slice selected for the 90° pulse [24, 25].

Preliminary in vivo measurements of diffusion coefficients have been published [13], but, except for the FEER sequence, none of the flow sensitive schemes have been used in a larger number of patients. In general, the clinical use of MR phase imaging schemes for quantitation of flow is at a very early stage.

3.1.5 Spin-Phase Effects: Summary

In the preceding sections we have seen that motion produces changes in spin phase relative to stationary spins (coherent intravoxel motion, Table 3.1). This phase can be measured and used to obtain qualitative or quantitative flow information. If different motions occur within a single voxel (incoher-

Table 3.1. Distinction of various motion types by amplitude and phase imaging and even-echo refocusing

Motion type	Amplitude change	Phase change	Even-echo refocusing
Coherent Bulk flow or motion	no	yes	no
Incoherent Flow with flow profile	yes	yes	yes
Perfusion in straight capillaries	yes	yes	yes
Perfusion in curved capillaries	yes	yes	partly
Diffusion	yes	yes	no

ent intravoxel motion), the variation in phase within the voxel also produces changes in signal amplitude, because only the net magnetization vector of a voxel can be measured, and it is a vector sum of all the spin magnetization vectors within that voxel. This is one of the two reasons why most blood vessels and the cardiac chambers appear without intravascular signal on MR SE images. Incoherent intravoxel motion occurs due to the flow profile in large vessels and the cardiac chambers but also due to blood flow in small vessels with a variable course in a single voxel and due to diffusion of spins. It can be subdivided according to Table 3.1. Hence, it is possible in principle to measure perfusion and diffusion in tissues, and some results have been obtained supporting this notion. As will be seen in Sect. 3.5, motion also produces artifacts which sometimes severely degrade MR images, particularly of the upper abdomen and the thorax, if cardiac triggering is not used. There are several tricks and techniques which can reduce these artifacts (Sect. 3.6), but the best method is fast imaging in respiratory apnea. In the next sections, the other major category of blood flow effects, the so-called time-of-flight phenomena, and their effect of MR images will be discussed.

3.2 Slice Transition or "Time-of-Flight" Phenomena

Slice transition or "time-of-flight" phenomena result from the fact that moving spins can enter or leave the imaged slice while a basic pulse sequence is applied. Such effects occur only if blood flow occurs with a component perpendicular to the imaged slice, which shall be assumed to be the xy-plane as in the previous sections. Hence, the flow is in the z-direction, and to simplify the discussion, we assume it to be strictly perpendicular to the xy-plane. Slice transition phenomena are closely related to slice thickness s, echo time TE, repetition time TR, flow velocity v_{zo}, and the position of a slice within a stack of slices, if multislice imaging is done.

Consider a volume element of the size of a voxel which moves with a constant velocity v_{zo}. If it moves a distance z during a time t, the following relation holds

$$v_{zo} = z_0/t \tag{3.1}$$

With a slice thickness of typically 5–10 mm, two situations have to be considered. If blood moves so fast that it leaves the slice between the nutation

pulse and the refocusing pulse in an SE experiment, signal loss results. This phenomenon has been termed "high-velocity signal loss". However, if blood flows so slowly that part of it is replaced by blood from the outside of the stack of slices, which has not been saturated and hence is still fully magnetized, strongly increased intravascular signal may result. This phenomenon is called flow-related enhancement.

3.2.1 High-Velocity Signal Loss

If spins leave the imaged slice in a time $nTE - TE/2$ after the 90° nutation pulse, that is, before the slice-selective 180° refocusing pulse which is responsible for the n-th echo, they cannot participate in the refocusing process. Hence, they continue to defocus and contribute very little signal at the

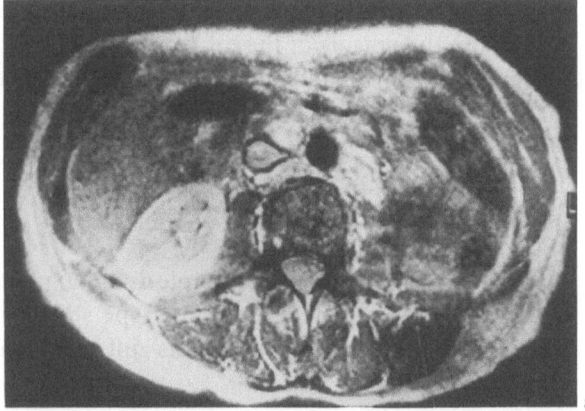

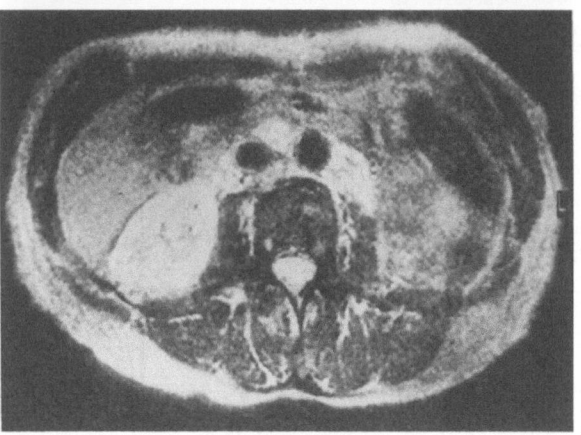

Fig. 3.11a–b. Transverse first (**a** 2000/30 ms) and second (**b** SE 2000/60 ms) echo SE image. Note intravascular signal on first echo, which disappears on second echo because spins have left the slice. This cannot be a spin-phase phenomenon, because one would then expect an increase in signal intensity on the second echo image

n-th echo. According to Eq. 3.1, the velocity above which this effect occurs is given by

$$v_{zo} \geq s/(n - 1/2)TE \tag{3.2}$$

For smaller velocities not the entire blood leaves the slice under consideration, but only a fraction $g_n = v_{zo}(n - 1/2)TE/s$. The signal measured at the n-th echo is then reduced to

$$
\begin{aligned}
M_{xy} &= (1 - g_n)M_{xyo}(TR)\exp(-nTE/T2) \\
&= (1 - g_n)M_{zo}[1 - \exp(TR/T1)]\exp(-nTE/T2)
\end{aligned}
\tag{3.3}
$$

according to Eq. 1.29, where $0 \leq g_n \leq 1$. As a result, the magnetization decreases to zero as a linear function of the velocity. An example of this phenomenon is shown in Fig. 3.11. In gradient echo imaging, the situation is different, because no slice-selective refocusing pulse is needed. Hence, spins undergoing the initial α nutation pulse will contribute to the signal no matter how far away from the slice they have moved.

For relatively slow velocity, there is not only signal loss due to spins moving out of the slice; other spins from the outside of the examined volume also enter the slice, resulting in flow-related enhancement.

3.2.2 Entry Slice Phenomena

During imaging, the stationary protons are exposed to repetitive pulse sequences of the type shown in Fig. 1.29. In most sequences, TR is not very long compared with the T1 of blood (≈ 800 ms, Table 1.2), and the spins in the sample under study cannot fully remagnetize before the next 90° nutation pulse is sent into the system in an SE experiment and even more so before the next α pulse in a gradient echo experiment. If blood moves with a velocity v_{zo} perpendicular to a slice or a stack of slices taken in the xy-plane, part of the blood in the slices close to the surface of the stack is replaced by blood from the outside of the imaged volume, which is still fully magnetized: it has not been exposed to the repetitive nutation pulses (Fig. 3.12). The net magnetization of the vessel within the slice(s) is thereby increased, as shown in Fig. 3.12, giving rise to the so-called flow-related enhancement. How strong an effect this is depends again on the slice thickness s, the repetition time TR, and the flow velocity v_{zo}. The fraction g_{TR} of the blood which is replaced within TR is given by

$$g_{TR} = v_{zo}TR/s \tag{3.4}$$

Hence, the net magnetization at the next nutation pulse is given by the magnetization of the blood previously exposed to a nutation pulse and the blood which has entered the slice fully magnetized:

$$M_z(TR) = M_{zo}\{(1 - g_{TR})[1 - \exp(-TR/T)] + g_{TR}\} \tag{3.5}$$

This effect becomes important when a substantial fraction of the blood in the slice is replaced during the repetition time TR, i.e., when

$$v_{zo} \approx s/TR$$

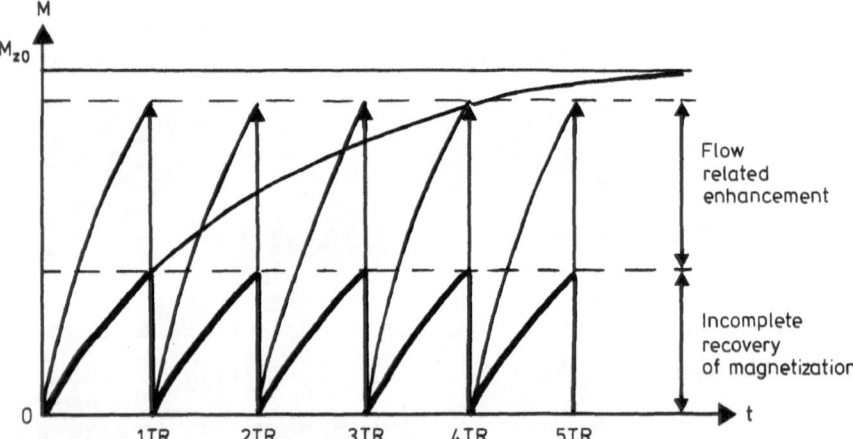

Fig. 3.12. Stationary spins show a "saw tooth" like magnetization M_z in SE experiments due to the 90° nutation pulses, which at each TR destroy the M_z magnetization completely. If in an interval TR some fully magnetized spins enter the slice, "flow related enhancement" occurs. The magnetization is increased up to a maximum of M_{zo}, which corresponds to the situation, where all spins in the slice have been replaced by fully magnetized spins. In gradient echo experiments, the situation is similar. However, since there the nutation pulse is less than 90°, the M_z magnetization is not completely destroyed, thus the saw tooth would have to be plotted on top of a constant M_z magnetization

For typical values of TR and *s* these velocities are some cm/s; at higher velocities, high-velocity signal loss supervenes. The dependence of the magnetization on flow velocity is obtained by combining Eqs. 3.4 and 3.5 for SE experiments, because at the 90° pulse the entire magnetization in the z-direction $M_z(TR)$ is flipped into the xy-plane and equals M_{xyo}. Thus, M_{xy} is given by

$$M_{xy}(v_{zo}, TR, TE)$$

$$= (1 - g_n)M_{zo}\{(1 - g_{TR})[1 - \exp(-TR/T1)] + g_{TR}\}$$
$$\exp(-nTE/T2)$$

$$= [1 - (n - 1/2)v_{zo}TE/s]M_{zo}$$
$$\{(1 - v_{zo}TR/s)$$
$$[1 - \exp(-TR/T1)] + v_{zo}TR\}\exp(-nTE/T2)$$
$$\tag{3.6}$$

As can be seen, this function is quadratic in the velocity v_{zo} and exhibits a maximum. The function is shown in Fig. 3.13 for $s = 5$ mm, TE = 30 ms and TR = 700 ms.

Entry slice phenomena are very prominent for gradient echo imaging. On the one hand, little signal is available from stationary tissues because of the short repetition times TR of 30-100 ms most often used. On the other hand, blood, with its high proton density, has a high signal intensity when fully magnetized, and from the above calculations we know that the blood in the slices is completely replaced even for small velocities. High-velocity signal loss does not occur, because there is no slice-se-lective refocusing pulse necessary in gradient echo imaging, even though there is still some signal loss due to spin-phase phenomena, unless flow compensation techniques are used (Sect. 1.4.9).

When a stack of slices is imaged, slice transition phenomena become somewhat more complex. As the blood moves from the outside of the stack into it, it starts to undergo the nutation pulses; thus, slices deeper in the stack will not obtain fully magnetized blood. How far fully magnetized spins can be carried into the stack depends on the slice thickness, the interslice gap, and the direction in which the slices in the stack are read relative to the flow direction. To simplify matters, we assume that the sequence in which the slices are read parallels the direction of flow. The flow profile inside a vessel is responsible for the fact that spins in the central part of the vessel are carried into the stack faster than the spins close to the vessel wall. If the entry sides of the slices are a distance q apart, the fully magnetized spins flowing with a velocity v_{zo}, reach the j-th slice after a time

$$t = (j - 1)q/v_z \tag{3.7}$$

after passing the entry side of the first slice. Spins which cover a distance jq, after the j-th and before the (j+1)-th slice, undergo their respective nutation pulses and contribute their full magnetization to the signal measured in the (j+1)-th slice, because they reach the (j+1)-th slice undisturbed by RF pulses [26]. The further into the stack the slice is, the faster the blood has to flow to arrive in time to enhance the signal in that slice. However, if the velocity is too high, high-velocity signal loss occurs. Thus, entry slice phenomena cannot be observed too far into the stack of slices. For a slice thickness $s = 7$ mm, a distance q of 10 mm, an echo time TE = 30 ms, and a time of 100 ms between the readout of neighboring slices total signal loss occurs for velocities of approximately 45 cm/s and higher (Eq. 3.2). Blood which arrives at the second slice between the refocusing pulse of the first slice (at 15 ms) and the nutation pulse for the second slice at 100 ms produces signal enhancement. The minimum velocity for this is 1 cm/85 ms according to Eq. 3.7, that is, 12 cm/s, below the limit for high-velocity signal loss (Fig. 3.14). Apparently, this is also true for the third and the fourth slice in the stack, which can be reached with velocities of 24 and 36 cm/s respectively, but due to the flow profile in the vessel, the region of spins coming from the outside of the stack becomes progressively smaller (Fig. 3.14). For slices further into the stack, high-velocity signal loss su-

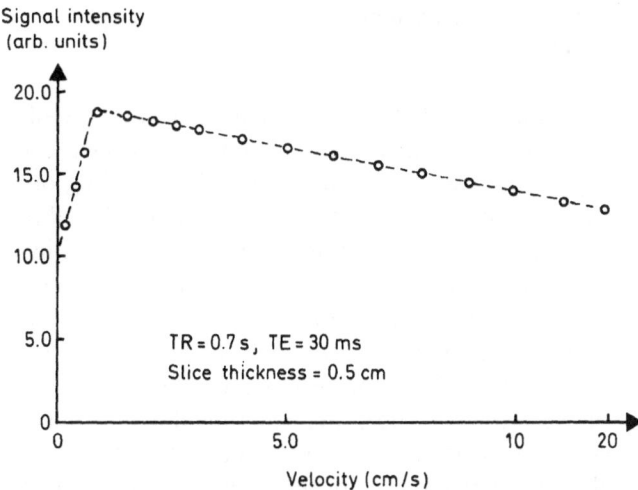

Fig. 3.13. Computer simulation of the signal intensity (in arbitrary units) as a function of flow velocity for the parameters TR = 700 ms, TE = 30 ms, and slice thickness s = 5 mm using Eq. 3.6. Note that there is a maximum in the curve for a flow of about 1 cm/s

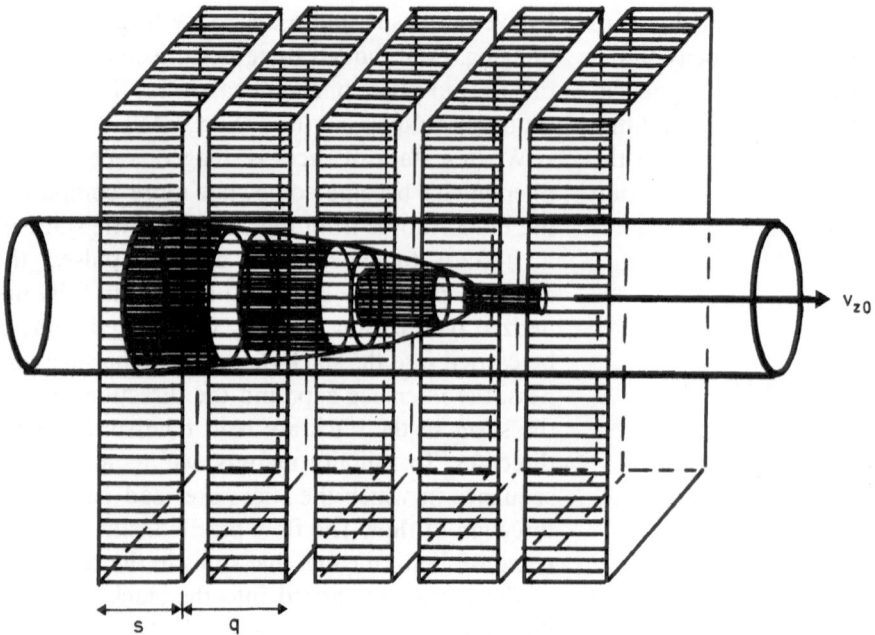

Fig. 3.14. A vessel courses perpendicularly through a stack of slices. Note, that the parabolic flow profile in the vessel means that smaller and smaller cylinders within the vessel contain spins from the outside of the stack. This explains why in deeper slices only a central signal-containing zone persists

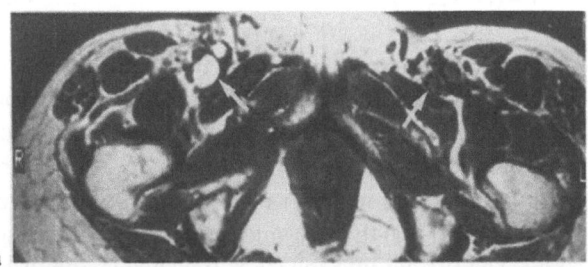

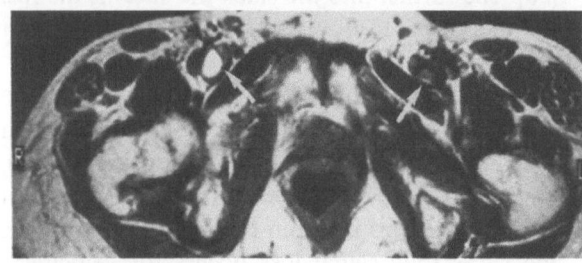

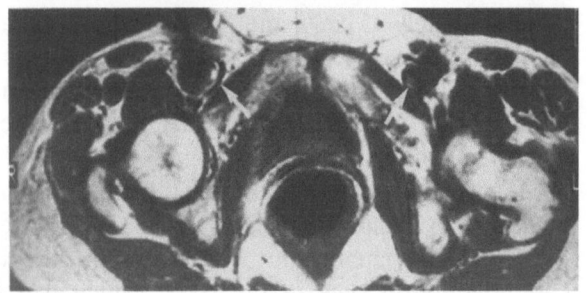

Fig. 3.15a–c. Entry slice phenomenon *(arrows)* observed in the femoral veins in a stack of transverse slices through the pelvis (SE 500/30 ms, slice separation 18 mm, slice thickness 7 mm). **a** Entry slice at the bottom of the slice stack; **b, c** more cranial slices. Note that the signal enhancement becomes progressively more central in the vessel

pervenes. In fact, the situation is somewhat more complicated, because the nutation pulse also moves into the stack and is not always applied to the first slice. Thus, higher velocities may still produce enhancement, but since the slice-select gradient is also applied during this process, spin-phase phenomena are also active in suppressing signal. Figure 3.15 shows an example of an entry slice phenomenon in the femoral veins of a patient.

3.2.3 Flow Measurements Using Time-of-Flight Effects

The principle of flow measurements using time-of-flight phenomena is simple. Spins in a slice are tagged by a 90° pulse, but rather than reading out the same slice, a slice downstream is read. Signal in this slice comes only from the tagged spins, which have moved the distance between the excited and the read slice. Since the time between tagging and readout is known, the velocity of flow can be determined. By varying the distance or excitation time between the two slices, the experiment can be made sensitive to arbitrary flow velocities [27]. If the same slice is excited and read, flow-related enhancement and high-velocity signal loss occur according to Eq. 3.6. Signal intensity in the vessel may thus be used, in principle, to measure the velocity [28, 29]. In practice, this does not work because the signal intensitiy to velocity relation is not unique (Fig. 3.13) and because spin-phase phenomena also influence intravascular signal intensity.

Special sequences producing a displacement of flowing spins relative to nonmoving spins along one axis of a function image are more promising because the velocity measurement does not rely on the absolute value of the signal intensity. Several schemes have been proposed but will not be described in detail [10, 30, 31].

3.3 MR Angiography

It was noted previously than in the arterial vessels there are strong intravascular variations in signal intensity on conventional SE images, when diastole and systole are compared (Sect. 3.1.2). Furthermore, gradient echo images produce very strong intravascular signal, particularly if flow-compensated sequences are used (Sects. 3.1.2 and 3.2.2). These phenomena have been used to produce images similar to those seen in angiography.

If two identical MR images that may have a large slice thickness are acquired, one in systole, where arterial flow is maximum, and one in diastole, where arterial flow is minimum, and the two images are subtracted, all structures that have the same signal intensity on both images will disappear. The only structures that vary in intensity are the arteries; thus, the subtraction image shows angiography-like qualities, except that the veins do not show strongly because of lack of pulsatile flow [32]. The method appears to work well in the periphery, and good definition of arterial structures in the legs has been accomplished [33]. Problems arise in the abdomen, where respiration and peristalsis prevent the two images to be subtracted from being identical. Artifacts similar to those in X-ray digital subtraction angiography appear, though these artifacts can be kept smaller, because the two images can be acquired in interleaved fashion. Still, the time difference of acquisition will be equal to TR. A further problem is to make the TRs for the diastolic and systolic images as close to each other as possible, so that static structures exhibit exactly the same signal intensity. This is not possible in general, due to the sinus arrhythmia encountered in the ECG RR interval (Sect. 4.1). Thus, this method, even though it is interesting, is unlikely to find any future use.

Gradient echo images, particularly the ones for which flow-compensated gradients are used, produce intravascular signal stronger than that of any other tissue. MR angiography can therefore be per-

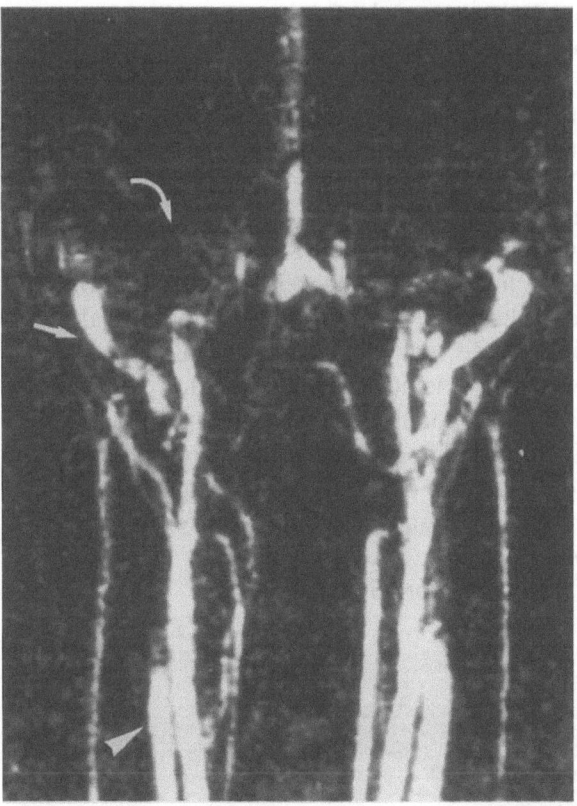

Fig. 3.16. MR angiographic display of the large vessels in the head and neck. The arteries and the veins are seen simultaneously (internal carotid: *straight arrow*, jugular vein: *arrowhead*). Note dephasing-dependent signal dropout in areas of sharp-bends like the intrapetrosal area of the carotid *(curved arrow)*. (Courtesy of Philips, Eindhoven)

formed using such sequences. In contrast to the procedure described in the previous paragraph, high signal is present in any vessel and even at high flow velocities. Rather than using images in systole and diastole and subtracting them, in this type of angiography two sequences, one flow-sensitive and the other flow-insensitive, are used and subtracted, as they exhibit large differences in intravascular signal intensity. Thus, instead of using physiologically determined intensity variations to produce the two images to be subtracted, different pulse sequences are used to generate the two images. An example of an MR angiogram is shown in Fig. 3.16. High-resolution images of the head vessels using this method have been published [34]. However, these methods are only now being installed on MR imagers, so no experience regarding the achievable spatial resolution or the clinical usefulness has been accumulated.

3.4 Pulsations of the Cerebrospinal Fluid Induced by Cardiac Motion

It has long been recognized that cardiovascular pulsations are transmitted to the cerebrospinal fluid [35, 36]. It is therefore not surprising that flow phenomena are observed not only in the cardiovascular system, but also in the CSF channels. Whether this phenomenon is due to cyclic expansions of the choroid plexus, to direct transmission of arterial pulsations to the ventricles, or to transmission of venous pulse waves is not entirely clear. However, because the total amount of CSF formed per hour is relatively low (approximately 25 ml/h [37]), the flow void has to be due to the to-and-fro motion of CSF in, e.g., the aqueduct rather than to unidirectional pulsatile flow caused by pulsatile production of CSF in the choroid plexus.

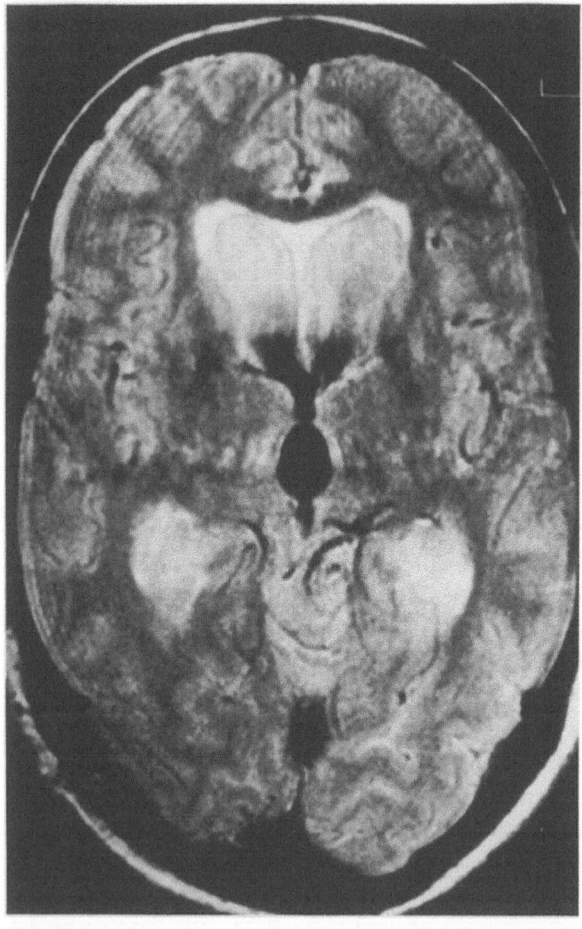

Fig. 3.17. Transverse section (SE 1800/30 ms) through the brain. Note the grayish appearance of the CSF in the lateral ventricles. In the region of the foramina of Monroe and the third ventricle there is total lack of signal, because in this region there is to-and-fro motion of the CSF induced by the cardiovascular pulsations, resulting in flow-related signal loss

The effects of CSF flow phenomena were first observed in the aqueduct of Sylvius, where, due to the narrowness of the channel, the highest flow velocities are expected [38]. Variations in the MR appearance of the CSF flow void were established early on by cardiac-gated MR studies [39]. In addition to producing variations in the signal intensity of the CSF spaces on MRI (Fig. 3.17), the pulsations also cause image artifacts [40], particularly in the neck region in analogy to blood flow artifacts from vessels [41, 42] (Sect. 3.5). They can be markedly reduced by cardiac gating (Sect. 4.1). A larger clinical series suggests that the appearance of the signal differentiates normal patients from patients with chronic, communicating normal-pressure hydrocephalus, who show a more pronounced flow void, and patients with atrophy, in whom the flow void is less pronounced [38]. Although the clinical usefulness of CSF circulation studies with nuclear medicine methods is well established, more extensive experience with MRI has to accumulate to demonstrate its usefulness in assessing alterations in CSF circulatory function.

3.5 Image Artifacts Due to Physiologic Motion

3.5.1 "Ghost" Artifacts

Motion affects the phase of moving relative to stationary spins. Since in 2DFT, phase encoding is used to spatially localize the signal in one dimension within the slice (let it be the y-axis in a transverse slice), additional variation of phases due to motion results in artifacts which are called "ghosts" [43]. The reason why these ghosts occur is simple to understand. When discussing phase encoding (Sect. 1.5.3), we saw that the systematic increase in the strength of the phase-encoding gradient results in a systematic increase or decrease of the phase of the pixel magnetization vectors, indentical for pixels in the same row. After n gradient steps, n data points are obtained for each row in the pixel matrix (Figs. 1.30 and 1.31), which fall onto a sine curve (Fig. 3.18). The frequency of this sine determines the position of the row. If the spins in a pixel happen to move at the same velocity whenever data are collected, this simply produces a phase shift of the curve (Fig. 3.18). For cardiosynchronous motion, this can be accomplished with ECG gating (Sect. 4.1). Respiratory, peristaltic, and swallowing motions vary in time, and these motions result in phase alterations which are different at each repetition of the pulse sequence. Then the measured

Abb. 3.18. Phase encoding results in a sine wave with different frequency for each row (or column) in the image. If in a pixel of such a row the spins are moving with the same characteristics for each repetition of, e.g., an SE sequence, the sine wave is simply phase-shifted, but its frequency and amplitude not changed. However, if motion is not synchronous with the cycle of data acquisition, the motion-induced phase changes are no longer constant and no perfect sine wave can be fitted through the points measured. Instead, the process of Fourier transformation (the second, remember!) yields several frequencies and a reduced amplitude from the pixel with the variable motion. Since the frequencies obtained code for position along the phase-encode direction, we find artifacts presenting as signal spread along the phase-encode direction

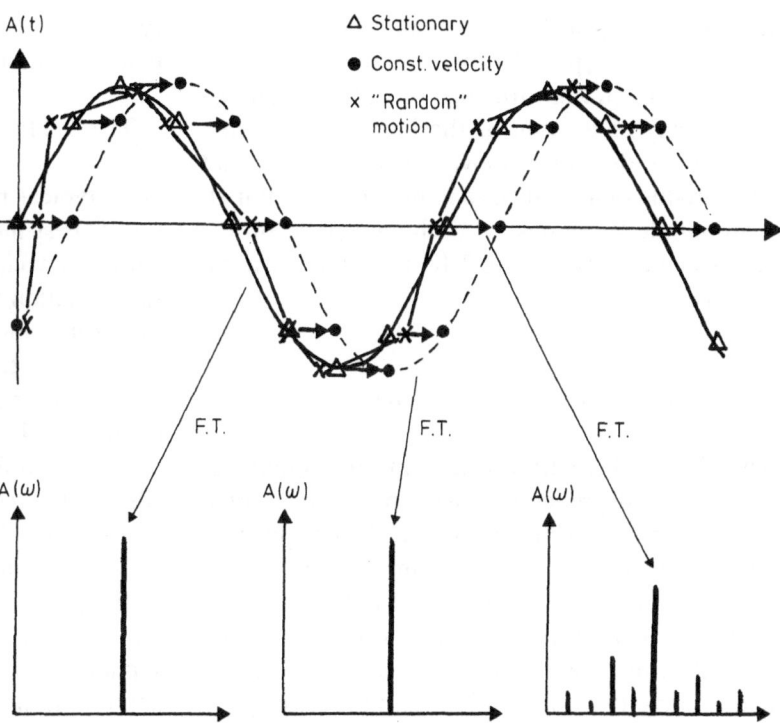

curve deviates from a simple sine function (Fig. 3.18). The data collected no longer fall onto a sine curve; the Fourier transformation now yields several frequencies and a reduced amplitude of the signal at the proper frequency. Since the frequency obtained from the second Fourier transform encodes for y-axis position, signal from a given row appears scattered along the phase-encode direction, and such image-artifacts are observed very frequently (Fig. 3.19).

Blood vessels are no problem in SE images, as long as they show no intravascular signal. For constant velocity flow, where intravascular signal appears under slow-flow conditions on SE images and for all velocities on gradient echo images, no detrimental interference with proper phase encoding occurs from the intravascular signal, because constant motion only phase-shifts the sine in Fig. 3.18. This is nearly the case for constant velocity venous flow found in the circulation not too close to the heart. However, pulsatile flow in the presence of intravas-

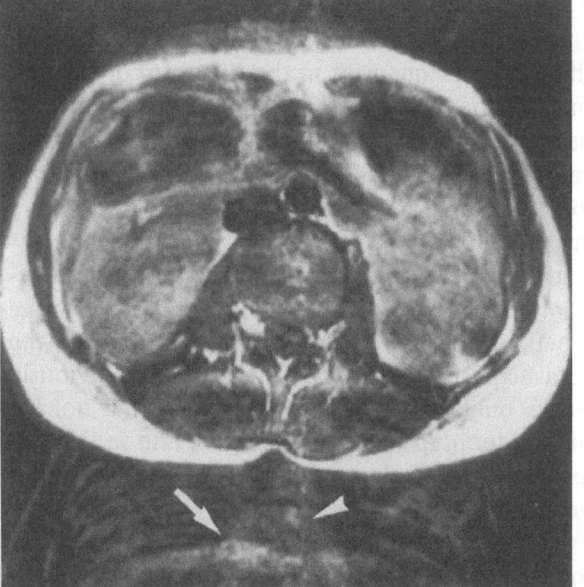

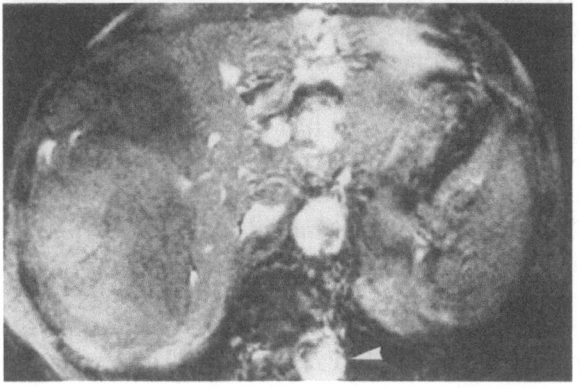

Fig. 3.19. a Ghosts along the phase-encode direction in an abdominal transverse image coming from respiratory motion, aortic pulsations, and peristaltic motion in an SE image (500/30 ms). Note reduplications of high signal intensity body fat contours due to respiration *(straight arrow)* and more scattered signal due to pulsatile motion of blood *(arrowhead)*. **b** In gradient echo images, which can be obtained in apnea, respiratory and peristaltic artifacts are absent, but artifacts from pulsatile aortic flow can be prominent, because the intravascular signal is very strong on gradient echo images

cular signal [44], such as slow pulsatile flow in SE images and all types of flow in gradient echo images, leads to strong variations in intravascular signal intensity as a result of the intravoxel incoherence effects described above. Then there are not only variable phase shifts, as in bulk motion, but also amplitude variations for each data point on the phase-encode curve of Fig. 3.18, resulting in vascular ghosts (Fig. 3.19).

3.5.2 Artifact Suppression Techniques

Remedies for these artifacts are most important, because image degradation caused by them is often severe. Several possibilities exist. If data acquisition can be synchronized to the pattern of motion, as with ECG triggering in the case of cardiac motion, the motion state of these moving structures will be nearly the same with each repetition. On the phase-encode curve this appears like constant velocity (or accelerated) motion, only phase-shifting the sine wave. The signal is not displaced in the image, and the phase shift is still a measure of the instantaneous motion state (Fig. 3.3). Uncontrolled phase shifts and variations in amplitude are nonexistent; thus, extra frequencies in the spectrum of the second Fourier transform and thus "ghost" artifacts have been removed. Respiratory gating was advocated in the early days of SE imaging, but it prolongs imaging times too much [45]. For respiratory artifact supression, the most promising techniques aside from fast imaging are methods which incorporate some knowledge of the relation between the repetition rate and the respiratory motion into the data acquisition strategy. This approach obviously works only for quasi-periodic motion, but not for the random-type peristaltic motion, and in this latter case fast-imaging techniques are the only solution to artifact removal.

The simplest technique for supressing respiratory (or cardiac motion) artifacts is as follows [46, 47]: In MR data acquisition, each subsequent phase-encode step is done not after the repetition time TR but after TR times the number of excitations (measurements, acquisitions) NEX. The principles of phase encoding dictate that the highest frequencies in the signal measured come from the rows placed furthest away from the center row of the image. Thus, signal variations modulated onto the phase-encode sine by motions such as respiration will generate ghosts the furthest away from the image center and thus the image itself, if they have the highest frequency possible. This is the case if the respiratory motion has a period TP, which is approximately twice TR, times the number of excitations

$$TP \approx 2\,TR\,NEX \qquad (3.8)$$

With typical respiratory periods of 4 s, this condition is best met for TRs of approximately 1000 ms with two excitations, which is easy to achieve. The same relation also holds for the vascular ghosts due to cardiac motion in non-triggered gradient echo images of the upper abdomen. Here, TR is 50–100 ms and NEX if possible only 1, but TP, now being the RR interval, is 600–1000 ms.

A more sophisticated incorporation of the knowledge on the respiratory cycle into data acquisition is the so-called ROPE technique (respiratory ordered phase encoding) [48]. With this technique, the value of the phase-encoding gradient is determined such that adjacent values of the gradient are sampled in similar respiratory phases. The result is that the signal variations due to respiration produce low-frequency oscillations or only a monotonic increase or decrease on top of the phase-encode sine function. In this way, ghosts can also be made to disappear, but rather than being placed far away from their proper position, they now closely approach the position where the signal comes from and thus lead to minimal blurring.

As stated, vascular ghosts occur only if intravascular signal is present. If such signal can be minimized, ghosting is minimized. One major source of such signal is the wash-in of fully magnetized spins (entry slice phenomena: Sect. 3.2.2) from the outside of the imaged stack of slices. Artifacts can be drastically reduced in SE imaging if the spins in the volumes adjacent to the imaged stack are also repetitively subjected to a 90° pulse; this demagnetizes the spins which will eventually be carried into the slice stack [49]. The additional pulse added onto a sequence like the one in Fig. 1.29 is shaped such that only spins to the left and the right of the slice stack are excited. This spoiler pulse is sent into the system after each recorded (multi-) echo train rather than after each TR, hence with a very short repetition time. This reduces the persisting magnetization of the inflowing spins strongly.

3.5.3 Spatial Misregistration

Slowly flowing blood sometimes shows signal which is not intravascular but is placed outside the anatomic confines of the vessel. This phenomenon is most readily observed when vessels course

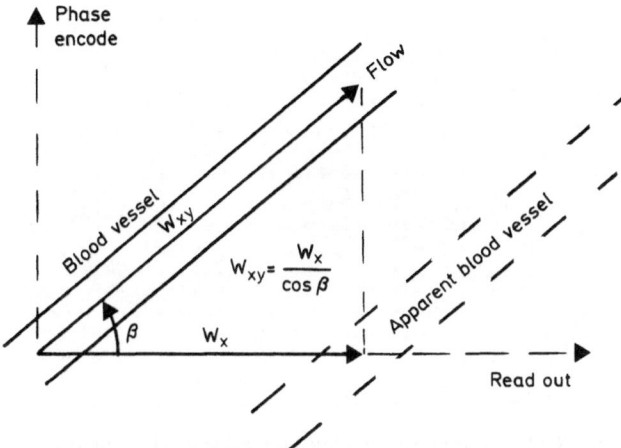

Fig. 3.20. Spatial misregistration. A vessel coursing obliquely in the imaging plane with a angle β carries spins whose position in the phase encode direction is fixed at the beginning of the pulse sequence. The position along the readout direction is measured only at the echo time, after the spins have moved a distance w_{xy}. The result is an apparent shift of intravascular signal out of the vessel by a direction w_x

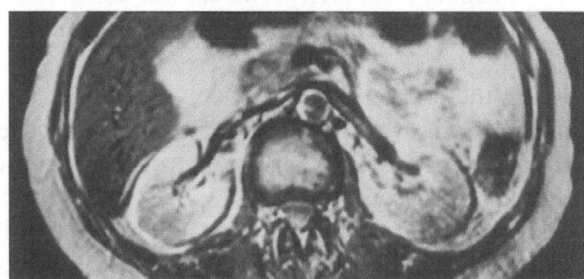

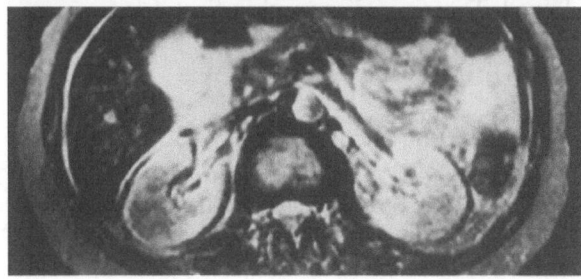

Fig. 3.21a, b. Spatial misregistration observed on a transverse section at the level of the renal veins. Note very little intravascular signal on the first echo image (**a**). On the second echo image (**b**), the signal is displaced towards the vertebral body, thus appearing outside the vessel and indicating flow towards the inferior vena cava

obliquely within the imaged plane. It can be understood by looking at the pulse sequence schematic of Fig. 1.29. Note that the phase encode gradient G_y, which we once more assume to lay along the y-direction, is switched on shortly after the 90° pulse, thus recording the position of a spin along the y-direction. However, the read process, and therefore the spatial localization along the x-direction, occurs

only at the echo, several tens of milliseconds later. For oblique motion within the plane the situation depicted in Fig. 3.20 arises. The spins flowing in the vessel are y-position encoded, then move until the n-th echo occurs, where the imaging process fixes the x-position. The result is a shift of intravascular signal in the direction of flow along the read axis (Fig. 3.20). In the renal veins, this flow is central, and with a left-right read direction the displacement is towards the vertebral bodies. If the spin has moved a distance w_{xy} between the phase-encode process and the echo (which is approximately the echo time at the n-th echo nTE), and the vessel subtends an angle β with the read axis, intravascular signal is found displaced by a distance w_x. w_x and β can be measured on the image, hence the velocity of blood in the vessel is found to be

$$v_{xy} = w_x/(nTE \cos \beta) \qquad (3.9)$$

Spatial misregistration [11] is therefore another way of obtaining velocity information, related to slice-transition velocity determinations in the sense that the velocity is determined by distance and time measurements rather than by the direct measurement of velocity, as is the case with spin-phase phenomena. Figure 3.21 is an example of spatial misregistration at the level of the renal veins, where this phenomenon is most often observed. The phenomenon ist usually observed on second echo images only, because intravascular signal is needed for the effect to be observed at all, and this is stronger on even echoes due to rephasing, and because the time delay between phase encode and read times for the second is twice that for the first echo, doubling the displacement (Eq. 3.9).

3.6 The Recognition of Flow Phenomena in Clinical Practice

We have seen in the previous sections that the understanding of MR flow phenomena is not as simple as one would hope. However, to understand cardiovascular function studies and the potential of MRI to obtain such information, a thorough understanding of motion and flow phenomena is mandatory. In the daily practice of MR image interpretation a certain level of familiarity with flow phenomena is also required. The clinician wants a definitive answer from the diagnostician on whether a vessel contains thrombus or slow flow, and the diagnostician should be able to distinguish pathologic solid structures such as lymph nodes from slow blood flow in vessels. This is not always easy, as clinical experience shows [50]. Despite the complexity of understanding flow phenomena, some simple qualitative rules can be given for unequivocally detecting the presence of a perfused vascular lumen vs. a solid structure.

1. A structure containing no signal on a SE image is a blood vessel with flowing blood, a air- or compact bone-filled space, or a metal artifact. If in proper anatomic location, it must be a perfused vessel, even if other methods using contrast media for vessel specification such as angiography do not show this vessel.
2. If signal is present in the anatomic region of a vessel, it is due to either slow flow or thrombus on SE images. In SE images with short echo times and in gradient echo imaging, high intravascular signal intensity occurs also for higher blood flow velocities.
3. There are several qualitative criteria for identifying high signal intensity as coming from flowing blood:
   a) Variations of signal intensity in studies gated to the cardiac cycle are due to flow.
   b) Ghost artifacts over a bright structure on an image are due to blood flow in that structure (Sect. 3.5, Fig. 3.19).
   c) Central signal in a vessel with a surrounding dark rim is due to flow resulting from the strong dephasing of spins along vessel walls. If the vessel is close to the surface of the stack of imaged slices, it can be the result of an entry slice phenomenon, where spins are washed only into the central portion of the slice due to higher central velocity.
   d) If the dark rim disappears on second echo and the vessel is filled with signal, this is a result of even-echo rephasing and thus a result of blood flow not consistent with stasis.
   e) If signal is present on first and absent on second echo, this is a washout phenomenon and thus is due to flow (Fig. 3.11).
   f) If there is central intravascular signal loss in a vessel but bright signal peripherally, this can be a washout phenomenon where the central spins move out of the slice more quickly than the peripheral ones. However, this can be observed in thrombosis as well, where the hemoglobin in the blood clot shows different metabolic states (Fig. 3.22). In this case, no firm diagnosis can be established.
   g) If the qualitative criteria cited above are equivocal, the decision whether there is flow or

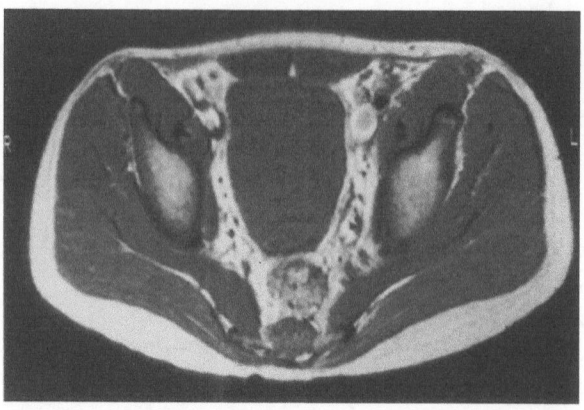

Fig. 3.22. Thrombosis in a left femoral vein, showing central signal decrease with a bright vascular rim. The rigth femoral vein has a similar appearance but contains slow flow rather than thrombosis (diagnosis was confirmed with Doppler ultrasound and angiography examinations)

thrombus in the vessel has to rely on the determination of T2 values (Sect. 3.1.2) or on phase imaging (Sect. 3.1.1). The clinical usefulness of these two methods is discussed in Chap. 5.

Using these criteria, and possibly the quantitative methods, intravascular signal can be distinguished from thrombosis or other solid structures close to the anatomic confines of a vessel such as lymph nodes with certainty. Flow phenomena are usually better identified if certain imaging rules are followed. These are discussed in Sect. 4.1.

References

1. von Schulthess GK, Augustiny N (1987) Calculation of T2 values versus phase imaging for the distinction between flow and thrombus in MR imaging. Radiology 164: 549–554
2. van Dijk P (1984) Direct cardiac NMR imaging of heart wall and blood flow velocity. J Comput Ass Tomogr 8: 429–436
3. Wedeen VJ, Rosen BR, Chesler D, Brady TJ (1985) MR velocity imaging by phase display. J comput Ass Tomogr 9: 530–536
4. White EM, Edelman RR, Wedeen VJ, Brady TJ (1986) Intravascular signal in MR imaging: use of phase display for differentiation of blood-flow signal from intraluminal disease. Radiology 161: 245–249
5. Nayler GL, Firmin DN, Longmore DB (1986) Blood flow imaging by cine magnetic resonance. J Comput Ass Tomogr 10: 715–722
6. Klipstein RH, Firmin N, Underwood SR, Nayler GL, Rees RSO, Longmore DB (1987) Colour display of quantitative blood flow and cardiac anatomy in a single magnetic resonance cine loop. Brit J Radiol 60: 105–111
7. Longmore DB (1987) Plenary lecture on cardiovascular imaging. SMRM New York

8. Underwood SR, Firmin DN, Mohiaddin RH et al. (1987) Cine magnetic resonance imaging of valvular heart disease. Book of abstracts, SMRM New York

9. Axel L (1984) Blood flow effects in magnetic resonance imaging. AJR 143: 1157-1166

10. Wehrli FJ, Shimakawa A, MacFall JR, Axel L, Perman W (1985) MR imaging of venous and arterial flow by a selective saturation-recovery spin echo (SSRSE) method. J Comput Ass Tomogr 9: 537-545

11. von Schulthess GK, Higgins CB (1985) Blood flow imaging with MR: spin-phase phenomena. Radiology 157: 687-695

12. Kucharczyk W, Brant-Zawadski M, Lemme-Plaghos L et al. (1985) MR technology: effect of even-echo rephasing on calculated T2 values and T2 images. Radiology 157: 95-101

13. Le Bihan D, Breton E, Lallemand D, Grenier P, Cabanis E, Laval-Jeantet M (1986) MR imaging of intravoxel incoherent motions: application to diffusion and perfusion in neurologic disorders. Radiology 161: 401-407

14. Ahn CB, Lee SY, Nalcioglu O, Cho ZH (1987) The effects of random directional distributed flow in nuclear magnetic resonance imaging. Med Phys 14: 43-48

15. Duewell S, Wüthrich R, Buck A, von Schulthess GK (1988) Signal loss in intravoxel incoherent motion: evaluation of different perfusion types and pulse sequences. SHRM book of abstracts 221

16. von Schulthess GK, Fisher MR, Higgins CB (1985) Pathologic blood flow in pulmonary vascular disease as shown by gated magnetic resonance imaging. Ann Int Med 103: 317-323

17. Moran PR (1982) A flow velocity Zeugmatographic interlace for NMR imaging in humans. Mag Res Imaging 1: 197-203

18. Bryant DJ, Payne JA, Firmin N, Longmore DB (1984) Measurement of flow with NMR imaging using a gradient pulse and phase difference technique. J Comp Ass Tomogr 8: 588-593

19. O'Donnell M (1985) NMR blood flow imaging using multiecho, phase-contrast sequences. Med Phys 12: 59-64

20. Moran PR, Moran RA, Karstaedt N (1985) Verification and evaluation of internal flow and motion. True magnetic resonance imaging by the phase gradient modulation method. Radiology 154: 433-441

21. Pettigrew RI, Dannels W, Galloway JR et al. (1987) Quantitative phase-flow MR imaging in dogs using standard sequences: comparison with in vivo flowmeter measurements. AJR 148: 411-415

22. Pettigrew RI, Dannels W (1987) Use of standard gradients with compound oblique angulation for optimal quantitative MR flow imaging in oblique vessels. AJR 148: 405-409

23. Nayler GL, Firmin DN, Longmore DB (1986) Blood flow imaging by cine magnetic resonance. J Comput Ass Tomogr 10: 715-722

24. Hennig J, Müri M, Friedburg H, Brunner P (1988) Quantitative flow measurement with MR imaging in clinical routine using the fast Fourier flow technique. Radiology 166: 239-240

25. Marks A, Feinberg DA (1986) Flow measurements in blood vessels. RSNA book of abstracts

26. Valk PE, Crooks LR, Kaufman L, Roos MS, Orthendahl DA, Higgins CB (1986) Blood flow in magnetic resonance imaging: correlation of image appearances with spin echo phase shift and signal intensity. AJR 146: 913-939

27. Singer JR, Crooks LE (1983) Nuclear magnetic resonance blood flow measurements in the human brain. Science 221: 654-656

28. Kaufman L, Crooks LE, Sheldon PE, Rowan W, Miller T (1982) Evaluation of NMR imaging for detection and quantification of obstructions in vessels. Invest Radiol 17: 554-560

29. Kaufman L, Crooks LE, Sheldon PE, Hricak H, Herfkens R, Bank W (1983) The potential impact of nuclear magnetic resonance imaging on cardiovascular diagnosis. Circulation 68: 251-257

30. Wehrli FW, Shimakawa A, Gullberg GT, MacFall JR (1986) Time-of-flight MR flow imaging: selective saturation recovery with gradient refocussing. Radiology 160: 781-785

31. Shimizu K, Matsuda T, Tsunetaro S et al. (1986) Visualization of moving fluid: quantitative analysis of blood flow velocity using MR imaging. Radiology 159: 195-199

32. Wedeen VJ, Meuli R, Edelman RR et al. (1985) Projective imaging of pulsatile flow with magnetic resonance. Science 230: 946-949

33. Meuli RA, Wedeen VJ, Geller SC et al. (1986) MR gated subtraction angiography: evaluation of lower extremities. Radiology 159: 411-418

34. Du Moulin CL, Hart HR jr (1986) Magnetic resonance angiography. Radiology 161: 717-720

35. Bering EA jr (1955) Choroid plexus and arterial pulsations of cerebrospinal fluid: demonstration of the choroid plexuses as a cerebrospinal fluid pump. Arch Neurol Psychiatr 73: 165-172

36. Du Boulay GH (1966) Pulsatile movements in the CSF pathways. Br J Radiol 39: 255-262

37. Citrin CM, Sherman JL, Gangarosa RE, Scanlon D (1987) Physiology of the CSF flow-void sign: modification by cardiac gating. AJR 148: 205-208

38. Bradley WG, Kortman KE, Burgoyne B (1986) Flowing cerebrospinal fluid in normal and hydrocephalic states: appearance on MR images. Radiology 159: 611-616

39. Bergstrand G, Bergström M, Nordell B et al. (1985) Cardiac gated MR imaging of cerebrospinal fluid flow. J Comput Ass Tomogr 9: 1003-1006

40. Schultz CL, Alfidi RJ, Nelson AD, Kopiwopda SY, Clampitt ME (1984) The effect of motion on two-dimensional Fourier transformation magnetic resonance images. Radiology 152: 117-180

41. Rubin JB, Enzmann DR (1987) Imaging of spinal CSF pulsation by 2DFT MR: significance during clinical imaging. AJR 148: 973-982

42. Enzmann DR, O'Donahue JO, Rubin JB, Shuer L, Cogen R (1986) CSF pulsations within nonneoplastic spinal cord cysts. AJR 161: 717-720

43. Schultz CL, Alfidi RJ, Nelson AD, Kopiwoda SY, Clampitt ME (1984) The effect of motion on two-dimensional Fourier transformation magnetic resonance images. Radiology 152: 117-121

44. Perman WH, Moran PR, Moran RA, Bernstein MA (1986) Artifacts from pulsatile flow in MR imaging. J Comput Ass Tomogr 10: 473-483

45. Lewis CE, Prato FS, Drost DJ, Nicholson RL (1986) Comparison of respiratory triggering and gating techniques for the removal of respiratory artifacts in MR imaging. Radiology 160: 803-810

46. Axel L, Summers RM, Kressel HY, Charles C (1986) Respiratory effects in two-dimensional Fourier transform MR imaging. Radiology 160: 795-801

47. Haake EM, Lenz GW, Nelson AD (1987) Pseudo-gating:

elimination of periodic motion artifacts in magnetic resonance imaging without gating. Mag Res Med 4: 162–174

48. Bailes DR, Gilderdale DJ, Bydder GM, Collins AG, Firmin DN (1985) Respiratory ordered phase encoding (ROPE): a method for reducing respiratory motion artifacts in MR imaging. J Comput Ass Tomogr 9: 835–838

49. Felmlee JP, Ehmann RL (1987) Spatial presaturation: a method for suppressing flow artifacts and improving depiction of vascular anatomy in MR imaging. Radiology 164: 559–564

50. von Schulthess GK, Weder W, Goebel N, Buchmann P, Gadze A, Augustiny N, Largiader F (1988) 1.5 T MRI, CT, sonography and scintigraphy in hyperparathyroidism. Eur J Radiology, 8, 157–164

Chapter 4   Cardiac Morphology and Function
in Magnetic Resonance Imaging

MR is capable of producing cardiac images with great morphological detail. However, for proper cardiac MRI, image acquisition with ECG triggering has to be used. The currently available MR techniques still require data acquisition over many cardiac cycles to generate images, but these images are of good quality because acquisition of a single image "line" takes only 20–40 ms; thus, "stopped-motion" images are obtained, even though they are acquired over many cardiac cycles. From patients with cardiac arrhythmias good images cannot be acquired, as proper repetitive triggering to the same phase in the cardiac cycle is not guaranteed. However, a rapid, 40-ms MRI technique producing real-time images has been described [1] recently, based on echo planar imaging [2]. At this time, this method is not available for broader use.

In Chaps. 1 and 3 we discussed the unique sensitivity of MRI to flow and motion, and the effects observed as a result of this motion sensitivity were described. In Chap. 3 we took more of a "passive" viewpoint, developing an understanding and guidelines on how to identify flow and motion phenomena and prevent related artifacts in routine MRI. In the next two chapters we will take a more "active" approach, specifically emphasizing the uses of flow and motion imaging in cardiovascular diagnosis with MRI. We thereby combine the uses of MRI to assess cardiovascular morphology and function. While Chap. 4 deals with the heart, Chap. 5 covers vascular MRI. However, an initial section is devoted to strategies used in imaging the cardiovascular system.

4.1 Special Imaging Techniques
in the Cardiovascular System
and Cardiovascular Imaging Strategy

Acquisition of an SE image requires at least 1 min of imaging time. This is much too long to permit a stopped-motion image of the heart, which requires a temporal resolution on the order of 20–40 ms [3].

Therefore, a technique which is well known under the term "ECG-triggered data acquisition" [4, 5] in nuclear cardiology has been used in MRI [6]. Since the acquisition of a single spin echo takes only 20–40 ms, a cardio-synchronous acquisition of such spin echoes will yield good MR images of structures moving in synchrony to the heart. This technique is mandatory for MRI of the heart and is highly recommended in most instances of vascular imaging. In addition to ECG triggering, it is important to pay attention to the order in which MR images are acquired in multislice imaging.

Furthermore, since the main axes of the heart do not coincide with the main axes of the human body, in some application of cardiac MR imaging it may therefore prove to be advantageous to acquire sections which are angulated such that they are oriented orthogonal to the cardiac rather than the body axes. As MRI permits slice acquisition in all spatial orientations using electronic angulation, this is achievable without difficult patient positioning.

4.1.1 ECG Triggering in MRI

In this method, an ECG from the patient is recorded inside the magnet using three standard ECG electrodes connected to a transducer. The signal is sent outside the magnetic field area either by a light signal guided by a fiber-optic cable or by telemetry. The signal is used to synchronize data acquisition of the machine with the events of the cardiac cycle. Typically, the QRS complex is used as the signal (Fig. 4.1) which triggers the machine to start with data acquisition. The machine then idles, until the next QRS complex triggers the acquisition of the next pulse sequence with the phase-en-code gradient incremented, and so on, until all phase-encoding steps have been completed. The repetition time TR in ECG-triggered image acquisition is equal to the RR interval of the ECG and can no longer be chosen at will. In normals, the RR interval equals 600–1000 ms (cardiac frequency between 60 and

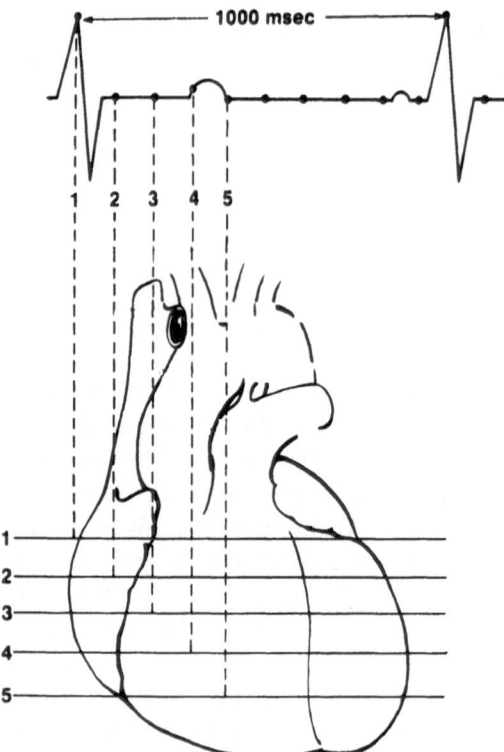

Fig. 4.1. Schematic representation of ECG-triggered data acquisition in MRI. The QRS complex of the ECG starts the machine, which acquires a spin echo for the first phase-encode gradient value and slice, then a spin echo for the first phase-encode gradient value and the second slice, and so on. The next QRS complex triggers the imager to acquire a spin echo with the second phase-encode gradient value for the first, second, etc. slices. This goes on until a spin echo with the last (i.e., 256th) phase-encode gradient value for the first, second, etc. slice has been recorded. The result is several slices at different anatomic levels in different phases of the cardiac cycle

Table 4.1. Order of slice acquisition in an ECG-triggered permutation sequence

Order of slice acquisition in sequence study number					Approximate time after QRS[a]		Approximate phase of cardiac cycle
1	2	3	4	5	1st echo	2nd echo	
1	2	3	4	5	50	80	end-diastole
2	3	4	5	1	150	180	early systole
3	4	5	1	2	250	280	mid-systole
4	5	1	2	3	350	380	end-systole
5	1	2	3	4	450	550	early diastole

[a] Dual SE sequence with echo times of 30 and 60 ms, trigger delay 20 ms

100 BPM); thus, triggering at every heart beat yields T1 weighted images. T2 weighted images can still be obtained by triggering to every second, third, or fourth heart beat and acquiring a dual-echo SE sequence; but with ECG triggering, the TRs obtained are multiple integers of the RR interval. By delaying the data acquisition relative to the QRS complex, imaging of a slice can be accomplished in different phases of the cardiac cycle. Minimal delay will yield end-diastolic images. If the delay is increased, systolic and, with further increase, diastolic images are obtained (Sect. 2.1.1).

The multislice technique can also be used in the ECG-triggered mode, as shown in Fig. 4.1. Note that the slices taken at different anatomic levels are also taken during different phases of the cardiac cycle. However, since the sequence in which the slices of the stack are read can be chosen at will, the top slice does not necessarily have to be measured dur-

ing end-diastole. The fact than in multislice ECG-triggered imaging not only the anatomic position but also the phase of the cardiac cycle changes for each slice makes image interpretation more difficult, particularly if one looks for function information in addition to anatomic abnormalities (Fig. 4.2).

This drawback can be circumvented in SE imaging by using a so-called permutation triggered sequence. In this type of sequence, an ECG-triggered imaging run containing n slices is simply repeated n times, but the order in which the slices are acquired is permuted cyclically (Table 4.1), with the result that each anatomic level is imaged in each phase of the cardiac cycle [6, 7, 8] (Fig. 4.3). Obviously, such a sequence requires n times as long as a single ECG-triggered sequence and thus easily on the order of 30 min. It turns out that the best images of the heart and arterial structures are obtained in systole. There are two reasons for this: First, the blood is moving fastest in the ventricles and arteries during this time, producing the weakest intracardiac signal possible and thus the least image degradation by flow artifacts. Second, the normal cardiac sinus arrhythmia affects the later (diastolic) phases of the heart cycle more strongly than the systolic phases do (Sect. 2.1.1). As a result, the position of the cardiac structures varies more strongly in diastole than in systole with each repetition of the basic pulse sequence, therefore producing a more blurry image (Fig. 4.3).

A different strategy for cardiovascular function studies is possible with gradient echo imaging. Since here the TRs are small and on the order of 30–100 ms, a single slice can be excited several times during a cardiac cycle. For example, a single slice can be imaged during 20 phases of the heart cycle (Fig. 4.4). ECG triggering is still required, because phase encoding proceeds as usual and after

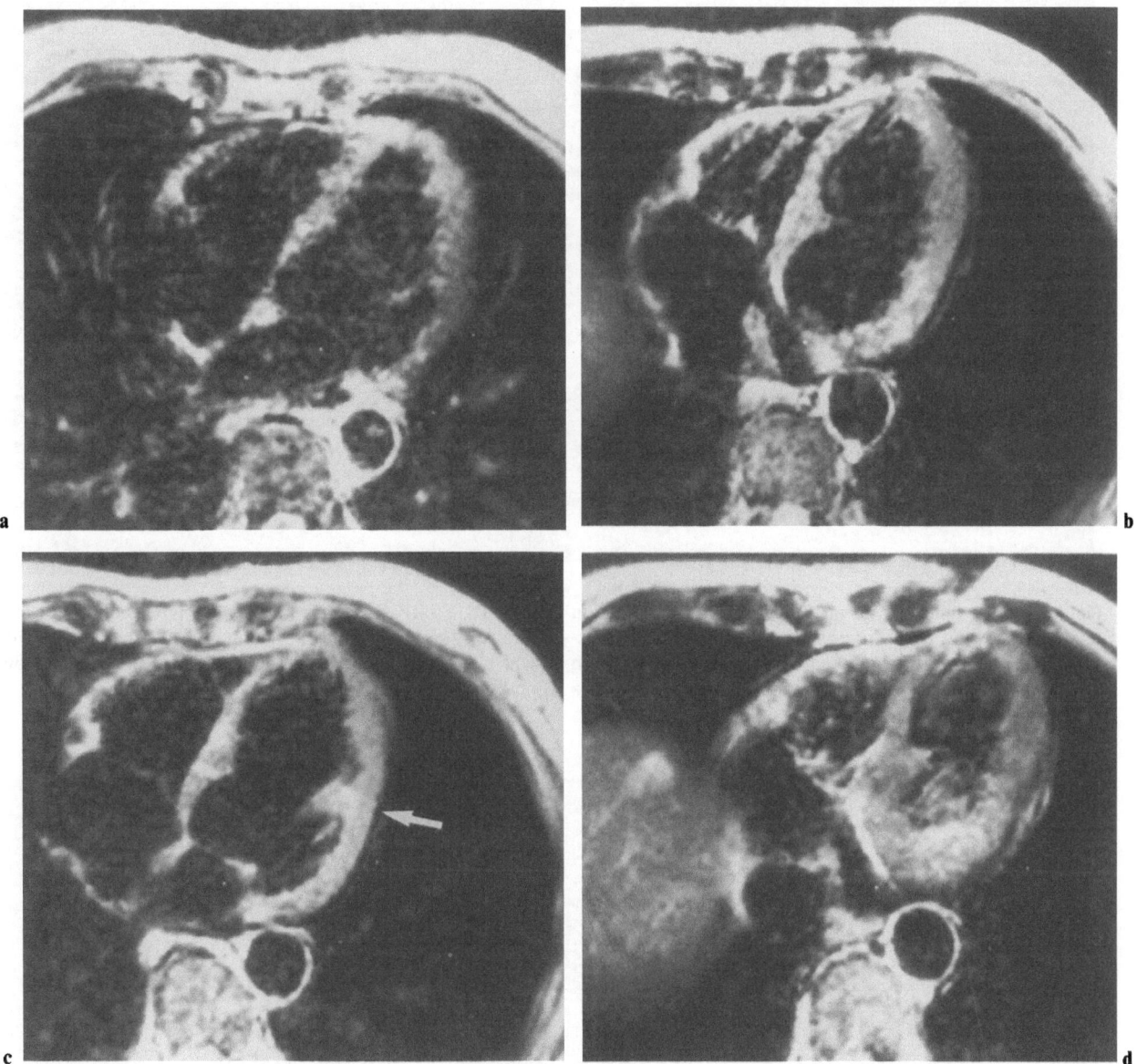

Fig. 4.2 a–d. Four ECG-triggered transverse images through the heart taken in four phases of the cardiac cycle and at four different anatomic levels, i.e., end-diastole, early systole, late systole, and end-systole/early diastole (cf. Table 4.1). End-diastole is recognized by the still-open mitral and tricuspid valves. Also note posterior papillary muscle *(arrow)*

each QRS complex its value is changed, if only one measurement at each gradient setting is performed. Obviously, the maximum number of cardiac phases which can be imaged depends again on the length of the RR interval. If this number is 20, 20 phases of the same slice, ten phases of two slices, five phases of four slices, and so on may be obtained.

The many images obtained in different heart phases from one slice are readily displayed in a movie format. With this format the wealth of flow information contained in the signal intensity variations of the flowing blood is best appreciated; thus, qualitative function analysis is done much more readily using the movie format.

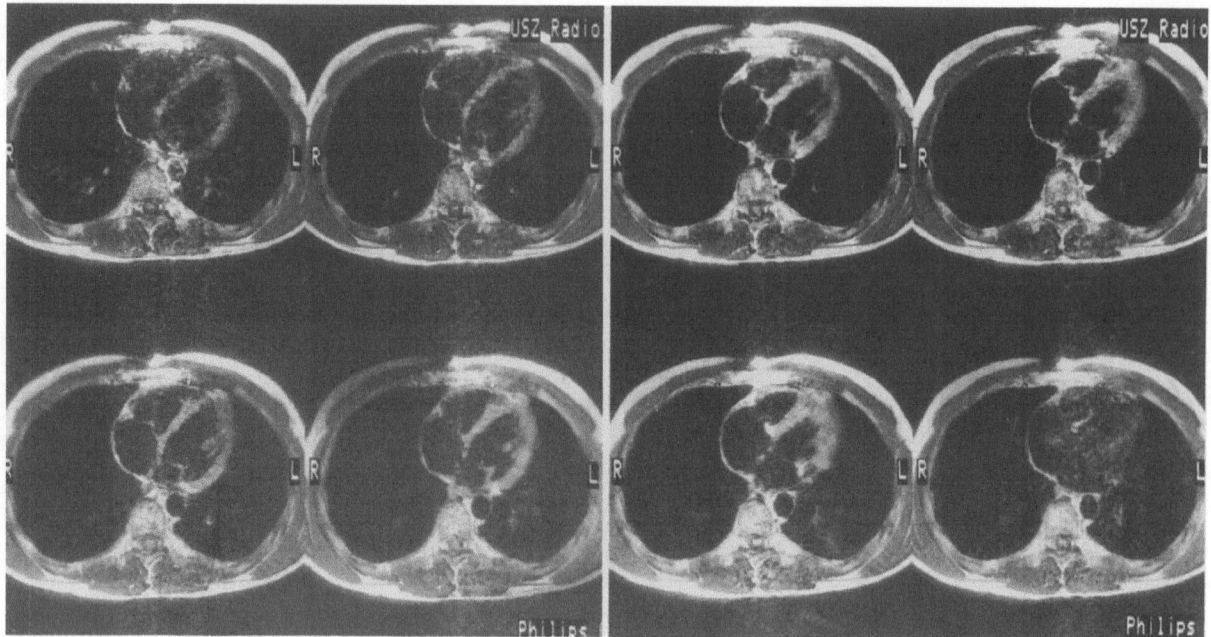

Fig. 4.3. Eight images from an ECG-triggered permutation sequence showing eight different cardiac phases at a transverse anatomic level through the mid-heart. The last image in this normal volunteer is blurred due to the sinus arrhythmia (HR ca. 60 BPM), which mostly affects the diastolic time intervals. Note the wall thickening and the anatomic details which can be identified. The left atrium is small in diastole and increases in size during systole

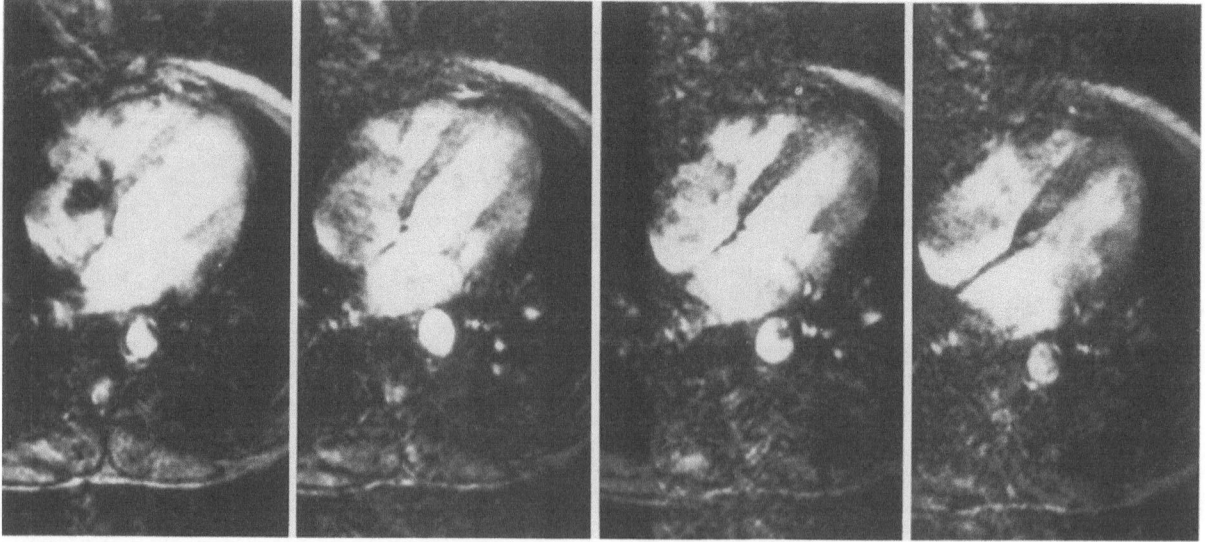

a–d

Fig. 4.4a–d. Four images from an ECG-triggered gradient echo sequence (GFE 34/20 ms, $\alpha = 40°$) showing end-diastole (ca. 50 ms after QRS), early (ca. 110 ms after QRS), and mid-systole (ca. 190 ms after QRS), and very early diastole (ca. 370 ms after QRS). Note that in this sequence the blood appears as the brightest structure, and slight variations in signal intensity are due to turbulence, which is more pronounced in the ventricles than in the atria. The mitral valve and its attachment to the inferior papillary muscle are seen, and the walls are noted to thicken markedly from diastole into systole. The mitral valve has opened up again in the last image

4.1.2 Angulation of Sections in Cardiac Imaging

Any oblique angulation of sections is possible with MRI; therefore, images parallel or perpendicular to the long axis of the heart may be obtained [9, 10]. For proper angulation, two initial views of the heart have to be obtained. The first may be a coronal scan, defining the angle of the long cardiac axis relative to the z-axis of the magnet (Fig. 4.5). The second orientation plane would then be taken as a transverse section, tilted by the previously determined angle around the anteroposterior (y-) axis. From this second scan the second angle is determined, and thus sections perpendicular (or parallel) to the long cardiac axis may be obtained (Figs. 4.5, 4.6). As software packages of the MR imagers become more sophisticated, the two angles needed to obtain such a section become more easy to determine, but presently, the advantages of obtaining long or short axis views are often not such that the extra time needed (approximately 10 min) to determine the two angles is worth spending.

4.1.3 Slice Ordering

When large blood vessels are present in MR images, as in most images of the neck, thorax, and abdomen, it is useful to pay attention to the order in which the slices in a stack in multislice imaging are acquired. This can help reduce blood flow artifacts [11] and makes it easier to identify intravascular signal as such. Furthermore, as stated above, the images containing the least amount of artifacts are the images acquired in cardiac systole. The following rules are useful and should be incorporated into a cardiovascular imaging strategy.

The order in which the slices are acquired should follow the direction of arterial flow. For example, in transverse imaging, abdominal sections should be acquired from top to bottom, whether ECG triggering is used or not, and the reverse should be done above the heart in the mediastinum or the neck. The heart is the structure with the strongest motion in the cardiovascular system; thus, if an area including the heart, i.e., the thoracoabdominal junc-

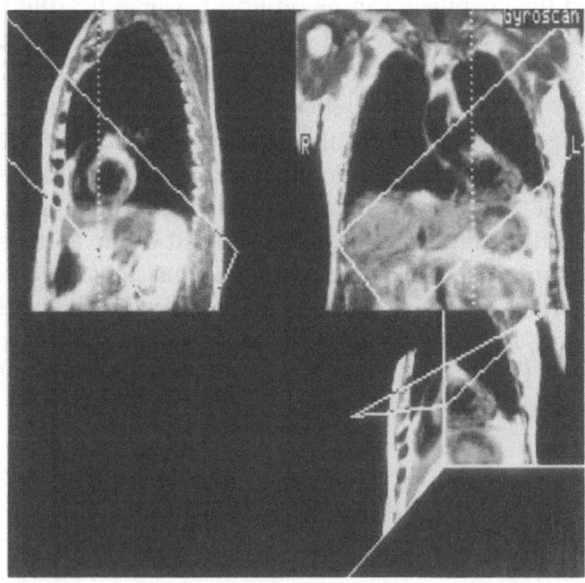

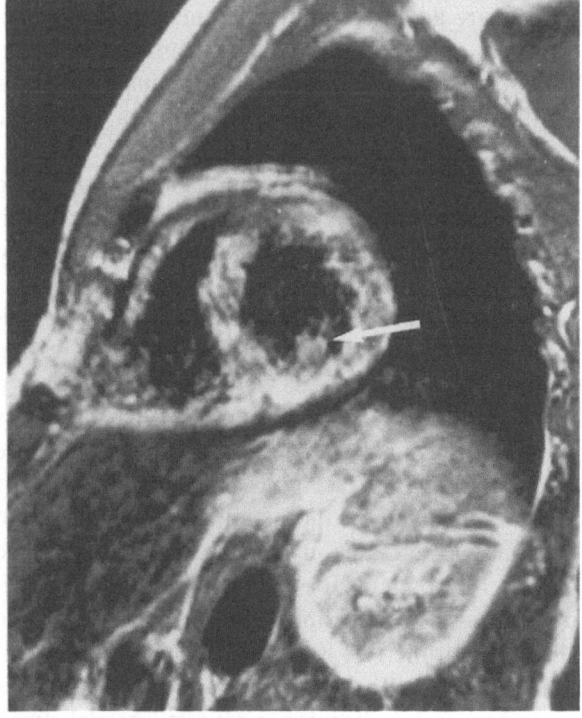

Fig. 4.5. Schematic representation of angle determination for oblique axis MRI of the heart. The spatial orientation of the heart is first defined using a coronal and a sagittal scan. Such a scan determines the inclination of the cardiac long axis relative to these planes. From these scans the angles are computed and a dual oblique image is obtained. (Courtesy of Philips, Eindhoven)

Fig. 4.6. ECG-triggered image perpendicular to the long axis of the heart of a normal volunteer. Note the quasi-circular shape of the left ventricle in this projection, familiar from thallium studies of the heart, and the papillary muscle (arrow). Acquisition of images in this orientation may be advantageous for volume determinations, because partial volume artifacts are minimized

tion, is imaged, care should be taken that the sections containing the heart fall into systole, where the best image qualitiy is obtained. Similar reasoning is used in coronal and sagittal imaging, where the early slices in an ECG-triggered study should be taken anteriorly and to the left, respectively, as it is these areas where the left ventricle lies.

4.1.4 Imaging Protocols

As when imaging other structures, it is mandatory to have proper imaging protocols in the cardiovascular system to minimize examination time. In examinations where the main emphasis is on morphological imaging, these protocols can be more clearly defined than when functional aspects are important, because there is considerably more experience with morphological imaging. When the suspected disease involves morphological alterations of vessels only, as is the case in congenital cardiovascular disease, images of good quality, often in several imaging planes, are required, but no variation of the pulse sequence may be used. If intravascular signal is observed and its significance cannot be interpreted readily, phase imaging is used or second echo images are acquired. Soft tissue masses require acquisition of T1- and T2-weighted images to distinguish between solid tumorous/inflammatory tissue, fluid, fibrous structures, and hematoma, as in the rest of the body. As stated in Sect. 4.1.1, T1- and T2-weighting have to be accomplished by triggering to every, every other, every third, or every fourth heart beat, since the RR interval equals the shortest possible repetition time in ECG-triggered studies.

Slice thickness and field of view have to be tailored to the disease entity under study. When using the body coil, the field of view should be kept at a reasonable size (> 35 cm) and the slice thickness should not be smaller than 5 mm for signal-to-noise considerations. Surface coils to examine the heart and the vessels of the thorax and abdomen have not been advocated, but in some cases they may be used in thin patients for the evaluation of retroperitoneal vessels. In defining the orientation of the slices, the prime rule is minimization of partial volume artifacts. Thus, the atrial septum requires transverse and, in its inferior aspects, coronal slices, the aortopulmonary window coronal or sagittal slices, and in dissecting aneurysms, care should be taken to cut perpendicularly to the dissection membrane. The thoracic aorta is often best imaged in a sagittal plane coinciding with the plane of the aortic arch, because sagittal (and coronal) images provide a larger field of view than transverse images, and it is advantageous to have at least one such view available. In the abdomen, the origin of the large vessels, particularly the renal arteries, is best seen on thin (5-mm) transverse images.

In coronal and sagittal images, the phase-encode direction has to be anteroposterior and left-right, respectively, to exclude backfolding of the lateral body parts into the image. In transverse images the phase-encode direction is usually chosen in the anteroposterior direction for the same reason. However, because of the body dimensions this is not mandatory, and occasionally, flow artifacts can be projected away from a structure of interest by interchanging read and phase-encode directions.

4.2 Normal Cardiac Morphology and Function in MRI

In this chapter we shall first discuss normal anatomy and function as imaged by MR. MRI is able to depict the cardiac walls in different phases of the heart cycle and shows the valves and the chamber lumina (Fig. 4.3). Furthermore, the motion of blood in the chambers can be observed. The pericardium is well visualized and the proximal parts of the coronary arteries can be identified. Figure 4.7 shows four anatomic slices taken using the standard trigger technique. In the top slice, the base of the heart with the aortic and pulmonary outflow tract is seen and the anatomic relation of the pulmonary outflow tract anterior and to the left of the aorta is established. The three lower sections are through various levels of the left and right ventricles and atria, showing details such as the papillary muscles and the moderator band in the apex of the right ventricle.

4.2.1 Cardiac Walls, Wall Thickness and Wall Motion

The cardiac walls are well depicted on ECG-triggered images of the heart, and on SE images they exhibit the gray tone typical for muscle tissue (Fig. 4.7). The left ventricular free wall is seen posteriorly and laterally. On lower anatomic sections (Fig. 4.7 c + d) the posterior papillary muscle is seen to protrude into the left ventricular chamber. The septum is seen separating the left from the right ventricular cavity and thins out towards the valve plane, where its membranous part can be identified. The left cardiac apex it is often seen to be sur-

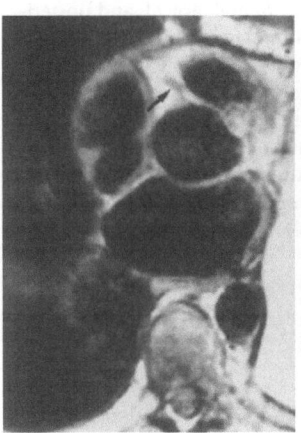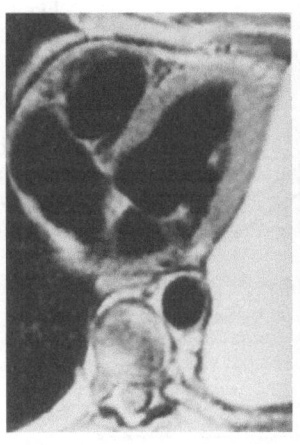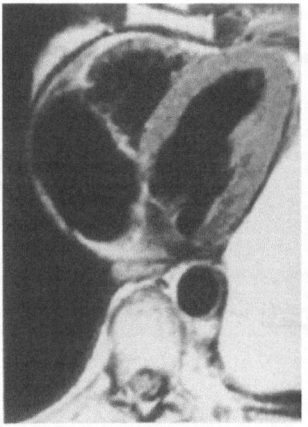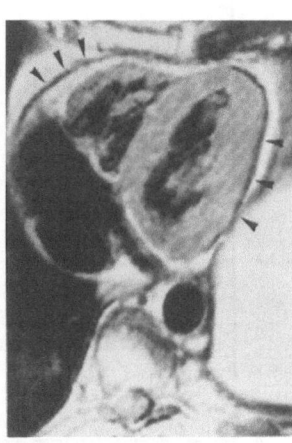

a–d

Fig. 4.7 a–d. Four transverse images through the aortic root and various levels of the heart in a patient with left-sided pleural effusion (SE ca. 800/30 ms, ECG-triggered). **a** Level of the aortic root (double line along left wall of left atrium is a chemical shift artifact); **b** level containing all four chambers, moderator band at the apex of the right ventricle, valves and **c** posterior papillary muscle, muscular and membranaceous interventricular and ventriculoatrial (Gerbode's) septum. **d** Level of junction of the coronary sinus and the right atrium. The right coronary is seen on two sections *(arrow)*. The pericardium appears as a dark line *(arrowheads)*. Posteriorly, the aorta and azygous vein are identified

rounded by liver tissue on transverse sections, as it abuts the diaphragm, and the abdominal contents rise somewhat cranially in the supine patient. Structures often identified in the region of the right cardiac apex correspond to the moderator band as it sweeps from the septum to innervate the right ventricular wall. The atria are well seen, the left atrium posterior and somewhat superior to the cardiac chambers. The right atrium lies to the right of the ventricles. The atrial septum, being a thin structure, is not always present in its entirety on transverse sections, as in its inferior part it curves towards the left. This fact has to be kept in mind when atrial septal defects are being imaged with MR. The cardiac walls are also well defined on gradient echo images (Fig. 4.4); however, here the wall border facing the chamber lumen is outlined by the strong signal of the blood pool rather than by the lack of signal seen in SE images.

Measurements of left ventricular muscle mass can be readily performed with MRI. There is no other imaging modality which can accurately determine this important parameter. Even though muscle mass is a morphological parameter, it reflects upon the myocardial work load. Studies in dogs, measuring LV muscle mass in end-diastole and in end-systole, show a very good correlation between the mass determined in vivo and the mass of the excised left ventricle [12].

The thickness of the left ventricular wall is readily assessed using MRI, due to its good anatomic definition. Quantitative measurements show that it is on the order of 7–9 mm in end-diastole. The wall is thinnest in the region of the septum. In normals the wall thickness has been measured as a function of the cardiac cycle [7, 13] and the results agree with data obtained by echocardiography [14]. The results of this study are shown in Fig. 4.8, where wall thickness is found to increase by roughly 50% from end-diastole to end-systole. Using such data, the percentage of regional wall thickening (Eq. 2.1) can be computed as a function parameter. Occasionally, problems can arise in the exact definition of the wall borders facing the left ventricular chamber, as stagnant blood between the trabeculae may show signal. When measuring the dimensions of the posterior wall, care has to be taken not to measure too close to the insertion of the inferior papillary muscle, which, when included, will produce erroneously high measurements. Using long and short axis views, regional wall motion can be assessed very much as in cine ventriculography [15]. However, because MRI is a tomographic method, much more accurate measurements can be obtained.

The instantaneous velocity of the ventricular walls can be determined either by looking at the position of the cardiac wall segments as a function of the cardiac cycle (distance/time method), or directly, by imaging spin-phase alterations. This latter method, applied to the heart, has been described by van Dijk [16], and its principle was discussed in Sect. 3.1.1. Even though qualitative information on wall motion can be obtained with this method at present (Fig. 3.3), specifically designed pulse sequences will have to be used for quantitative measurements. Assessment of regional wall motion is

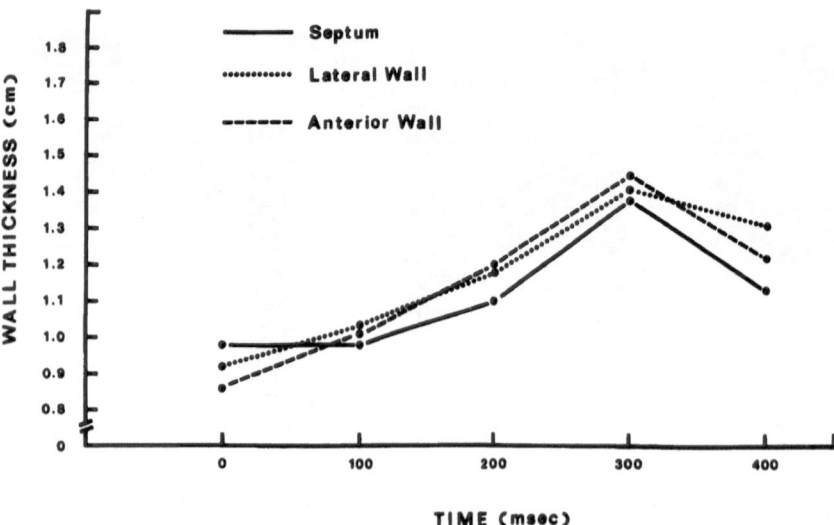

Fig. 4.8. Septal, apical, and posterior wall thickness plotted in five different phases of the cardiac cycle (average obtained from measurements in 9 normal individuals). The wall thickness is seen to increase by approximately 50% from end-diastole to end-systole (see also Figs. 4.3 and 4.4)

presently the domain of quantitative cine ventriculography, echocardiography and gated blood-pool scanning.

4.2.2 Chamber Volumetry

Since cardiac anatomy can be extremely well defined in all phases of the cardiac cycle with MRI, ventricular chamber volumetry permits one to measure quantities such as the end-diastolic (EDV), end-systolic (ESV), and stroke volumes (SV), as well as the ejection fraction (EF). These quantities have been measured with MRI either with the area-length method [17, 18] (Sect. 2.1.1) used in the evaluation of cine ventriculograms and echocardiograms, or with the volumetric information available in the tomographic method and used in nuclear medicine. Due to the rapidity of data acquisition, gradient echo image determination of the EF by volumetry of tomographic slices seems particularly promising [19, 20]. It has been shown that left and right ventricular stroke volumes can be determined with accuracy in MRI and that they are close to equal [21], as they should be. The ability to determine stroke volumes is a precondition for the determination of shunt volumes by any method evaluating congenital heart disease.

4.2.3 Valvular Motion

Valve motion can be observed on MR images even though the fact that valves are thin structures makes them not optimal for imaging with an ECG-triggered technique; real-time echocardiography is at an advantage, here.

The mitral and tricuspid valves are readily noted on systolic transverse images, when they are in a closed position (Figs. 4.3, 4.4, 4.7), but the valve leaflets are not identified in diastole (Figs. 4.3, 4.4). The presence of the valve leaflets can also be inferred from the flow phenomena occurring around them in gradient echo imaging. The cusps of the aortic valve in their closed position can be seen on diastolic images, but they are noted less frequently on transverse than on coronal images due to their oblique position. The tricuspid valve is rarely seen, as it is oblique to all usual imaging planes.

Patients with prosthetic heart valves can be imaged with MRI without danger [22] except perhaps in the case of infected valves with periannular leaks. The metallic parts produce the artifacts typical of metallic implants [23]. As a consequence, the areas in the vicinity of the metallic valvular parts cannot be assessed.

4.2.4 Coronary Arteries

The coronary arteries can be identified in their proximal parts in many patients. When imaging is done with the intention to identify the proximal coronaries using sections perpendicular to the aortic root, they can be identified in almost all patients [24] (Fig. 4.9). The right coronary is often seen in its course in the right atrioventricular groove on transverse sections (Fig. 4.7). However, care has to be taken not to confound cardiac veins with the coronary arteries, particularly along the course of the left coronary branches. With gradient echo imaging there is considerable hope that the coronaries can be visualized well, because there is a positive, rather than the negative vascular contrast which is found

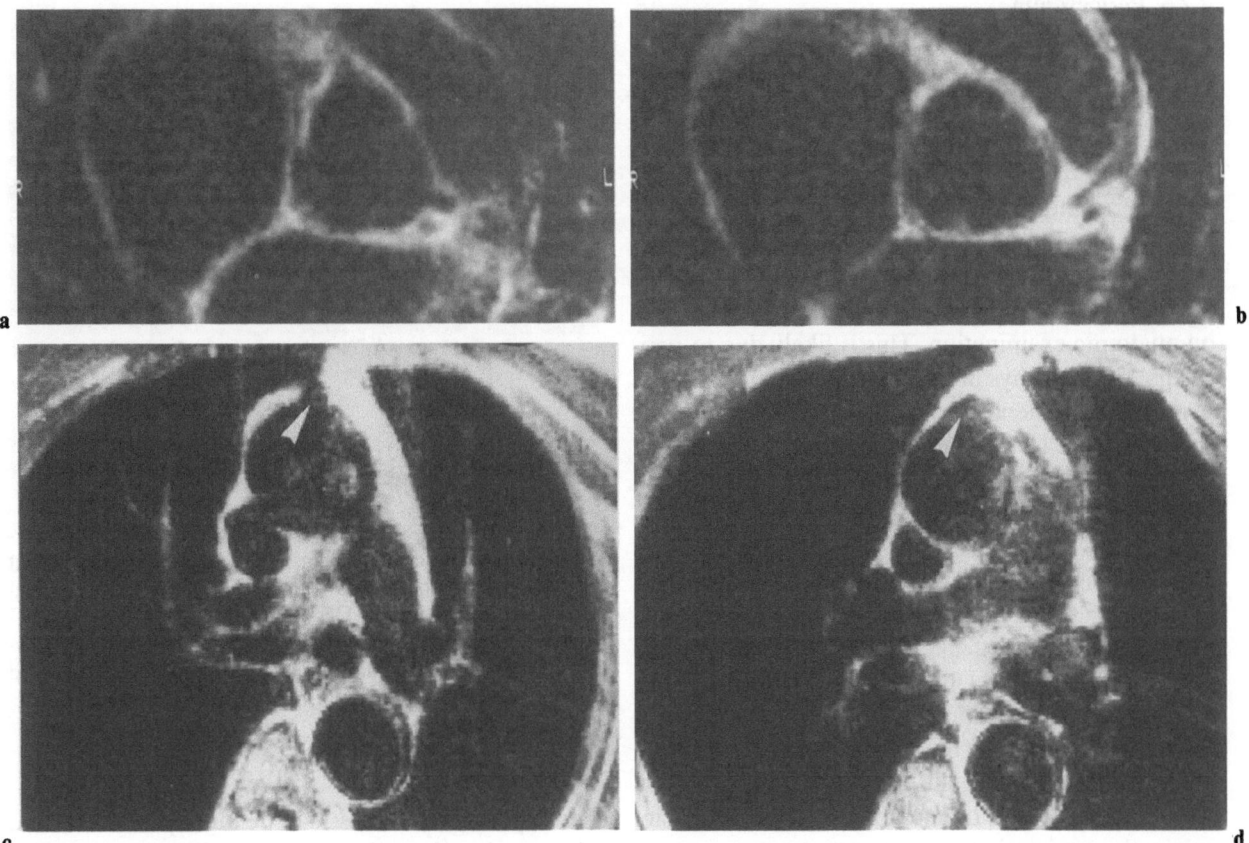

a   b

c   d

Fig. 4.9. a, b Sections through the root of the aorta, demonstrating the right coronary artery and the bifurcation of the left main coronary artery into circumflex and left anterior decending coronary arteries *(arrow)* (SE ca. 800/30 ms, ECG-triggered. **c, d** Sections showing a bypass graft leaving the proximal aorta and descending towards the left *(arrowheads)*

in SE imaging. Hence, partial volume effects are expected to interfere less with vessel identification (Fig. 4.10). Venous coronary bypass grafts are detected with a frequency in the range of 85% on SE images, whereas internal mammary bypasses are seen with a frequency of less than 50% [25]. The appearance of a bypass as a structure without signal is at the same time an indication of its patency. Flow velocity measurements in coronary arteries and bypass grafts have been reported using the FEER sequence [26], but a larger patient series awaits completion.

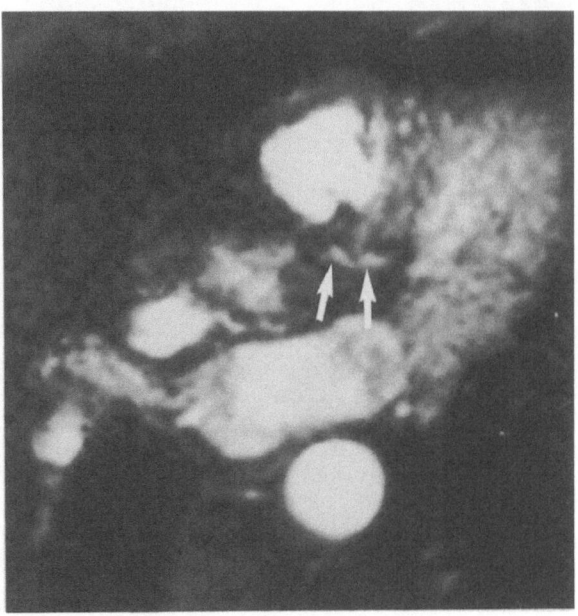

Fig. 4.10. Gradient echo imaging through the base of the heart of a normal volunteer, showing the left main coronary artery and the bifurcation with positive rather than negative contrast

4.2.5 Pericardium

MRI is an excellent method for identifying the pericardium, which is consistently visualized in the retrosternal area in front of the right ventricle (Fig. 4.7). It is less consistently visualized in other areas surrounding the heart, but always appears as a structure without signal, owing to its fibrous nature. Quantitative analysis has shown [27] that the normal pericardium appears wider in MRI than upon anatomic examination. This is likely due to pericardial fluid, always present in small quantities. The pericardium extends cranially behind the aortic root, where it forms a reflection, and a small area containing a pocket of pericardial fluid is often seen, even at transaxial levels above the right pulmonary artery. Another such pericardial recess lies anterior (Fig. 4.11), between the aortic and pulmonary roots, there often visualized as a signal-free triangular structure [28]. Interestingly, neither the pericardial fluid layer nor the fluid pockets in the recesses are seen to increase in signal intensity on T2-weighted images. This suggests that there is signal loss in the pericardial fluid due to constant flow occurring as a result of cardiac motion. In fact, signal in the pericardial space seems to appear only when an organizing process is present. The retro-

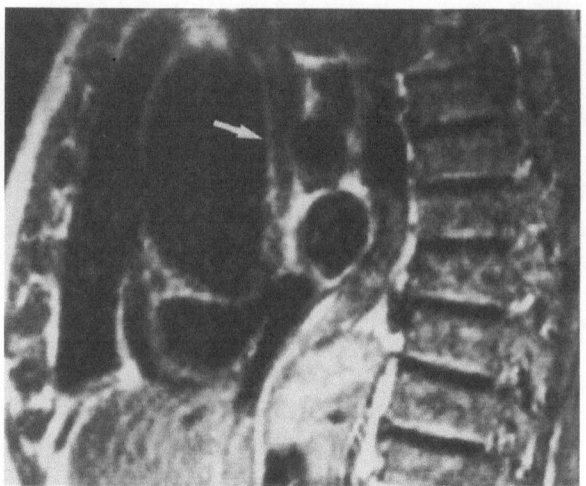

Fig. 4.12. Large retroaortic pericardial recess mimicking aortic dissection (SE ca. 650/30 ms, ECG-triggered). This patient was operated on because of an aortic dissection type B, diagnosed by angiography, CT, and MRI. In addition, MRI showed a "membrane" in the ascending aorta *(arrow)*. However, the presence of a dissection in the ascending aorta could be excluded upon operation. Repeat MRI showed the structure to be unaltered

aortic pericardial recess can be quite prominent and elongated and is directly apposed to the posterior wall of the ascending aorta. It may thus be mis-

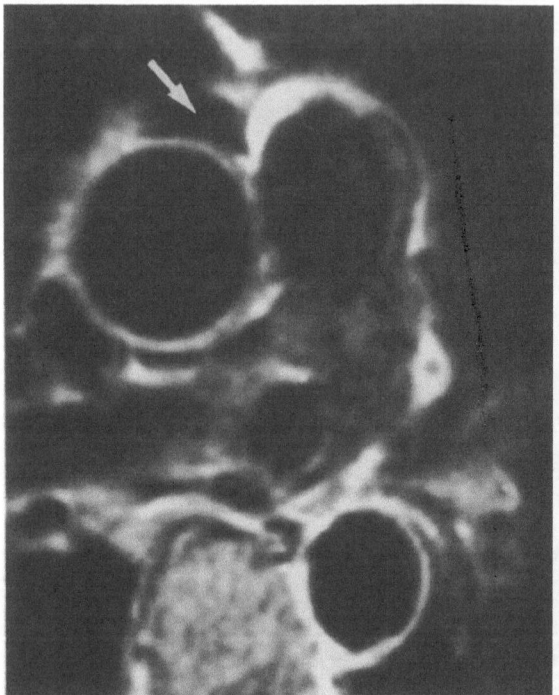

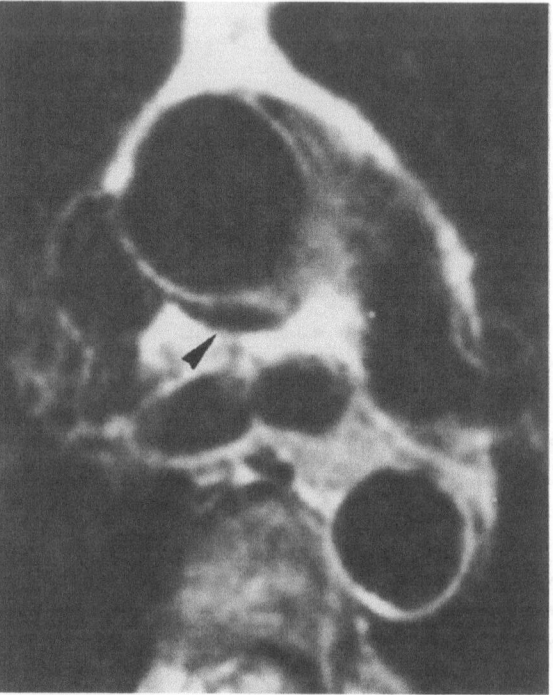

a   b

Fig. 4.11 a, b. The reflections of the pericardium around the roots of the aorta and pulmonary artery are known as pericardial recesses. Note triangular area anterior to and between aorta and pulmonary artery *(arrow)* and behind the aorta *(arrowhead)*. This posterior pericardial recess sometimes can extend far cranially and even minic aortic dissection (Fig. 4.12). The signal void in the recesses is probably due to the motion of pericardial fluid (SE ca. 750/30, ECG-triggered)

taken for the false lumen of an aortic dissection (Fig. 4.12).

4.2.6 Normal Appearance of the Intracavitary Blood Pool

Being the largest blood filled structures and containing blood almost in constant motion, the cardiac chambers exhibit a variety of flow phenomena. The signal intensity variations of intracardiac blood contain physiologic and pathophysiologic information, and are of great interest in SE [8] and gradient echo images [29]. Based on the knowledge of flow phenomena presented in Chap. 3, we expect intracardiac signals to arise when the blood pool is stagnant. In contrast, areas of signal void occur in regions of steep velocity profiles, high flow velocities, and turbulence, which because of the size of the ventricles are present at relatively low flow velocities (Eq. 2.8). The difference in the appearance of the blood pool between SE images and gradient echo images is a gradual one: gradient echo images exhibit much more signal under the same flow conditions.

The occurrence of signal in the left ventricle and atrium obtained in one study of nine normals, using permutation ECG-triggered SE imaging, is given in Table 4.2 [8]. Note that in most subjects ventricular signal occurs in end-diastole and extends into early systole, particularly in the anteroapical region. On the other hand, little signal is observed in the area of the mitral valve. The higher the heart rate, the less intracardiac signal is present, because ventricular ejection and filling alternate incessantly, whereas in subjects with slower heart rates (≤ 75 BPM), the late diastolic phase becomes prolonged and a longer period occurs, where the intraventricular blood pool is stagnant (Sect. 3.1.1). Of the nine subjets in the study cited above, the two with a heart rate above 75 BPM showed no intraventricular signal in any phase of the cardiac cycle.

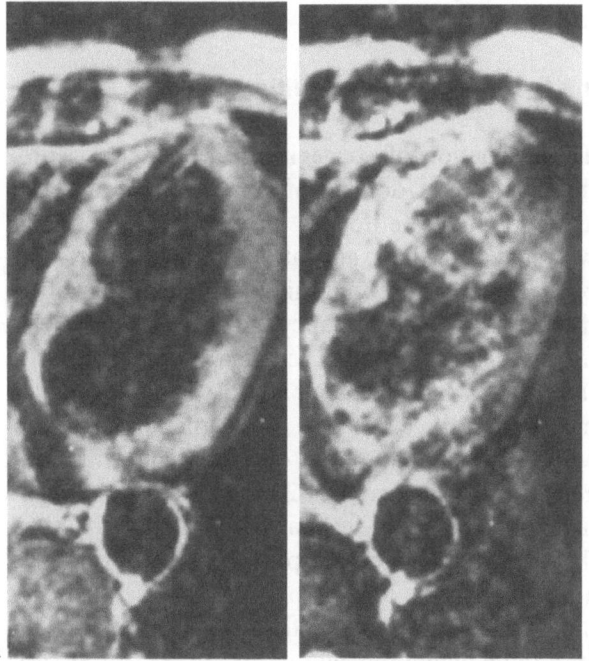

a   b

Fig. 4.13 a, b. First and second echo ECG-triggered images of the heart. (SE ca. 850/30, 60 ms, ECG-triggered). There is total signal void in the left ventricle on first echo. On second echo, much of the left ventricular cavity is filled with signal. This phenomenon is normal and is due to the even-echo rephasing phenomenon

As expected, intraventricular signal increases on second echo images (Fig. 4.13) due to the even-echo rephasing phenomenon (Sect. 3.1.2). Signal intensity variations in the left atrium are opposite to the ventricular signal intensity variations. The signal is highest towards end-systole, when the atrium is filled and inflow into the atrium subsides, and lowest during diastole, when inflow into the left ventricle takes place. The presence of intravascular signal in the right ventricle and right atrium parallels that of the left chambers. However, for reasons probably related to ventricular geometry or pressures, the intracavitary signal on SE images is less pronounced.

On gradient echo images, areas of rapid jetlike flow show signal loss due to turbulence (Fig. 4.4). This occurs in the aortic region during early to midsystole. Similarly, the most marked signal loss in the right cardiac chambers occurs during the times of rapid flow across the tricuspid and pulmonary valves and again in the valvular areas. Superposition of gradient echo (FEER) images sensitized to flow onto anatomic ECG-triggered SE images has been accomplished [30], appearing very much like color Doppler maps simultaneously depicting cardiovascular morphology and function.

Table 4.2. Intracavitary signal on second-echo images in nine healthy individuals

Cardiac region	Frequency (%)				
	End-diastole	Early systole	Late systole	End-systole	Early diastole
Left ventr.					
Septum	22	0	0	0	0
Ant. apical	66	66	22	11	32
Posterior	44	33	11	0	0
Valve area	11	0	0	0	11
Left atrium	0	11	77	77	33

4.3 Pathologic Cardiac Morphology and Function in MRI

4.3.1 Congenital Abnormalities

The evaluation of congenital heart disease is predominantly the domain of echocardiography and angiography. The former method is particularly well suited for the examination of infants. For obvious reasons, severe congenital heart disease is often discovered in early infancy, and the role of MRI in this field has been a secondary one. The large field of view and the good soft tissue contrast help, however, in the evaluation of complex disease, and MRI is a valuable tool in older patients with congenital heart disease [31, 32, 33]. Much of the diagnostic process in congenital heart disease relies on the identification of morphological abnormalities alone (Fig. 4.14). MRI is particularly useful in the diagnosis of atrial septal defects (Fig. 4.15), which tend to be diagnosed later in life [34, 35, 36]. A case report on the diagnosis of absent left pericardium with MRI has been published [37].

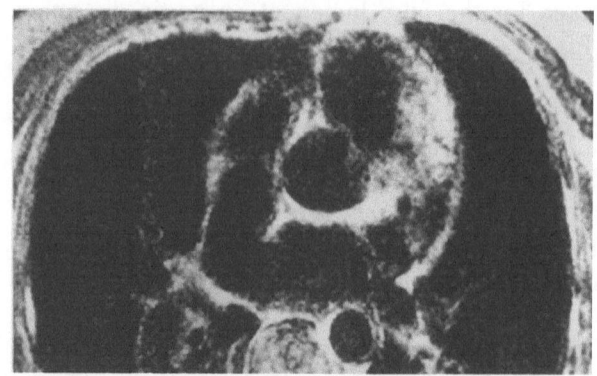

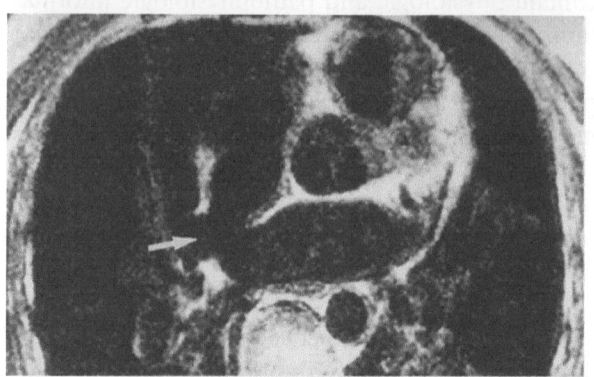

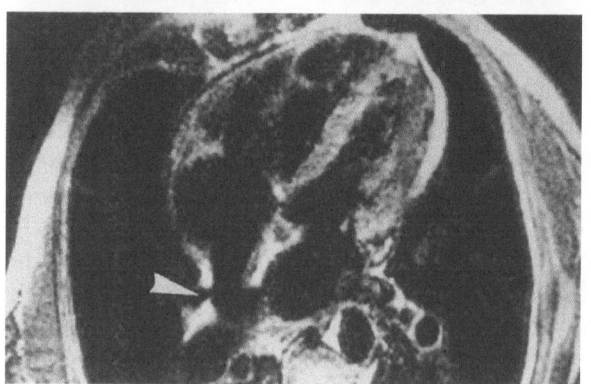

Fig. 4.15 a–c. Atrial septal defect of the sinus venosus type with anomalous connection of the right superior pulmonary vein to the right atrium. On the transaxial scans (**a** and **b**, SE ca. 850/30 ms, ECG-triggered) the atrial septal defect is noted together with a large right superior pulmonary vein *(arrow)*. **c** On a section parallel to the long axis of the heart a four-chamber view also shows the defect *(arrow-head)* and the right superior pulmonary artery

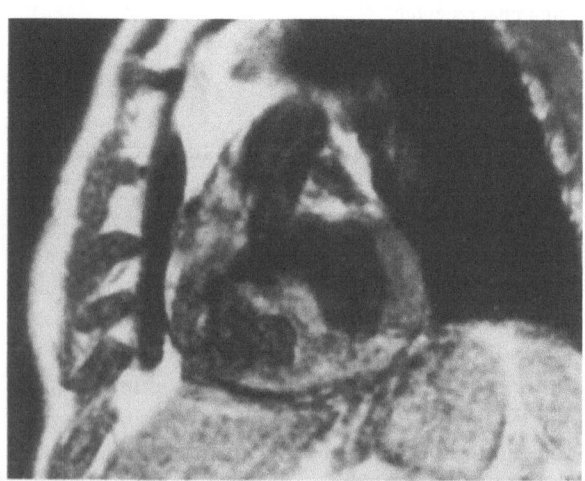

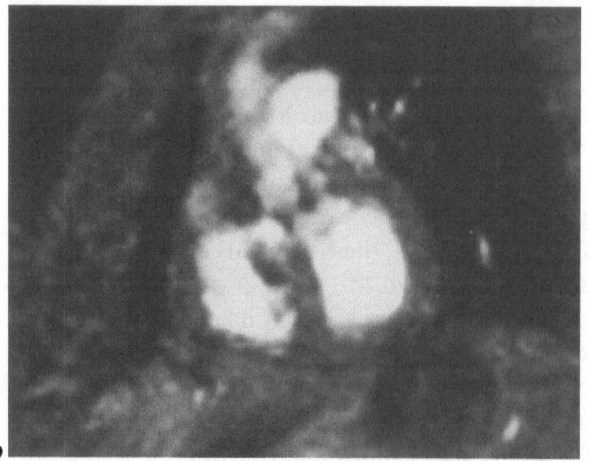

◄ **Fig. 4.14 a, b.** Aneurysm in the membranous part of the septum with small ventricular septal defect (shunt <10% echocardiographically). **a** The SE image (SE ca. 900/30 ms, sagittal, angulated) clearly shows the aneurysm, but no certainty can be obtained regarding a VSD. **b** The corresponding gradient echo image (GFE 35/21 ms, α = 40°, ECG-triggered) shows an area of signal loss in the right ventricle close to the defect during systole. This corresponds to the turbulent jet resulting from the left-right shunt

Function information obtainable with MRI includes the determination of shunt volumina [38, 39], the pulmonary vascular resistance, which is an important parameter of postoperative outcome (Sect. 5.2.1), and possibly pressure drops across stenoses. To our knowledge, this last application has not yet been implemented with MRI, but it could probably be implemented in analogy to echocardiographic methods [40].

Fig. 4.16a-e. Chronic infarction in a patient with a large anteroseptal infarction. **a** The extreme thinning of the septal and anterior wall is noted on the transverse SE image (SE ca. 750/30 ms, ECG-triggered) together with a enlarged left ventricular cavity. Muscle mass is maintained in the unaffected posterior region. **b** On a sagittal angulated gradient echo scan (GFE 35/21 ms, $\alpha = 40°$, ECG-triggered), a small turbulent "puff" is noted going into the ascending aorta, but aortic signal loss is not as marked as in normals, suggesting poor cardiac output. On transverse gradient echo images (**c-e**) (GFE 35/21 ms, $\alpha = 40°$, ECG-triggered), angulated to be parallel to the long axis of the heart, little variation in the signal intensity of the blood is noted from early systole (**c**) into early diastole (**e**). This is an expression of slow ventricular filling. A small vortex, shedding from the anterior mitral valve leaflet, is observed after mitral valve opening *(arrow)*

4.3.2 Coronary Artery Disease

Coronary artery disease has been evaluated extensively with MRI, even with the experimental use of contrast agents to enhance ischemic or infarcted myocardial regions.

The morphological changes due to myocardial infarction are often obvious. Chronic infarction shows areas of wall thinning and aneurysmatic dilatations [41] (Fig. 4.16), and the region of scarring shows, as expected from the signal intensity behavior of fibrous tissue, no increase in signal intensity on T2-weighted images. However, smaller chronic infarctions cannot be seen [42]. Acute myocardial infarction results in myocardial edema formation. This edema can be identified as a region in the ventricular wall which increases in signal intensity with progressively heavier T2 weighting [43]. The increase in signal intensity is an early sign occurring between 3 and 5 h after the acute event, as shown in dog studies [44]. Correlation between anatomic infarct size and size as defined by the region of altered signal intensity is excellent [45]. Upon reperfusion of an infarct, signal intensity in the jeopardized

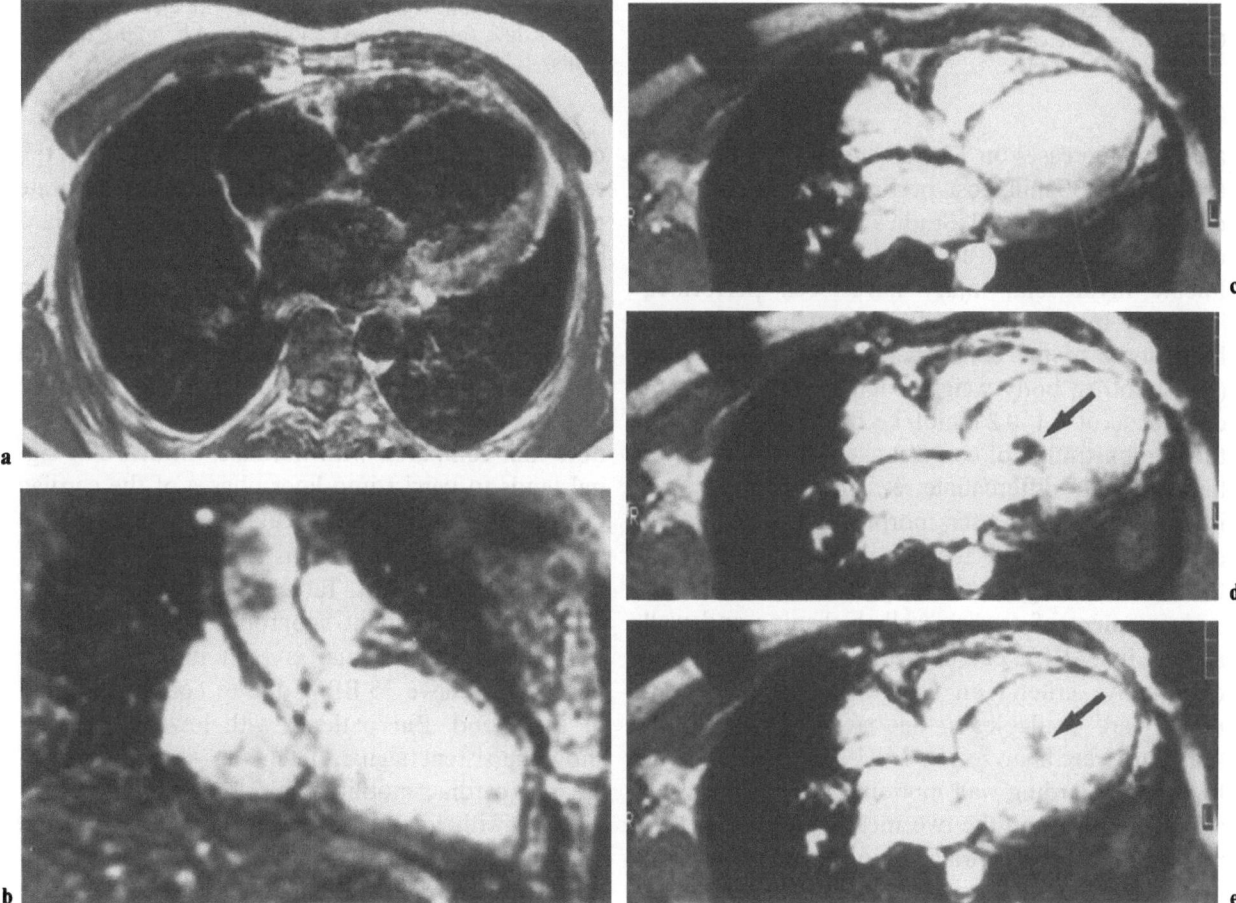

Table 4.3. Presence of intraluminal signal on second-echo images (%)

Cardiac region (of patients)	Phase			Heart rate (mean ± SD bpm)
	End-diastole	Early systole	Late systole	
Left atrium				
Volunteers (n = 12)	0	0	60	66.3 ± 11.8
CCM* (n = 10)	0	67	67	77.9 ± 11.1
Infarction (n = 19)	50	27	25	70.3 ± 12.1
Left ventricle				
Volunteers				
Septal	17	0	0	
Ant.-apical (n = 12)	67	42	0	66.3 ± 11.8
Posterior	17	8	0	
Valve area	0	0	0	
CCM				
Septal	20	20	30	77.9 ± 11.1
Ant.-apical (n = 10)	20	60	70	
Posterior	0	20	20	
Valve area	0	10	0	
Infarction				
Septal	16	16	16	
Ant.-apical (n = 19)	27	27	29	70.2 ± 12.3
Posterior	10	16	16	
Valve area	5	10	5	

CCM, Congestive cardiomyopathy

Table 4.4. Intraventricular second-echo signal in patient subgroups (%)

Subgroup characterization by variations and region	End-diast.	Early syst.	Late syst.	Heart rate (mean ± SD bpm)	No. of pat. or regions
Infarction and CCM					
HR > 75					
Septal	19	6	0		
Ant.-apical	0	13	19	84.4 ± 7.3	13
Posterior	0	0	25		
Heart rate < 75					
Septal	25	25	25		
Ant.-apical	31	37	56	63.9 ± 5.9	16
Infarction					
EF < 30%, aneurysms: 8/9					
Septal	22	22	22		
Ant.-apical	33	33	44	73.6 ± 13.0	9
Posterior	22	22	22		
EF > 30%, aneurysms: 5/10					
Septal	10	10	10		
Ant.-apical	20	30	10	66.5 ± 9.8	10
Posterior	0	10	10		
Dysfunctional region					
Septal	20	20	20		5
Ant.-apical	15	31	46		13
Posterior	0	0	20		5

Note: The group with myocardial infarction and CCM is subdivided into those patients with heart rates (HR) greater than or less than 75 beats per minute (bpm). The group with recent infarctions is divided into those with ejection fractions (EF) < 30% (nine patients) and those with > 30% (ten patients)

area also increases on T2-weighted images, and this as early as 30 min post perfusion of an area occluded for 60 min [46]. Studies using paramagnetic contrast agents such as gadolinium-DTPA to delineate myocardial injury have been performed [47, 48]. In these animal experiments relatively high doses of the contrast agent have been used (0.5 mmol/kg body weight compared with a standard dose of 0.1-0.2 mmol/kg body weight). With the administration of contrast agent it was found to be possible to differentiate reversible from irreversible ischemia [49]. So far, morphological changes in coronaries go undetected, the spatial resolution of the method being insufficient [24].

Assessment of cardiac wall thickening and wall motion by MRI is possible, and early results using quantitative criteria on wall thickening and wall motion are available. In one study [15], 105 wall segments were analyzed by MRI and cine ventriculography regarding wall motion abnormalities. The agreement between the two methods was 95%. Direct measurement of wall motion using spin-phase methods, although possible and published for a few

cases [50], awaits clinical trials. Ejection fraction determinations by gradient echo MRI are accurate using cine ventriculography as the gold standard [19].

The behavior of intravascular signal has been evaluated in a study on ECG-triggered SE images in 19 patients with myocardial infarction and ten patients with congestive cardiomyopathy [8]. The findings are given in Tables 4.3 and 4.4. In Table 4.3 note that compared with normals, intracardiac signal tends to persist into later phases of the cardiac cycle in patients with ventricular dysfunction. There are probably several reasons for this, and in order to separate the factors, Table 4.4 represents an analysis of several patient subgroups. As in normals, little intracavitary signal is seen in patients with heart rates above 75 BPM due to constant motion of the blood. But patients with lower heart rate show persistent signal, likely as a result of decreased cardiac motility. This is definitely true in patients with low ejection fractions. However, the conclusion that there is more signal adjacent to a dysfunctional wall is fallacious, because blood in that area may still move tangentially to the wall and with a large spatial variation in velocity, thus producing signal loss. Differentiation between cardiac thrombi and slow flow is possible in most cases [51, 52]. No study evaluating intravascular signal using gradient echo images in a similar patient group is available at present, but the fact, that in these images, signal and signal intensity variations over the cardiac cycle are almost always present suggests that such an analysis will be of great interest.

4.3.3 Other Cardiomyopathies

Limited experience exists in the evaluation of cardiomyopathies other than that due to coronary artery disease. Wall motion abnormalities are present [15]

and intracavitary blood flow abnormalities exist as in coronary cardiomyopathy (Table 4.3) [8]. Even in the case of hemochromatosis, where the iron deposition in the liver leads to a total signal loss in this organ [53] (Fig. 4.17), similar changes in the heart have not been noted.

Animal studies done in order to evaluate the potential of MRI to detect early changes in transplanted hearts have been done with success [54]. The use of Gd-DTPA to more clearly indicate a rejection reaction in human subjects has so far yielded inconclusive results [55].

4.3.4 Valvular Disease

Conventional SE images are not very useful in evaluating valvular disease for the reasons cited in Sect. 4.2.3, and there is no question that echocardiography is the method of choice for the morphological and functional evaluation of the heart valves.

There are indications for MRI examinations in valvular diseases. Evaluation of the morphology of the base of the heart to demonstrate perivalvular infectious changes or sequelae thereof can be accomplished well with MRI, as is shown in a case of perivalvular pseudoaneurysm formation [56] (Fig. 4.18). Volumetric measurements to assess the left and right ventricular ejection fractions as well as the left-to-right ventricular stroke volume ratio have been performed on patients with aortic and mitral regurgitation and correlate well with angiography and radionuclide ventriculography [57].

In gradient echo imaging the situation may be different, because it has been well documented that turbulence-induced signal loss occurs due to the jet-type flow across stenotic or insufficient valves [29]. A series of such varying flow patterns across a stenosis is shown in Fig. 4.19, even though it is clear that such variations are much better appreciated in movie format. This type of imaging bears the potential of providing an assessment of the severity of valvular disease and will possibly yield estimations of valvular orifice surface area like those obtained with echocardiography.

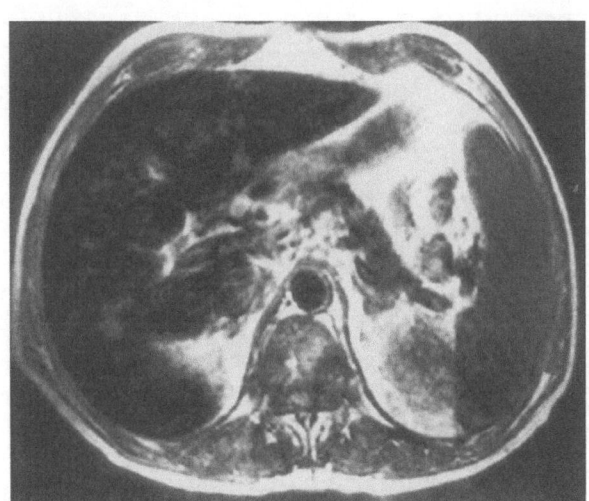

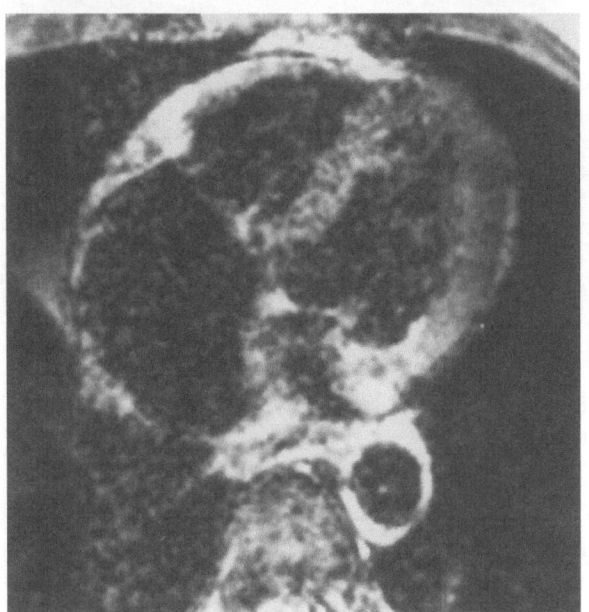

Fig. 4.17. a Transverse SE image through the liver (SE, ca. 850/30 ms) in a patient with primary hemochromatosis. Note the total lack of signal in the liver and the dark-appearing pancreas. **b** A transverse image through the heart shows relatively low cardiac signal intensity, suggesting that there is also some iron deposition in the heart muscle

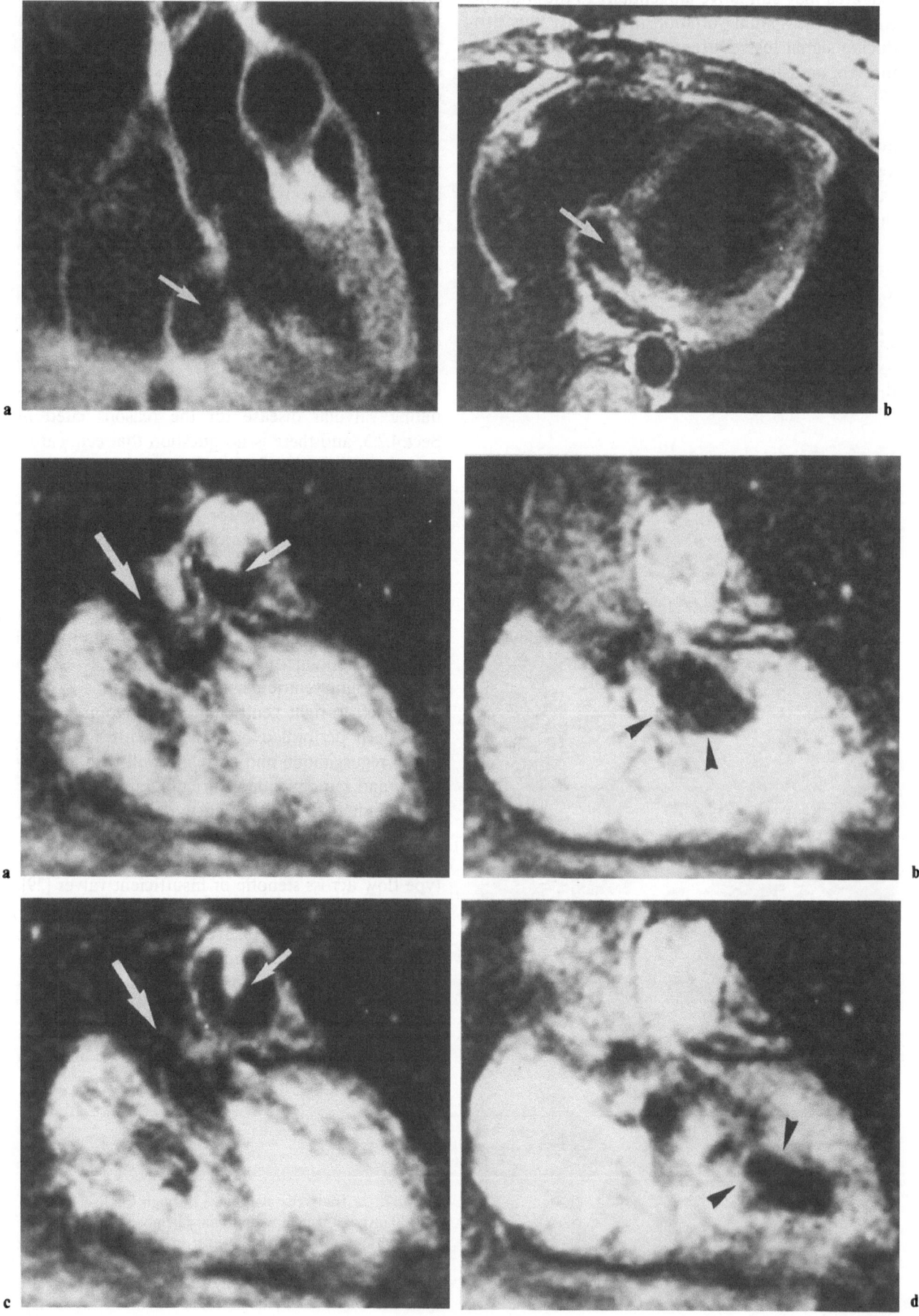

◄ **Fig. 4.18 a, b.** Sterile, perivalvular pseudoaneurysm in a patient who, 2 years prior to imaging, suffered from a infected mitral valve. **a** Note the cavity between the left ventricle and right atrium on a coronal scan (SE ca. 950/30 ms), which is void of signal, thus containing rapidly flowing blood *(arrow)*. **b** On a transverse SE image, the pseudoaneurysm is seen to be in an anteroinferior position relative to the left atrium *(arrow)* and anterior to the coronary sinus *(arrowhead)*

◄ **Fig. 4.19 a-d.** Flow patterns in four phases of the cardiac cycle in a patient with aortic insufficiency, imaged with a gradient echo sequence (GFE 26/15 ms, α = 40°, ECG-triggered). **a** Note the signal loss in the aortic root and the inferior portion of the pulmonary arterial trunk during early systole *(arrows)*. **b** Later in systole, the aortic and pulmonary signal loss becomes more extensive. **c, d** In diastole, an area of signal loss moves rapidly from the aortic valve to the apex of the left ventricle *(arrowheads)*. This is due to the turbulent regurgitative jet of aortic insufficiency

4.3.5 Other Acquired Cardiac Disease

The other larger group of cardiac diseases studied so far by MRI are cardiac and paracardiac masses [58]. Ample evidence exists that for these relatively rare tumors MRI is well suited and, because of its superior anatomic delineation of such masses, is often more definitive in the diagnosis than echocardiography [59]. MRI is well suited to demonstrating the presence or absence of such a mass (Fig. 4.20) suspected on a conventional chest roentgenogram, and in some instances one is able to make a specific diagnosis, as in the case where the mass is a vascular enlargement or frank aneurysm (Fig. 5.17). Pericardiac cysts can also be diagnosed with confidence, and the author is aware of several cases where either a left atrial tumor detected by echocardiography was excluded by MRI or the diagnosis of a lipomatous degeneration of the atrial septum was made (Fig. 4.21). Several studies have appeared on this subject [60], also comparing CT with MRI [61]. However, the diagnosis of cardiac and paracardiac masses is a morphological one; function information is of importance only when such a mass leads to obstruction or compression of the cardiac chambers.

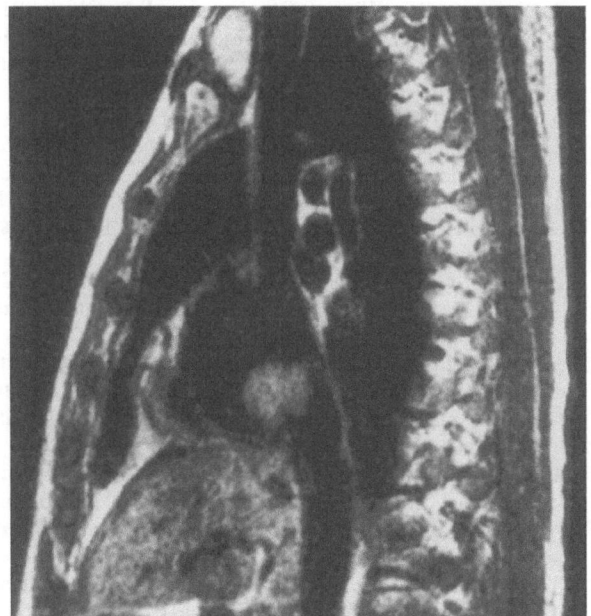

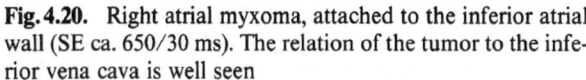

Fig. 4.20. Right atrial myxoma, attached to the inferior atrial wall (SE ca. 650/30 ms). The relation of the tumor to the inferior vena cava is well seen

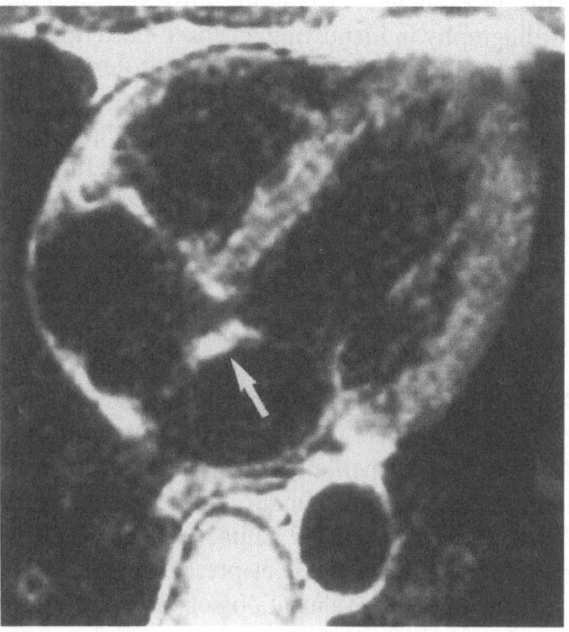

Fig. 4.21. Lipomatous degeneration of the atrial septum *(arrow)*. This SE image (SE ca. 830/30 ms, ECG-triggered) shows merely a somewhat prominent portion of the atrial septum, protruding into the left atrium. This patient was referred for MRI to rule out a left atrial mass which was suspected during echocardiography

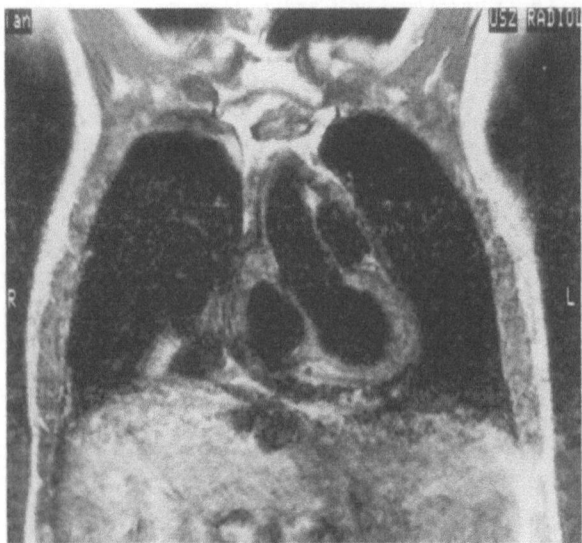

Fig. 4.22. Thickening of the pericardium noted on a coronal image (SE ca. 750/30 ms, ECG triggered) in a patient who had had mediastinal radiation therapy 3 years previously for the treatment of Hodgkin's disease. This patient presented with the symptoms of constrictive pericarditis, which was thought to be due to radiation fibrosis

4.3.6 Pericardial Disease

Like echocardiography, MRI is able to detect pericardial disease. Effusions and pericardial thickening can be recognized well and the quality of the effusion evaluated. It is more sensitive than echocardiography in identifying localized posterior pericardial effusions [62]. A hemopericardium can be distinguished from clear pericardial fluid and fibrinous material, as in the case of fibrinous pericarditis [62]. The method appears to be very useful in the evaluation of constrictive pericardial [63] (Fig. 4.22) and epicardial disease.

4.3.7 Summary

Much experience in MR imaging of the heart has been accumulated over the past few years, and MRI is clearly superior to CT in this area. However, most of the information presently obtainable by MRI can be more easily gained with echocardiography. Therefore, there is at present no great clinical need for MR examinations of the heart, except possibly in the evaluation of cardiac and paracardiac masses, adult congenital heart disease, and pericardial disease. With the advent of the new gradient echo techniques, their optimization, and software packages easier to handle, the role of MRI in the evaluation of cardiac morphology and function

will no doubt increase considerably. This is due to the fact that the combined morphological and function imaging possible with MRI, as with Doppler sonography, is a perfect match for the needs encountered in the evaluation of the heart.

References

1. Rzedzian RR, Pykett IL (1987) Instant images of the human heart using a new, whole-body MR imaging system. AJR 149: 245–250
2. Mansfield PG, Morris P (1982) NMR imaging in biomedicine. Academic Press, New York
3. Green MV, Ostrow HG, Douglas MA et al (1974) High temporal resolution ECG-gated scintigraphic angiocardiography. J Nuc Med 16: 95–98
4. Berger HJ, Zaret BL (1981) Nuclear cardiology (second of two parts). New Engl J Med 305: 855–865
5. von Schulthess GK, Pfeiffer A, Horst W (1983) Vergleich zweier Computertomogramme zur Bestimmung globaler und regionaler Auswurffraktionen aus der EKG-gesteuerten Herzbinnenraumszintigraphie. Nuc Comp 14: 118–119
6. Crooks LR, Barker B, Chang H et al (1984) Magnetic resonance imaging strategies for heart studies. Radiology 153: 459–465
7. Fisher MR, von Schulthess GK, Higgins CB (1985) Multiphasic cardiac magnetic resonance imaging: normal regional left ventricular wall thickening. AJR 145: 27–30
8. von Schulthess GK, Fisher MR, Crooks LE, Higgins CB (1985) Gated MR imaging of the heart: intracardiac signals in patients and healthy subjects. Radiology 156: 125–132
9. Dinsmore RE, Wismer GL, Lewvine RA, Okada RD, Brady TJ (1984) Magnetic resonance imaging of the heart: positioning and gradient angle selection for optimal imaging planes. AJR 143: 1135–1142
10. Feiglin DH, George CG, MacIntyre WJ et al (1985) Gated cardiac magnetic resonance structural imaging: optimization by electronic axial rotation. Radiology 154: 129–132
11. von Schulthess GK (1987) Blood flow. In: Higgins CB, Hricak H (eds) MR imaging of the body. Raven Press, New York
12. Caputo GR, Tscholakoff D, Sechtem U, Higgins CB (1986) Measurement of canine left ventricular mass using MR imaging. AJR 148: 33–38
13. von Schulthess GK, Fisher MR, Higgins CB (1985) Multiphasisch getriggerte NMR-Bildgebung zur Beurteilung der regionalen linksventrikulären Myokardfunktion beim Menschen. Schweiz. Med. Wochenschrift (Abstract)
14. Lieberman AN, Weiss JL, Jujdutt BL et al (1981) Two-dimensional echocardiography and infarct size: relationship of regional wall motion and thickening to the extent of myocardial infarction in the dog. Circulation 63: 739–746
15. Underwood SR, Rees RSO, Savage PE (1986) Assessment of regional left ventricular function by magnetic resonance. Br Heart J 56: 334–340
16. van Dijk P (1984) Direct cardiac NMR imaging of heart wall and blood flow velocity. J Comput Ass Tomogr 8: 419–436
17. Stratemeier DJ, Thompson R, Brady TJ et al (1986) Ejection fraction determination by MR imaging: comparison with left ventricular angiography. Radiology 158: 775–777

18. Buckwalter KA, Aisen AM, Dilworth LR, Nancini GBJ, Buda AJ (1986) Gated cardiac MRI: ejection fraction determination using the right anterior oblique view. AJR 147: 33-37
19. Utz JA, Herfkens RJ, Heinsimer JA (1987) Cine MR determination of left ventricular ejection fraction. AJR 148: 839-843
20. Sechtem U, Pflugfelder PW, Gould RG, Cassidy MM, Higgins CB (1987) Measurement of right and left ventricular volumes in healthy individuals with cine MR imaging. Radiology 163: 697-702
21. Longmore DB, Underwood SR, Hounsfield GN et al (1985) Dimensional accuracy of magnetic resonance in studies of the heart. Lancet; June 15: 1360-1362
22. Soulen RL, Budinger TF, Higgins CB (1985) Magnetic resonance imaging of prosthetic heart valves. Radiology 154: 705-707
23. Augustiny N, von Schulthess GK, Meier D, Bösiger P (1986) Magnetic resonance imaging (MRI) of large metallic implants at 1.5 Tesla. J Comput Ass Tomogr
24. Paulin S, von Schulthess GK, Fossel E, Krayenbuehl HP (1987) MR imaging of the aortic root and the proximal coronary arteries AJR 145: 665-670
25. Gomes AS, Lois JF, Drinkwater DC jr, Corday SR (1987) Coronary artery bypass grafts: visualization with MR imaging. Radiology 162: 175-179
26. Longmore DB (1987) MR: an opportunity for cardiology. Plenary lecture SMRM, New York
27. Sechtem U, Tscholakoff D, Higgins CB (1986) MRI of the normal pericardium. AJR 147: 239-244
28. McMurdo KK, Webb WR, von Schulthess GK, Gamsu G (1985) Magnetic resonance imaging of the superior pericardial recesses. AJR 145: 985-988
29. Sechtem U, Pflugfelder PW, White RD et al (1987) Cine MR imaging: potential for the evaluation of cardiovascular function. AJR 148: 239-246
30. Klipstein RH, Firmin DH, Underwood SR et al (1987) Colour display of quantitative blood flow and cardiac anatomy in a single magnetic resonance cine loop. Brit J Radiol 60: 105-111
31. Higgins CB, Byrd BF III, Farmer DW, Osaki L, Silverman NH, Cheitlin MD (1984) Magnetic resonance imaging in patients with congenital heart disease. Circulation 70: 851-860
32. Didier D, Higgins CB, Fisher MR, Osaki L, Silverman NH, Cheitlin MD (1986) Congenital heart disease: gated MR imaging in 72 patients. Radiology 158: 227-235
33. Guit GL, Bluemm R, Rohmer J et al. (1986) Levotransposition of the aorta: identification of segmental cardiac anatomy using MR imaging. Radiology 161: 673-679
34. Jacobstein MD, Fletcher BD, Goldstein S, Riemenschneider TA (1985) Evaluation of atrioventricular septal defect by magnetic resonance imaging. Am J Cardiol 55: 1158-1163
35. Dinsmore RE, Wismer GL, Guyer D et al (1985) Magnetic resonance imaging of the interatrial septum and atrial septal defects. AJR 145: 697-703
36. Diethelm L, Dery R, Lipton MJ, Higgins CB (1987) Atrial-level shunts: sensitivity and specificity of MR in diagnosis. Radiology 162: 181-186
37. Gutierrez R, Shackelford GD, McKnight RC, Levitt RG, Hartmann A (1985) Diagnosis of congenital absence of left pericardium by MR imaging. J Comput Ass Tomogr 9: 551-553
38. Underwood SR (1987) Functional studies of the cardiovascular system using magnetic resonance imaging. In: Functional studies using NMR. McCready VR, Leach M, Ell PJ. Springer, Berlin Heidelberg London New York Tokyo
39. Sechtem U, Pflugfelder P, Cassidy MC, Holt W, Wolfe C, Higgins CB (1987) Ventricular septal defect: visualization of shunt flow and determination of shunt size by cine MR imaging. AJR 149: 689-692
40. Hatle L, Angelsen B (1985) Doppler ultrasound in cardiology (2nd ed) Lea & Febiger, Philadelphia, p 101
41. Allgayer B, Rupp N, Bosiljanoff P, Reiser M, Lukas P (1986) Einsatzmöglichkeiten der Kernspintomographie bei Erkrankungen des Herzens. Fortschr Röntgenstr 144: 1-6
42. McNamara MT, Higgins CB (1986) Magnetic resonance imaging of chronic myocardial infarcts in man. AJR 146: 315-320
43. Fisher MR, McNamara MT, Higgins CB (1987). Acute myocardial infarction: MR evaluation in 29 patients. AJR 148: 247-251
44. Tscholakoff D, Higgins CB, McNamara MT, Derugin N (1986) Early-phase myocardial infarction: evaluation by MR imaging. Radiology 159: 667-672
45. Rokey R, Verani MS, Bolli R et al (1986) Myocardial infarct size quantification by MR imaging early after coronary artery occlusion in dogs. Radiology 158: 771-774
46. Tscholakoff D, Higgins CB, Sechtem U, Caputo G, Derugin N (1986) MRI of reperfused myocardial infarct in dogs. AJR 146: 925-930
47. McNamara MT, Higgins CB, Ehman RL, Revel D, Sievers R, Brasch RC (1984). Acute myocardial ischemia: magnetic resonance contrast enhancement with gadolinium-DTPA. Radiology 153: 157-163
48. Tscholakoff D, Higgins CB, Sechtem U, McNamara MT (1986) Occlusive and reperfused myocardial infarcts: effect of Gd-DTPA on ECG-gated MR imaging. Radiology 160: 515-519
49. McNamara MT, Tscholakoff D, Revel D et al (1986) Differentiation of reversible and irreversible myocardial injury by MR imaging with a without gadolinium-DTPA. Radiology 158: 765-769
50. Bachus R, Mueller E, Koenig H, Braeckle G, Weber H, Reinhardt ER (1987) Functional imaging using NMR. In: Functional studies using NMR. McCready VR, Leach M, Ell PJ. Springer, Berlin Heidelberg London New York Tokyo
51. Zeitler E (1986) Private communication
52. Dooms G, Higgins CB (1986) MR imaging of cardiac thrombi. J Comput Ass Tomogr 10: 415-420
53. Wuethrich R, Rhyner K, von Schulthess GK (1987) Correlation between MRI and serum parameters in the diagnosis of iron overload. SMRM, New York
54. Tscholakoff D, Aherne T, Yeh A, Higgins CB (1985) Cardiac transplantation in dogs: evaluation with MRI. Radiology 157: 697-702
55. van Voorthuisen A (1988) Plenary lecture SMRM San Francisco
56. Winkler ML, Higgins CB (1986) MRI of perivascular infectious pseudoaneurysms. AJR 147: 253-256
57. Underwood SR, Klipstein RH, Firmin DN et al (1986) Magnetic resonance assessment of aortic and mitral regurgitation. Br heart J 56: 455-462
58. Amparo EG, Higgins CB, Farmer D, Gamsu G, McNamara MT (1984) Gated MRI of cardiac and paracardiac masses: initial experience. AJR 143: 1151-1156
59. Go R, O'Donnell JK, Underwood DA et al (1985) Comparison of gated cardiac MRI and 2D echocardiography of intracardiac neoplasms. AJR 145: 21-25

60. Winkler M, Higgins CB (1987) Suspected intracardiac masses: evaluation with MR imaging. Radiology 165: 117–122
61. von Schulthess GK, McMurdo KK, Tscholakoff D, de Geer G, Gamsu G, Higgins CB (1986) Mediastinal masses: MR imaging. Radiology 158: 289–296
62. Sechtem U, Tscholakoff D, Higgins CB (1986) MRI of the abnormal pericardium. AJR 147: 245–252
63. Soulen RL, Stark DD, Higgins CB (1985) Magnetic resonance imaging of constrictive pericardial disease. Am J Cardiol 55: 480–484

Chapter 5 Vascular Morphology and Function in Magnetic Resonance Imaging

Vascular MRI requires special imaging procedures and strategies, similar to the ones used for cardiac MRI. These strategies were discussed in Sect. 4.1 and will not be reiterated here. In summary, ECG triggering is always beneficial, and in the thorax it is mandatory. Proper slice ordering is very useful, and familiarity with blood flow phenomena is needed for proper image interpretation.

5.1 Normal Vascular Morphology and Function in MRI

One of the most striking features of MR images is the excellent soft tissue/vessel contrast. This permits imaging without injection of contrast media for the delineation of vascular structures in contradistinction to CT imaging. Injected contrast media will produce enhancement of well-perfused tissues (Chap. 4), but due to the flow effects discussed in Chap. 3, there is still signal void in the large vessels in most SE images, despite the presence of contrast media. This fact must be emphasized. A vessel may be patent and perfused, thus showing as a dark structure on MRI, but not show on angiography or bolus CT because the flow of the injected contrast medium bypasses the region of interest through a collateral circulation. We shall first discuss MR imaging of the normal vasculature, and then the pathologic states of the arterial and venous systems. Very few clinical data are available on MRI of the microcirculation, and this will be discussed at the end of this chapter.

5.1.1 Normal Arterial Anatomy and Arterial Flow Phenomena

To look for morphological pathology with MRI, ECG-triggered SE images are almost exclusively used. Thus, the MR appearance of vascular anatomy is presented on such images rather than on gradient echo images. Depiction of the aorta and the

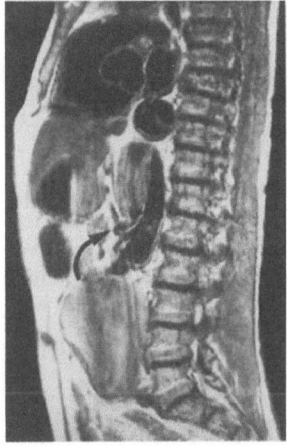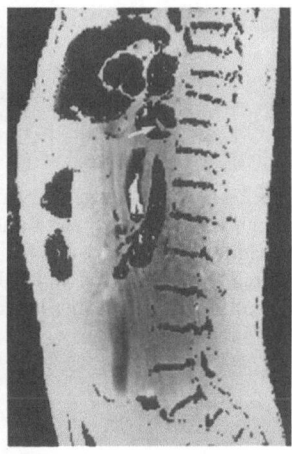

a, b

Fig. 5.1 a, b. Parasagittal amplitude (**a**) and phase (**b**) images (SE ca. 850/30 ms, ECG triggered) of a patient with aortic dissection. The normal anatomic findings in this patient are the nicely depicted sinus of Valsalva and the pulmonary outflow tract as well as the left atrium. Just below it, the descending aorta runs horizontally in a segment of extreme kinking. In it, a dissection membrane is identified (better seen on the phase image, *arrow*). The dissection is seen to continue into the abdominal aorta, where the false lumen ends in the celiac axis *(curved arrow)*. Further below is a true aneurysm. The central portion of this aneurysm and areas in the false lumen of the dissecting aneurysm are seen to contain slowly flowing blood on the phase image

great arterial vessels of the neck is well accomplished with MRI. The aortic root is best imaged with coronal or transverse angulated slices [1]. The sinus of Valsalva are seen as extensions in the most proximal part of the ascending aorta (Fig. 5.1), which appears as a circular structure on transverse images; behind it, the reflection of the pericardial sinus is often seen as a structure also void of signal (Sect. 4.2.5 and Figs. 4.11 and 4.12). With high field imagers, a crescent-like contour reduplication is frequently seen with its center perpendicular to the read axis (Figs. 1.34 and 5.18). This is not pathologic but a chemical-shift artifact (Sect. 1.5.5) and has to be recognized as such.

The aortic arch gives off the brachiocephalic artery and the left carotid artery, which on coronal

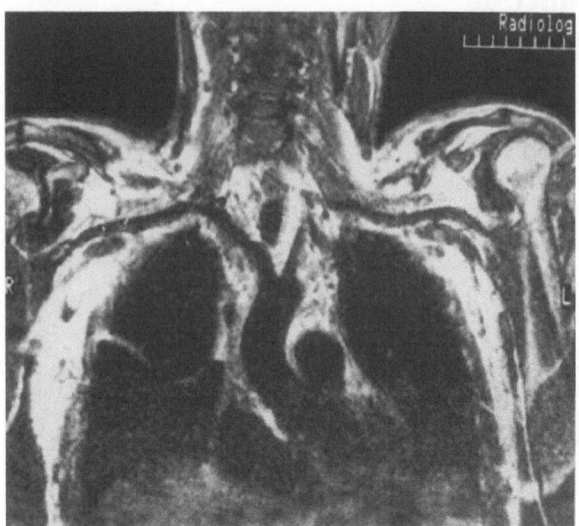

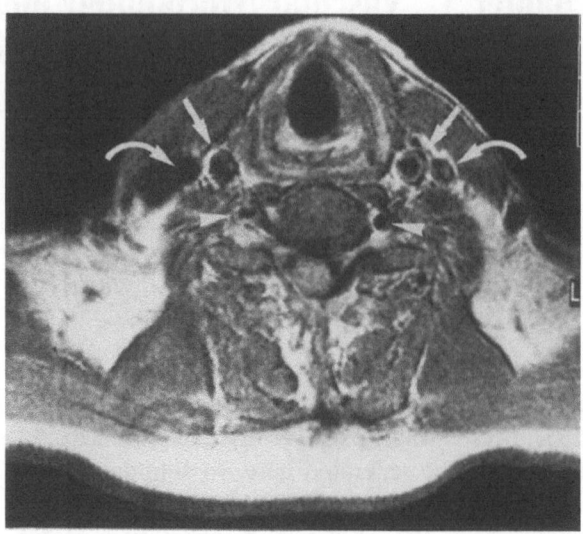

Fig. 5.2. Coronal image (SE ca. 750/30 ms, ECG triggered) through the ascending aorta and the pulmonary trunk. The branchiocephalic artery and the left carotid are seen to leave the arch region. The left and right subclavian course towards the axilla. Portions of the left carotid and jugular vein are identifiable on this scan

Fig. 5.3 Transverse section through the neck (SE 2000/30 ms) at the level of the larynx. The common carotid arteries *(arrows)*, the vertebral arteries *(arrowheads)*, and the jugular veins *(curved arrows)* are easy to identify. The right jugular vein is often larger than the left one

images often are found in the same plane. The left subclavian originates more posteriorly. The branching of the brachiocephalic artery is readily seen, and both subclavian arteries are seen to course over the apex of the lung into the arms (Fig. 5.2). On the large-field-of-view images needed to depict the shoulder region bilaterally (typically 40 cm), smaller arterial vessels are identified inconsistently. The carotid arteries, their bifurcations, and the vertebral arteries are usually seen without problem (Fig. 5.3) on transverse scans using a saddle-type head coil permitting imaging of the neck or a specialized head coil, and they are also seen on small-field-of-view (20–30 cm) body coil images.

The descending aorta is also well depicted on MR images in its left paramedian position next to the vertebral column. In many instances it is advantageous to obtain one scan in a sagittal plane, angulated such that it coincides with the plane of the aortic arch (Fig. 5.4). The entire thoracic aorta can then be seen within one or two sections. The esophagus is seen in close proximity to the descending aorta along its entire mediastinal course.

In the abdomen, the aorta is found to approach the midline in its retroperitoneal course. The celiac axis and occasionally its hepatic branch are noted (Fig. 5.4). The superior mesenteric artery is always seen and often can be identified in its caudal course

(Fig. 5.5); however, identification of the more distal and sometimes even intermediate portion is hampered by artifacts of peristaltic and respiratory motion. The renal arteries are almost always seen, but their aortic origin and the part of the right renal artery behind the inferior vena cava cannot always be positively identified. The inferior mesenteric artery is usually not seen. The common and external iliacs are always seen, as are the proximal portions of the internal iliac and the superficial femoral arteries (Fig. 5.6).

In the extremities, the large arteries are consistently visualized whenever high-resolution surface-coil image acquisition is used. This is done in most imaging from the knee down (Fig. 5.7) and in the entire arm. Branches even below the trifurcation of the popliteal artery can be seen when MR angiography techniques are used [2].

The main, right, and left pulmonary arteries are always seen (Fig. 5.8). As in CT, the right pulmonary artery most commonly appears transverse in its course, lying above the left atrium and anterior to the right main bronchus. The left pulmonary artery arches somewhat more cranially over the left main bronchus. The branches of the left and right pulmonary arteries are not identified in most instances, particularly if the image is gated to the systolic phases of the cardiac cycle, where no intralu-

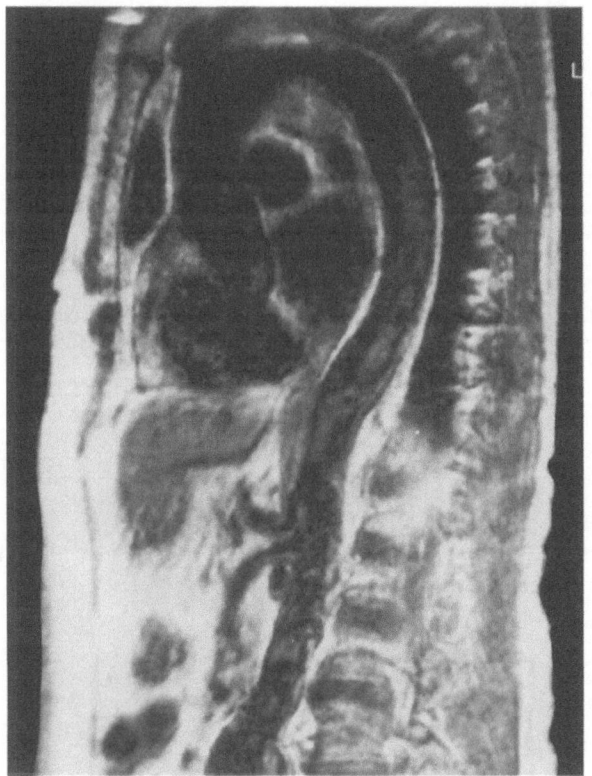

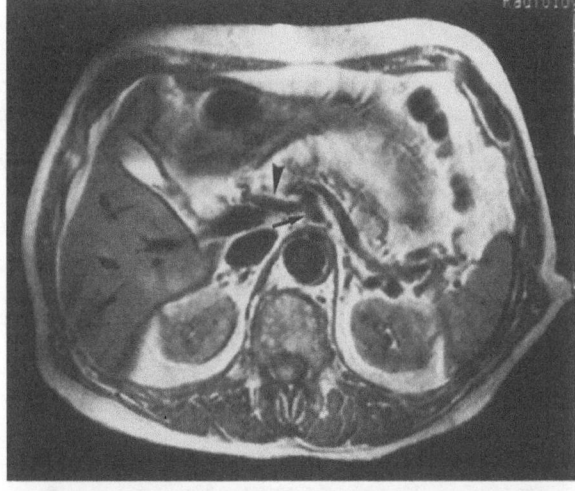

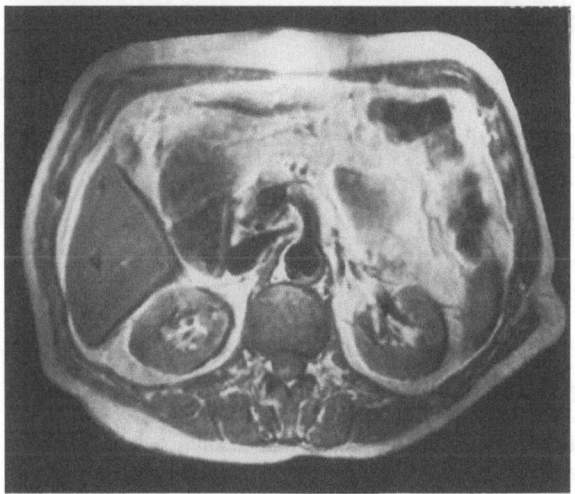

Fig. 5.4. Sagittal angulated scan (SE ca. 750/30 ms, ECG triggered) showing the entire thoracic and parts of the abdominal aorta. The celiac axis is seen to take off towards a cranial course, whereas the superior mesenteric artery turns caudally

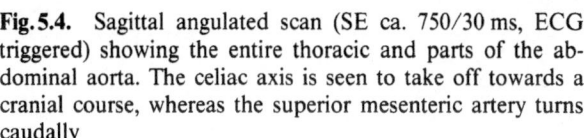

Fig. 5.5 a-c. Three transverse sections through the upper abdomen (SE 2000/30 ms). **a** At the origin of the celiac axis *(arrow)*, a short section of the hepatic artery is identified *(arrowhead)*. The venous structures seen in addition to the inferior vena cava are the portal and splenic veins. **b** One centimeter more caudad, the superior mesenteric artery is seen to leave the aorta. The confluent of the superior mesenteric vein and the splenic vein as well as the most proximal portion of the left renal vein are identified. **c** The superior mesenteric artery *(curved arrow)* lies next to the superior mesenteric vein. The distal portions of the renal arteries are seen. The left renal vein is prominent

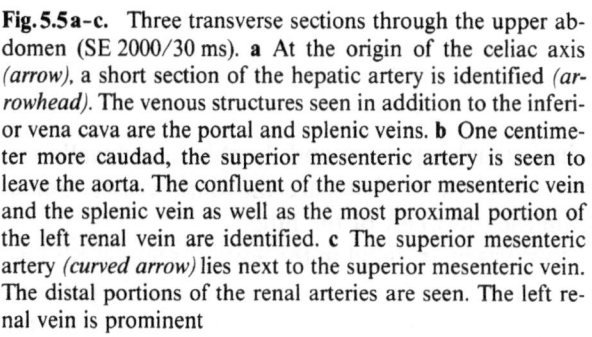

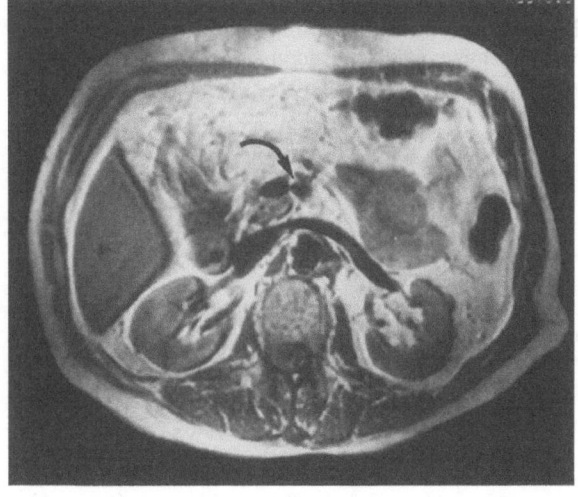

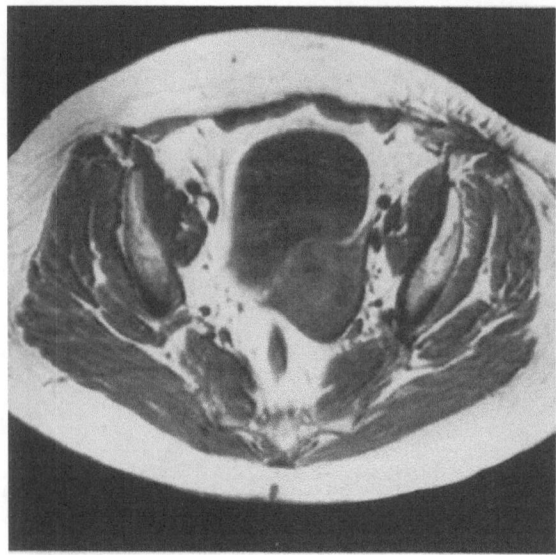

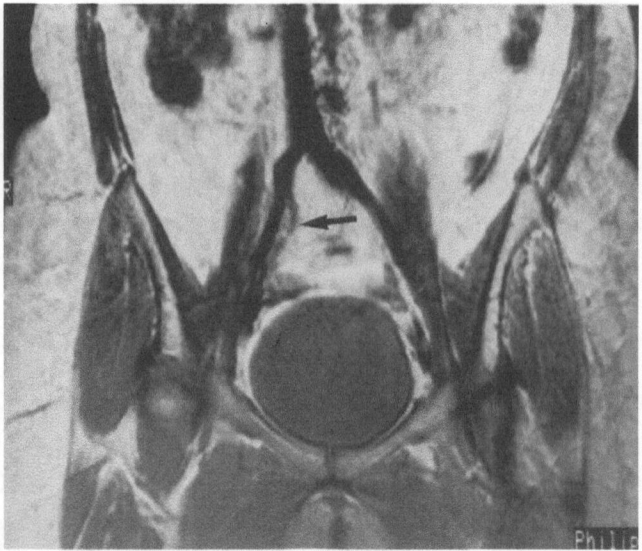

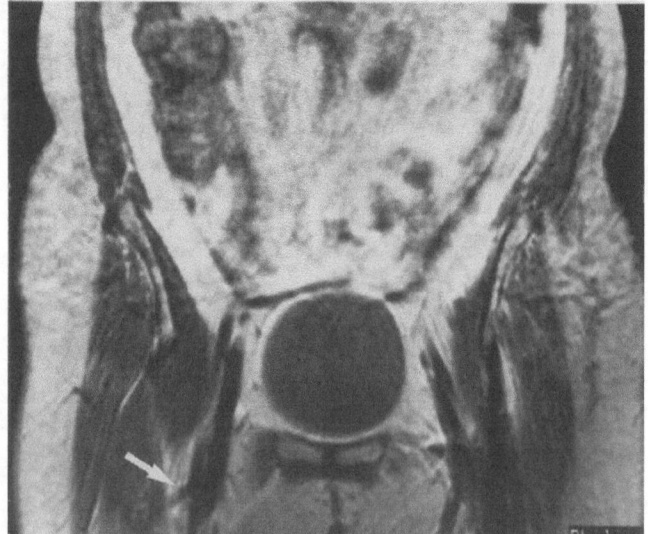

Fig.5.6a–c. Sections through the pelvis showing **a** the internal and external iliac vessels on a transverse (SE 900/30 ms) and **b** the aorta and common/external iliacs on a coronal (SE 1100/30 ms) scan. The right internal iliac artery is seen in its proximal portion *(arrow)*. **c** Slightly more anterior coronal scan. The femoral vessels can be seen, the artery lying lateral to the vein. Note origin of deep femoral artery on the right *(arrow)*

Table 5.1. Second-echo signal in the descending aorta in normals and patients

	Frequency (%)					Heart rate	*n*
	End-diast.	Early syst.	Late syst.	End-syst.	Early diast.		
Normals	100	11	0	0	0	66.3 ±11.8	12
CAD	100	32	16	–	–	70.3 ±12.1	19
CCM	100	50	0	–	–	77.9 ±11.1	10

CCM, Congestive cardiomyopathy

minal signal is present and the thin vessel walls are not sufficient to delineate the dark vessel lumen from the (dark) air of the lung.

Intravascular signal in the aorta is seen on SE images mostly in diastole in normals and in patients [3, 4] (Table 5.1), and the same holds true for the pulmonary arteries (Fig. 5.9). This is due to slow to stagnant and even retrograde diastolic blood flow (Fig. 2.3), which can be observed in normal healthy individuals and is a result of aortic compliance. In the branches of the aorta retrograde flow does not occur (Fig. 2.3), but diastolic blood flow is so slow that on SE images intravascular signal is also present. In gradient echo imaging the blood appears

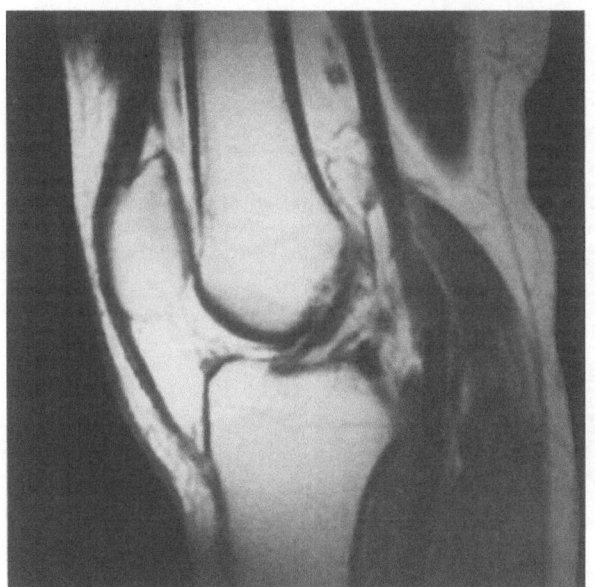

Fig. 5.7. Popliteal artery in a sagittal scan of the knee (SE 1000/30 ms)

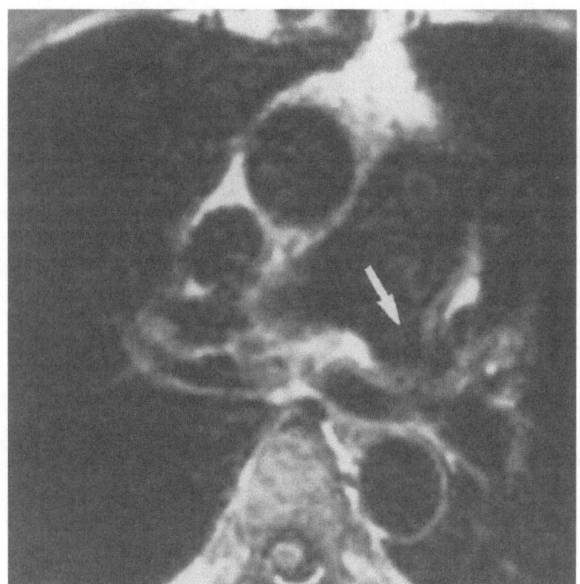

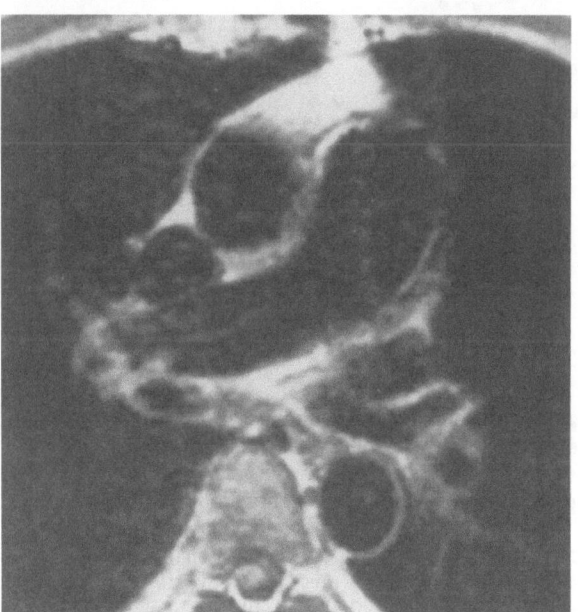

bright, even when flowing at high velocity. Only in the proximal portions of the aorta and pulmonary arteries does signal loss occur; it is due to turbulent motion of blood in these vascular segments (Fig. 5.10).

Quantitative analysis of blood flow in the aorta shows that there is a diastolic period of retrograde flow, and measurements of blood flow in the aorta of normals have been obtained and correlated with Doppler blood flow measurements [5, 6]. It has been suggested [7] that MRI will eventually be able to measure shear stress on vessel walls, which is known to play an important role in the genesis of arteriosclerotic disease.

Fig. 5.8a, b. Transverse sections through the mediastinum (SE ca. 750/30, ECG triggered). **a** The bifurcation of the main pulmonary artery. The left pulmonary artery arches over the left main bronchus *(arrow)*. **b** The right pulmonary artery follows a more or less straight course behind the ascending aorta and the superior vena cava

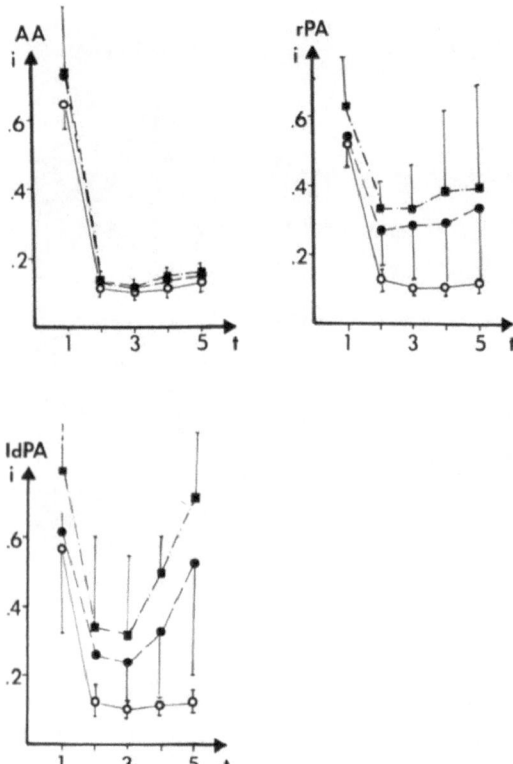

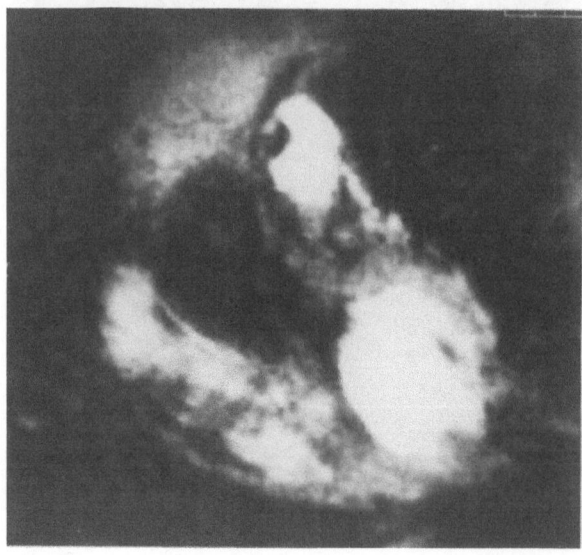

Fig. 5.9. Signal in the right pulmonary artery as a function of the cardiac cycle (*1*, end-diastole; *2*, early systole; *3*, mid-systole; *4*, end-systole; *5*, early diastole) measured on ECG-triggered transverse SE images in nine volunteers *(open circle)*, in nine patients with primary pulmonary arterial hypertension (PAH) *(full circles)* and a subgroup of five patients with systolic pulmonary artery pressures above 100 mm Hg *(full squares)*. Note the virtual absence of systolic signals in normals but the pansystolic presence of signal in patients with PAH. (Reprinted with permission from von Schulthess et al. [4])

Fig. 5.10 a, b. Coronal gradient echo sequence (GFE 34/16.1 ms, α = 40°, ECG triggered) through the left ventricle and the ascending aorta. **a** Strong LV and aortic signal in end-diastole. **b** In systole, the ejection of blood into the ascending aorta leads to turbulence, which manifests itself on this GFE image as signal loss in the proximal aorta

5.1.2 Normal Venous Anatomy and Venous Flow Phenomena

Like the larger arteries, the larger veins are well depicted by MRI and usually appear dark on SE images. The superior and inferior vena cava, the coronary sinus, and the innominate, subclavian, and jugular veins can be followed in their entire course. The anatomic separation between the left innominate vein and the ascending aorta is sometimes not visible; this is also true of the separation between the superior vena cava (SVC) (Fig. 5.11) and the

right pulmonary artery. This is a result of motion artifacts. The left and right jugular veins often exhibit a marked size difference, but this is normal (Fig. 5.3). In the abdomen, the venous structures identified are the inferior vena cava (IVC) in its entire course (Fig. 5.11), the hepatic and renal veins with the left renal vein in its course anterior to the aorta, the iliac vein, and the femoral veins. The larger veins of the portal system, i.e. the confluent of the superior mesenteric (Fig. 5.12) and the splenic vein, the splenic and portal veins, and some of their branches, are also well depicted. The superior mes-

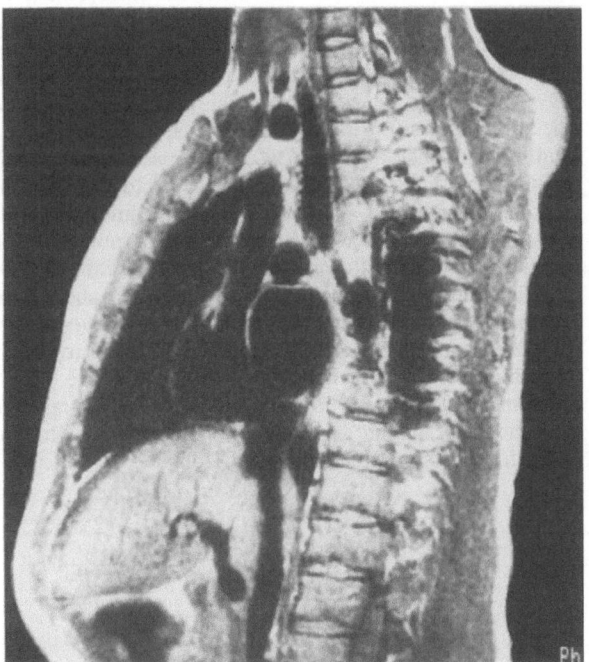

Fig. 5.11. Sagittal SE image (SE ca. 850/30 ms, ECG triggered) through the superior and inferior vena cava and the right atrium. Such sections are particularly useful in evaluating the extent of a thrombosis

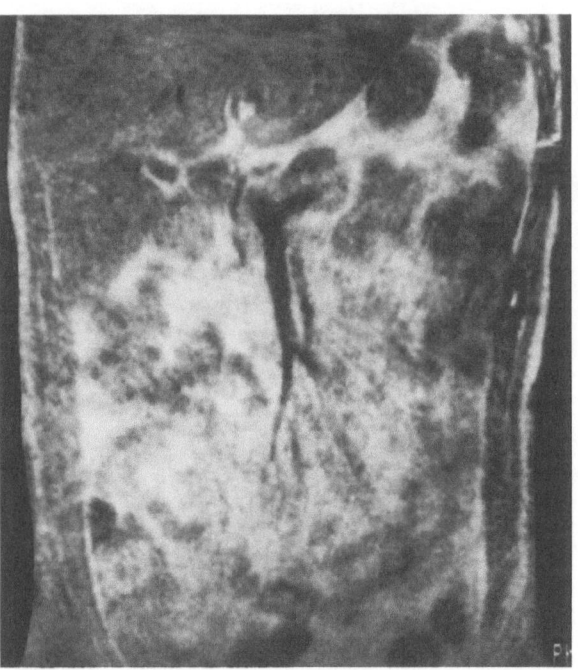

Fig. 5.12. Coronal section (SE 1100/30 ms) through the superior mesenteric vein and its confluent with the splenic vein. The superior mesenteric artery is also identified

enteric vein is usually also seen in its more distal portion, but motion artifacts obscure the abdominal venous structures, particularly the ones located intraperitoneally to a larger or lesser degree. Like the arteries, the veins in the extremities are well depicted, particularly when high-resolution imaging with the head coil or surface coils is done.

The larger veins have flow velocities of 10–20 cm/s and relatively steady flow conditions prevail. Intravascular signal thus normally occurs mostly as entry slice phenomenon and in dilated venous segments, such as in a large jugular vein. Some signal is normally observed on first-echo SE images in the renal veins, the hepatic veins, and the portal system. In these vessels rephasing phenomena (Sect. 3.1.2) are observed quite frequently, but strong rephasing is an expression of stasis of blood flow, which may be pathologic. The spatial misregistration effect can also be observed in renal, hepatic, and portal vessels (Sect. 3.5.3, Fig. 3.21). Quantitative blood flow measurements with MRI have been done experimentally in the dog and correlated with intraoperative flowmeter measurements for the IVC and the superior mesenteric veins, and good agreement has been found [8, 9].

5.2 Arterial Pathology

5.2.1 Congenital Malformations

Unlike many of the congenital cardiac malformations, arterial malformations are often discovered in adult life and are of no consequence to the health of the patient. Most of the anomalies are so-called ring anomalies occurring as a result of a pathologic regression of vascular sections of the double aortic arch present in early embryonic life (Fig. 5.13) [10]. Thus, their only importance for MRI (and other diagnostic imaging procedures) is their recognition and proper identification (Fig. 5.14). Occasionally, the malformation may produce clinical symptoms, as in the case of the aberrant right subclavian artery shown in Fig. 5.14. ECG-gated MR is a very effective means of imaging such anomalies, as indicated by several recent reports [11, 12]. One group of congenital anomalies, coarctation of the aorta, may become symptomatic only in adult life, and in these cases, evaluation by MRI also shows promise. The stenosis is represented well in sagittal angulated sections. The location of the stenosis relative to the neck vessels, the collateral circulation, and the

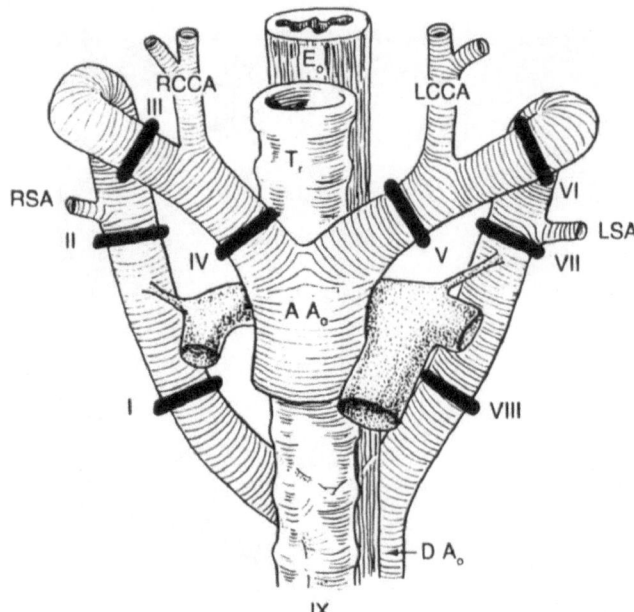

Fig. 5.13. Schematic representation of the embryonic development of the paired aortic arches with sites of potential interruption. The ascending aorta *(AA$_o$)* divides into a right and a left arch. The right arch gives rise to the common carotid artery *(RCCA)* and the right subclavian artery *(RSA)*, whereas the left arch gives off the left common carotid artery *(LCCA)* and the left subclavian artery *(LSA)*. The aortic arches unite behind the trachea *(Tr)* and esophagus *(E$_o$)* to form the descending aorta *(DA$_o$)* I, Normal; II, left aortic arch with aortic diverticulum; III, left aortic arch with an aberrant right subclavian artery; IV, left aortic arch with a aberrant right innominate artery; V, right aortic arch with a left aberrant innominate artery; VI, right aortic arch with an aberrant left subclavian artery; VII, right aortic arch with mirror image branching (rare); VIII, right arch with mirror image branching (rare); VIII, right aortic arch with mirror image branching (common); IX, double aortic arch (no interruption). (Reprinted with permission from Moss et al. [10])

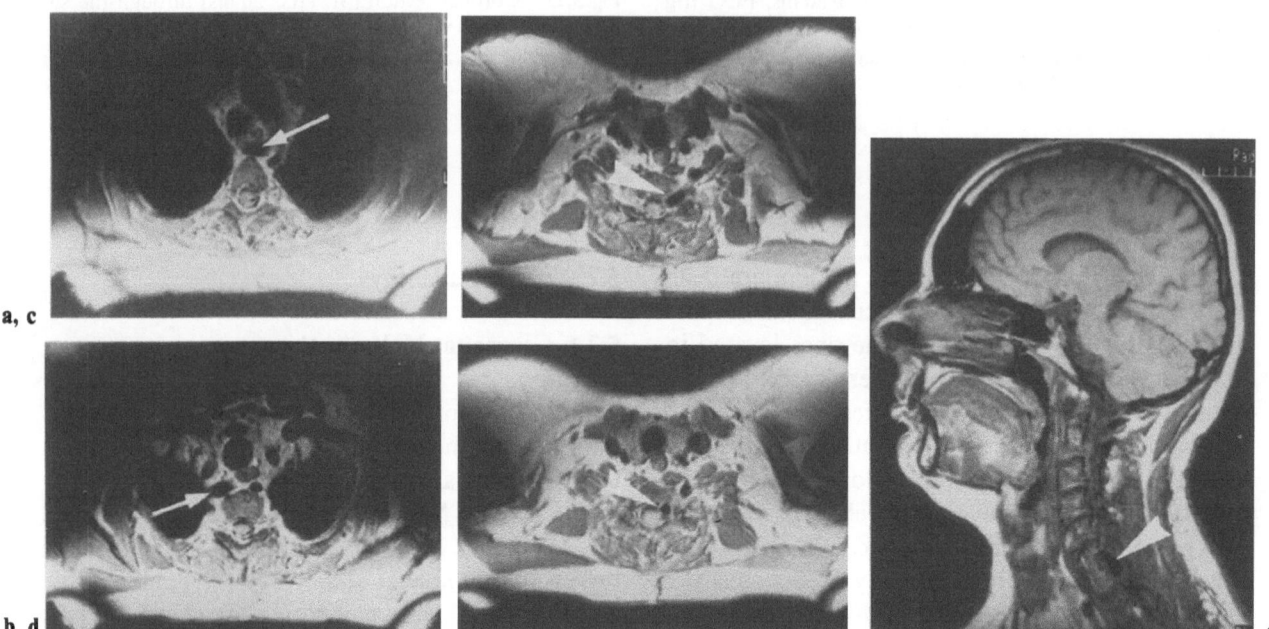

Fig. 5.14a–e. Congenital anomalous course of the subclavian in a patient with neurologic symptoms (SE ca. 900/30 ms, ECG-triggered). **a, b** There is a retroesophageal right subclavian artery *(arrow)* (type-III malformation in Fig. 5.13). **c–e** The left subclavian takes a course with a loop, with its most medial part abutting the spinal chord *(arrowheads)*

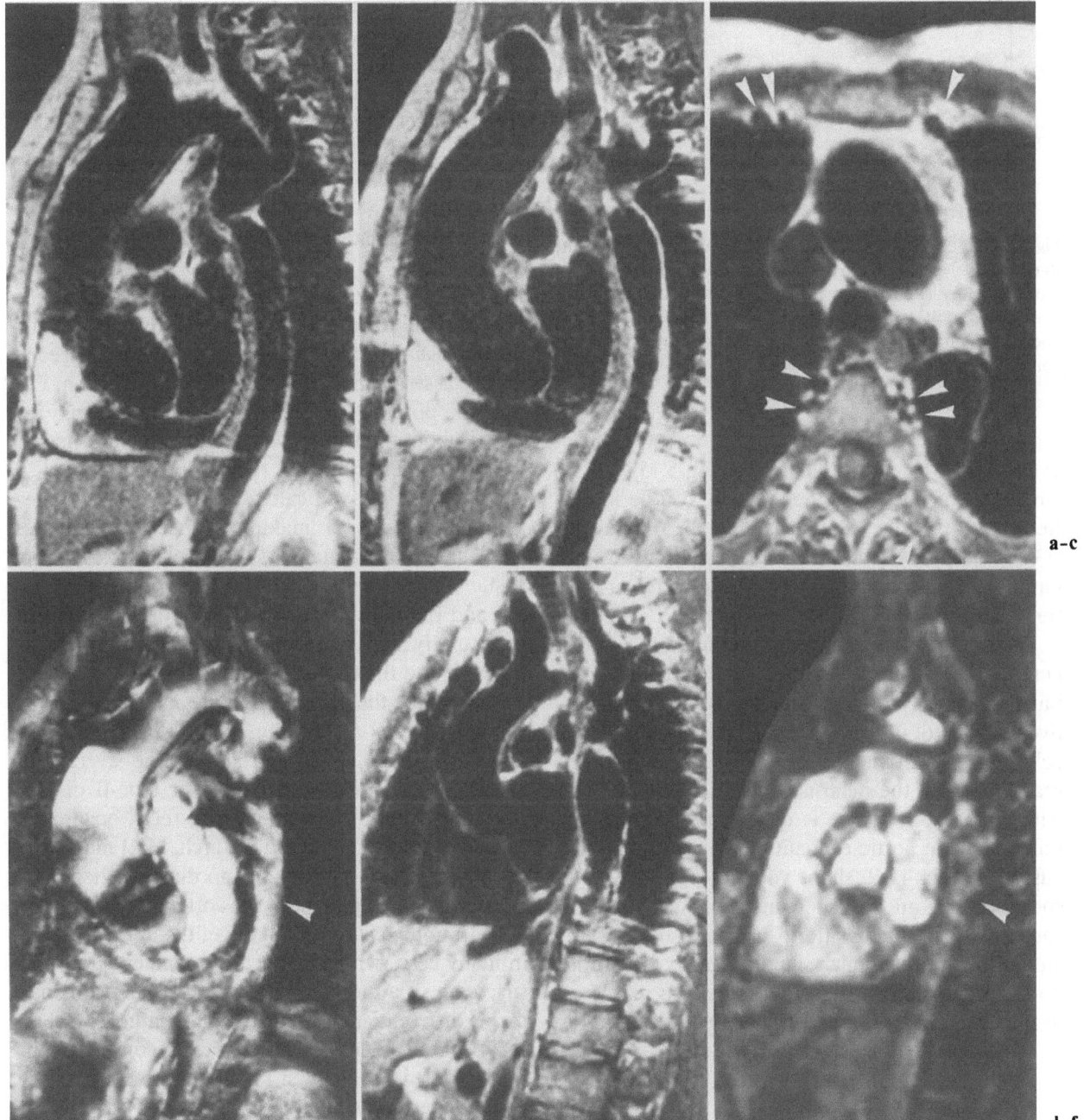

a-c

d-f

Fig. 5.15 a-f. Coarctation of the aorta. **a, b** Sagittal angulated sections (SE ca. 840/30 ms, ECG triggered) through the coarcation showing minimal poststenotic dilatation and prominent subclavian artery, which originates proximal to the stenosis. **c** Transverse image shows dilated internal mammaries and posterior mediastinal collaterals *(arrowheads).* **d** A gradient echo image (GFE 34/15 ms, $\alpha = 40°$, ECG-triggered) during systole shows little signal loss in the poststenotic segment, indicating that there is no turbulence. **e** Another patient with more marked poststenotic dilatation, **f** shows poststenotic signal loss on systolic gradient echo images *(arrowhead),* thus indicating different flow characteristics across the stenotic segments in these two patients

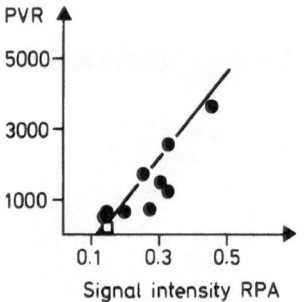

Fig. 5.16. Plot of the pulmonary vascular resistance (PVR) in dynes s cm^{-5} as a function of signal intensity in the right pulmonary artery (RPA) for nine patients *(closed circles)*. The *open square* represents the mean value for controls. Note the good correlation ($r = 0.89$). (Reprinted with permission from von Schulthess et al. [4])

extent of poststenotic dilatation (Fig. 5.15), all of which are of interest to the surgeon, can be identified. Postoperative restenosis may be monitored [13]. Similarly, MRI has been advocated in the evaluation of malformations of the pulmonary arterial tree [14].

Function studies analyzing flow patterns in congenital arterial malformations have not appeared, but it is conceivable that qualitative and quantitative analyses of intravascular signal loss on gradient echo images will yield information on the pressure gradient across the stenosis, similar to examinations with sonography. There is clearly poststenotic turbulent flow in aortic coarctation (Fig. 5.15). As discussed in Sect. 4.2.2, shunt volumes potentially associated with an arterial congenital malformation such as patent ductus arteriosus can also be evaluated. Since intravascular signal intensity is a function of flow velocity, and flow velocity is regulated in part by the peripheral vascular resistance, intra-

vascular signal intensity in the pulmonary arteries has been correlated to the peripheral pulmonary vascular resistance (PVR). Work done on patients with primary pulmonary hypertension [4] (Fig. 5.16, Table 5.2) was later extended to patients with the Eisenmenger complex due to congenital cardiac malformations [15].

5.2.2 Aneurysmatic Disease

Like CT, MRI is likely to become an important imaging tool for evaluating degenerative changes of the aorta and its large branches and for their preoperative assessment. Apnea imaging, practiced in CT but not possible in in MR SE examinations, reduces abdominal image artifacts and often makes CT still superior in this region. Furthermore, CT shows the vessel wall calcifications, which is sometimes important for making a specific diagnosis. MRI has the advantage of an excellent vessel/soft tissue contrast without application of contrast media and the multiplanar imaging capability. This is particularly useful in imaging aortic dissections in the arch and the thoracoabdominal junction region, because there the dissection flap can lay (Fig. 5.1) in a plane parallel to the transverse CT cuts and disappear as a result of partial volume averaging. Since the diagnosis of a type-A or type-B dissection, most crucial to the surgeon, relies on proper identification of the flap in the arch, MRI may soon become the method of choice to diagnose hemodynamically stable patients with aortic dissection.

Morphological MR imaging of the aorta is useful in many cases where on a chest roentgenogram the suspicion of a mediastinal mass arises and this has to be differentiated from vascular pathology (Fig. 5.17). The exellent soft-tissue vessel contrast without the need for contrast media makes MRI a very useful investigative method, particularly in younger patients, where bronchial carcinoma is an unlikely diagnosis and there is no need for optimal imaging of the lung tissues. Aneurysmatic dilatation of the ascending aorta, as it occurs in hypertensive disease and Marfan's syndrome [16], and post-traumatic aneurysms [17] can be diagnosed definitively and a dissection can be excluded.

Many reports on MRI of aortic dissection have appeared in the recent literature [18, 19]. On SE images, the dissection membrane appears as a bright structure separating the true and the false lumina (Fig. 5.18). The potential pitfalls of chemical shift artifacts or a large pericardial recess mimicking dissection have been pointed out (Figs. 1.34 and 4.12).

Table 5.2. Clinical data of nine patients with primary pulmonary hypertension (PAH)

Pa-tient	Age (years)/ sex	Blood pressure (mm Hg)	Cardiac output (l/min)	Pulm. arterial pressure (mm Hg)	Pulm. vascular resist. (dyness cm^{-5})
1	42/F	99/65	1.78	120/85	3685
2	24/F	126/64	8.38	131/46	706
3	48/F	132/78	3.50	88/34	1189
4	15/F	149/63	6.88	191/85	1395
5	34/M	137/80	3.19	163/71	2558
6	28/F	112/68	2.60	115/46	1660
7	54/F	140/80	4.70	75/15	612
8	31/F	86/52	4.44	81/42	308
9	24/M	102/44	11.6	93/38	426

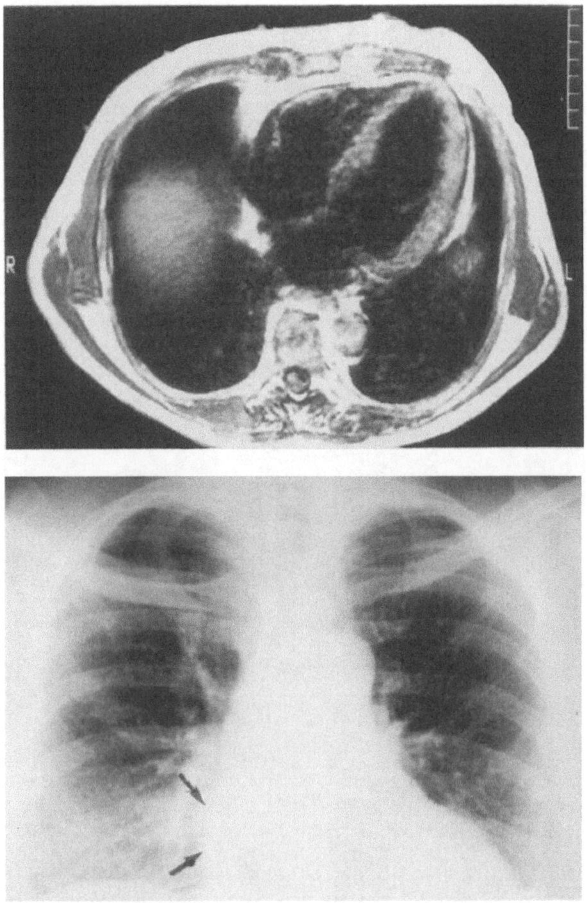

Fig. 5.17. **a** Right paracardiac mass in an other-wise asymptomatic patient. To rule out a tumor, an MR scan was performed. **b** Transverse section at the level of the lesion shows merely a somewhat prominent left atrium (SE ca. 950/30 ms, ECG-triggered)

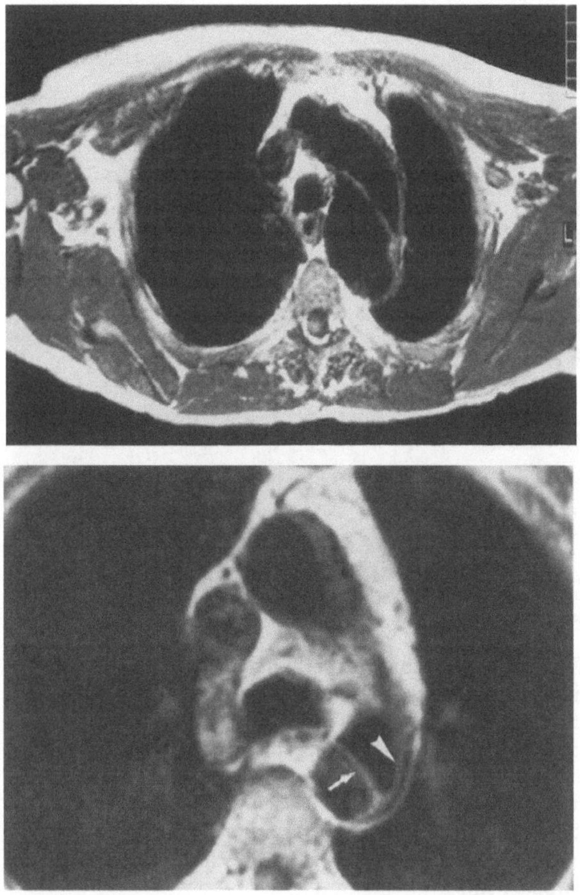

Fig. 5.18 a, b. Transverse section through the descending aorta (SE ca. 800/30 ms, ECG triggered) showing the dissection flap *(arrow)* as well as a chemical shift artifact *(arrowhead)* not to be confounded with a dissection membrane

Fig. 5.19. Coronal angulated scan through the descending ▶ aorta showing a narrow true lumen and a false lumen containing some thrombus in a patient with postpartum aortic dissection (SE ca. 750/30 ms, ECG triggered)

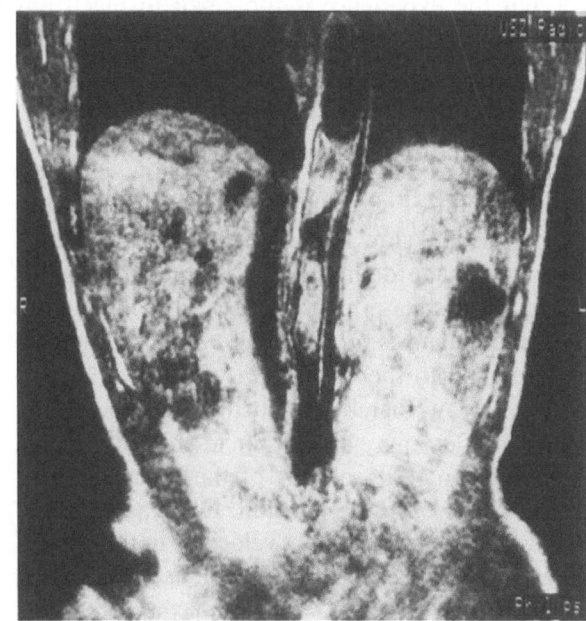

Due to the aortic kinking usually present in patients with dissecting aneurysm, it is rarely possible to image the entire thoracic aorta in just a few sections. The multiplanar imaging capability almost always permits visualization of the dissection flap (Fig. 5.1 and 5.19), and differentiation of type-A (Fig. 5.20) from type-B dissections, because the relation of the flap to the neck vessels is often best assessed on sections other than transverse (Fig. 5.21). As a result, extension of the dissection into one of the neck vessels may be better diagnosed with MRI than with CT. In cases of dissection to the level of or below the renal arteries (see below), MRI has to be

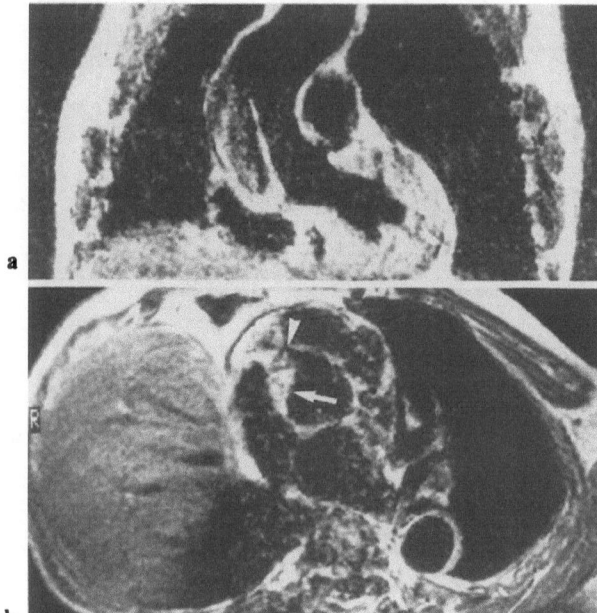

Fig. 5.20 a, b. Aortic dissection type A, originating in the noncoronary sinus. **a** Note signal due to slow flow behind the membrane in the false lumen in this coronal SE image (SE ca. 1000/30 ms, ECG triggered). **b** In a transverse image, electronically angulated to be perpendicular to the aortic root, the sinus of Valsalva are seen. Bright signal in the false lumen is seen *(arrow)* to extend up to the orifice of the right coronary artery *(arrowhead)*, and thus also involves the right coronary sinus

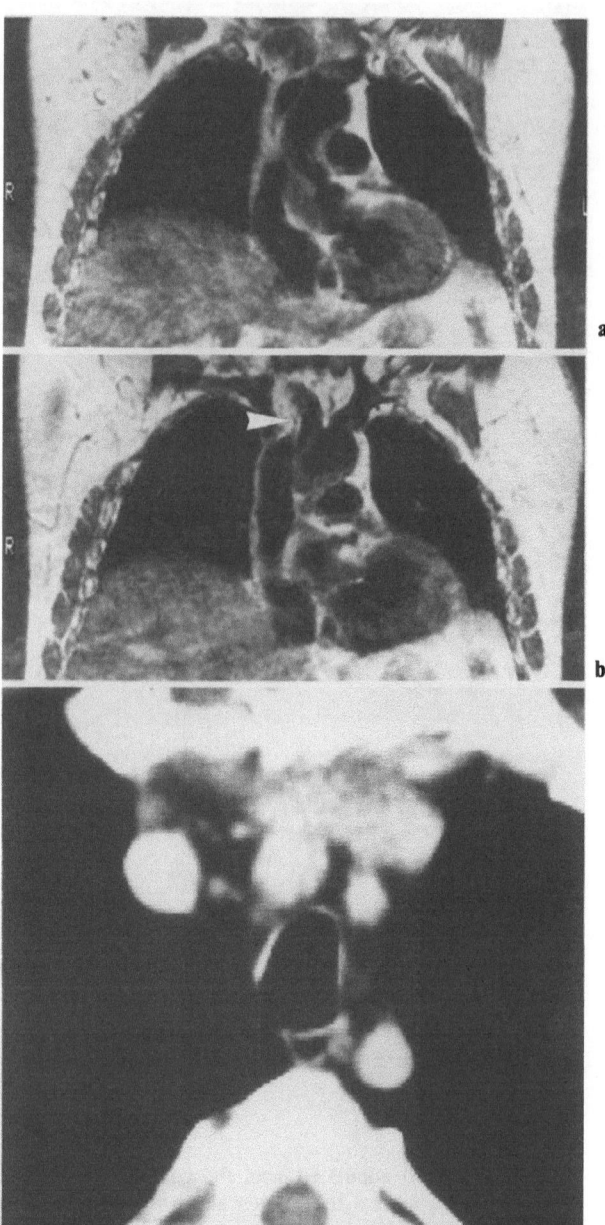

Fig. 5.21 a–c. Dissecting aneurysm type A (SE ca. 900/30 ms. ECG-triggered), **a** originating in the arch region and **b** involving the brachiocephalic artery in its most proximal portion *(arrowhead)*. **c** This involvement was not seen on the corresponding CT scan

chosen over contrast-enhanced CT in patients suffering from renal insufficiency, in order to exclude the possibility that the insufficiency is related to the aneurysm. Dissection in smaller vessels than the aorta, such as the carotids, has also been observed [20], but the experience is too small to reach any conclusion on the clinical usefulness of MRI in this setting.

Function information in dissection may be obtained from SE images, because the lumen containing the slower flow does often not show complete signal void [21] (Fig. 5.20). If the distinction between thrombosis and slow flow in one of the two lumina cannot be made definitively, T2-value calculations (Table 5.3) or phase images have to be obtained to make the diagnosis [22]. The false lumen shows signal proximal to the reentry (Fig. 5.1) when the reentry is narrow, thereby obstructing free flow. However, slow flow may also occur in the true lumen, depending on the geometry of the vascular channels in their narrowest portion. On gradient echo images, the differential flow velocities in the two lumina are also noted (Fig. 5.22) and, as with cardiac gradient echo imaging, best displayed using the

movie format. Thus, MRI yields information on the flow state in the lumina in aortic dissection.

The other large group of aneurysms are the true aneurysms, occurring mainly in the abdominal aorta and the iliac vessels. Since their diameter is an important determinant of when to operate and their extent has to be known to plan the operative procedure, imaging of these aneurysms is done preopera-

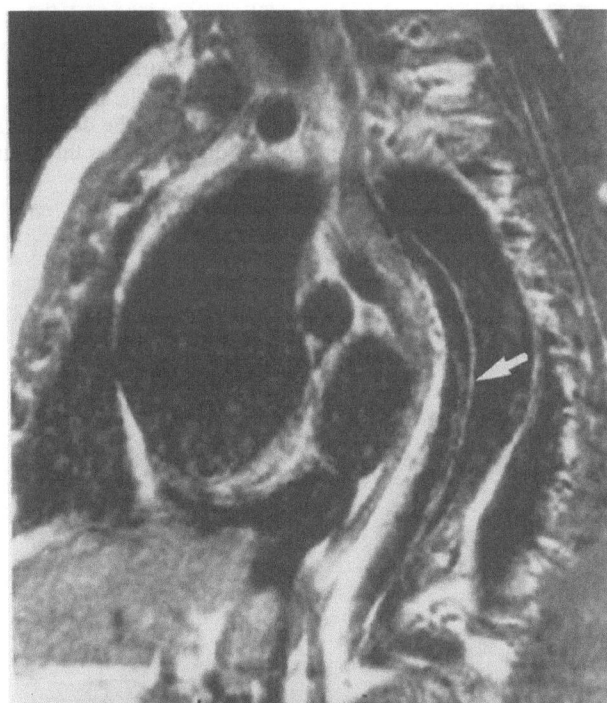

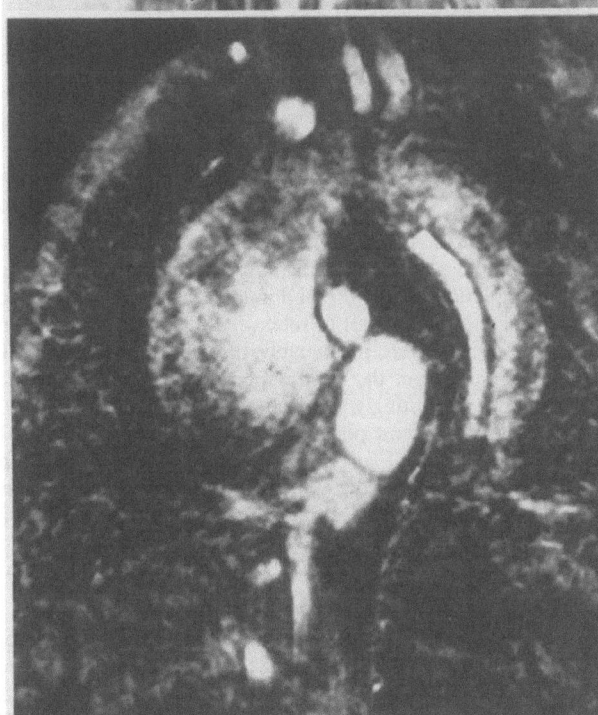

Fig. 5.22 a, b. Dissecting aortic aneurysm of the descending aorta (type B) and enormous aneurysmatic dialtation of the ascending aorta. **a** The image (SE ca. 700/30 ms, ECG triggered) shows the dissection flap in the descending aorta as a bright structure *(arrow)* and both lumina are void of signal. In the corresponding gradient echo image (GFE 34/21 ms, α = 40 ms, ECG-triggered) in mid-systole, the narrow channel exhibits less turbulent and thus probably slower flow than the wider channel, as can be inferred from the different signal intensities

tively, whenever the condition of the patient permits this. Angiography shows only the perfused, but not the thrombosed parts of the aneurysm; therefore, sonography and CT have become the main imaging methods for evaluating them. MRI has also been used. In this condition the advantage of MRI over CT is only its multiplanar imaging capability and the lack of need for intravenous contrast media application, but motion artifacts, which are particularly strong in the abdomen, and the inability to demonstrate small calcified areas are important drawbacks, which make CT still the method of choice in most cases, even though early published reports on MRI to evaluate the abdominal aorta were more optimistic [23, 24].

Various stages of aneurysmatic transformation of the aorta are well visualized. Plaques and thrombotic material on the wall can be identified (Fig. 5.23), but not calcifications, and again, care has to be taken, that a widening of the wall on one side of the aorta due to the chemical shift artifact is not read as a plaque (Fig. 1.34). As the aneurysm grows larger, several thrombotic layers are often seen, which we believe are due to variable paramagnetic effects of different stages and types of hemoglobin breakdown products (Sect. 1.3.3, Fig. 5.24). Since these thrombotic layers exhibit constant or decreasing signal intensity on T2-weighted images, differentiation of thrombotic from mycotic and inflammatory aortic aneurysms can be made, because the infected or inflammatory tissue increases in signal intensity on T2-weighted images (Fig. 5.25). However, unlike in CT, where the inflammatory aneurysm shows the calcifications in the vessel wall well inside the perimeter of the aneurysm, and thus can be diagnosed specifically, this is not possible with MRI (Fig. 5.26). As with dissecting aneurysms, the extent of involvement of the origin of the large abdominal vessels has to be known by the surgeon. This assessment is possible in MRI (Fig. 5.27), but in our experience, motion artifacts often degrade the images such that a definitive statement is not possible. Peripheral aneurysms (Fig. 5.28) and aneurysms formation at the sites of graft anastomosis can be demonstrated nicely using coronal or sagittal scans (Fig. 5.29), and MRI has been used successfully to evaluate infected grafts [25].

Function information in the evaluation of aneurysmatic disease is usually not necessary, but phase images may have to be obtained to positively identify the areas of thrombosis and slow flow (Fig. 5.29).

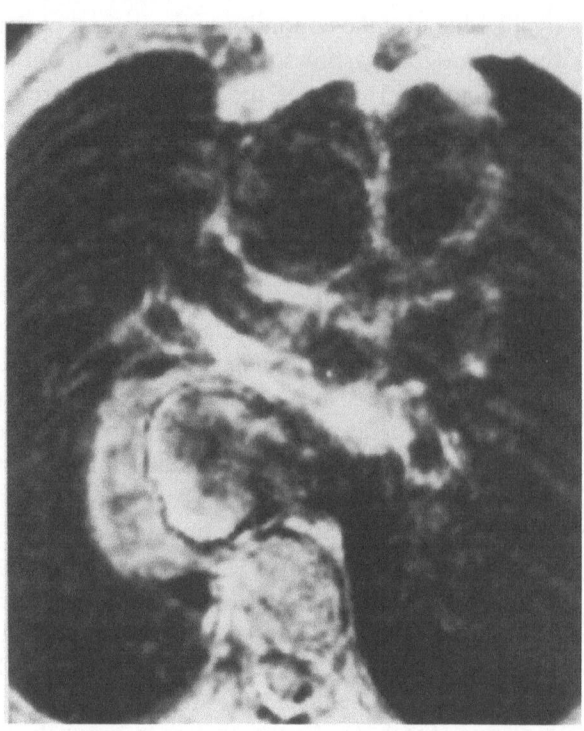

◄ **Fig.5.23.** Transverse image (SE ca. 900/30 ms, ECG triggered) in a patient with kinking of the thoracic aorta. Note the thrombus affixed to the right side of the vessel wall. In this case, slow aortic flow in this early systolic image can be distinguished from the thrombus because of the dark rim separating the flow signal from the thrombus and the central signal loss due to a slice transition phenomenon

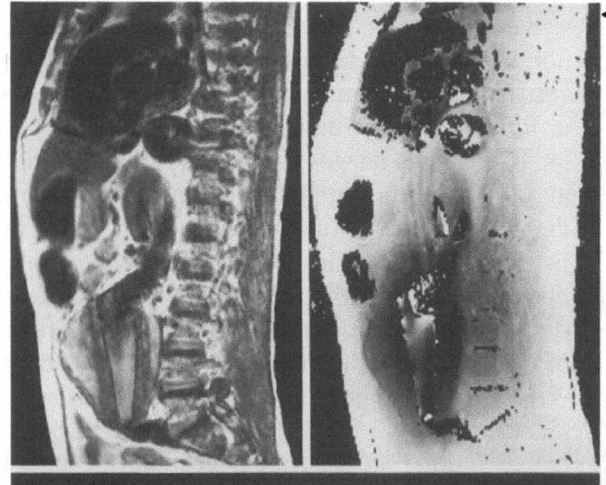

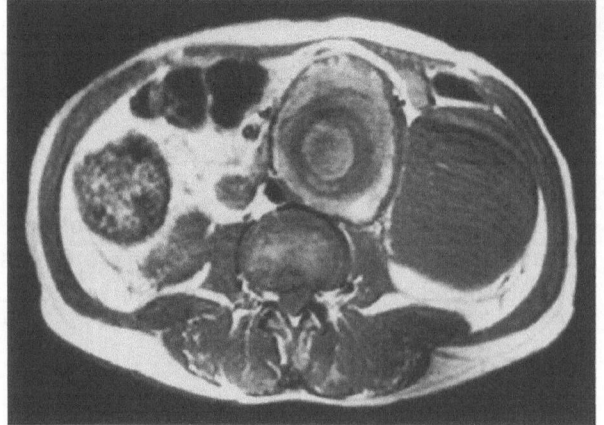

a, b

c

◄ **Fig.5.24a–c.** Images from the same patient shown in Fig. 5.1 (SE ca. 850/30 ms, ECG-triggered), who suffered from a dissecting and a true abdominal aortic aneurysm. **a** In the sagittal amplitude image, the abdominal aneurysm shows a funnel-shaped central part of relatively high signal intensity and surrounding layers presumably thrombotic in origin. **b** On the phase image, the central portion clearly contains slow flow, but interestingly, the thrombosed part of the aneurysm also has a different phase than the surrounding tissue. This may be a result of susceptibility effects. **c** Transverse amplitude image, again showing the slowly perfused central lumen and the surrounding thrombotic layers. In addition, the patient had a large left renal cyst

Fig.5.25a–c. Mycotic aneurysm of the right deep femoral ► artery in a young patient (age 18; note hematopoietic marrow in proximal femora). **a** On the transverse T1-weighted image (SE 500/30 ms), the aneurysmatic material appears dark. The signal void corresponds to the perfused lumen. **b** On a more T2-weighted coronal image (SE 2000/30 ms), the thrombotic material becomes bright, as is generally the case with infected material. **c** Corresponding angiogram, showing the relatively small perfused lumen of the aneurysm

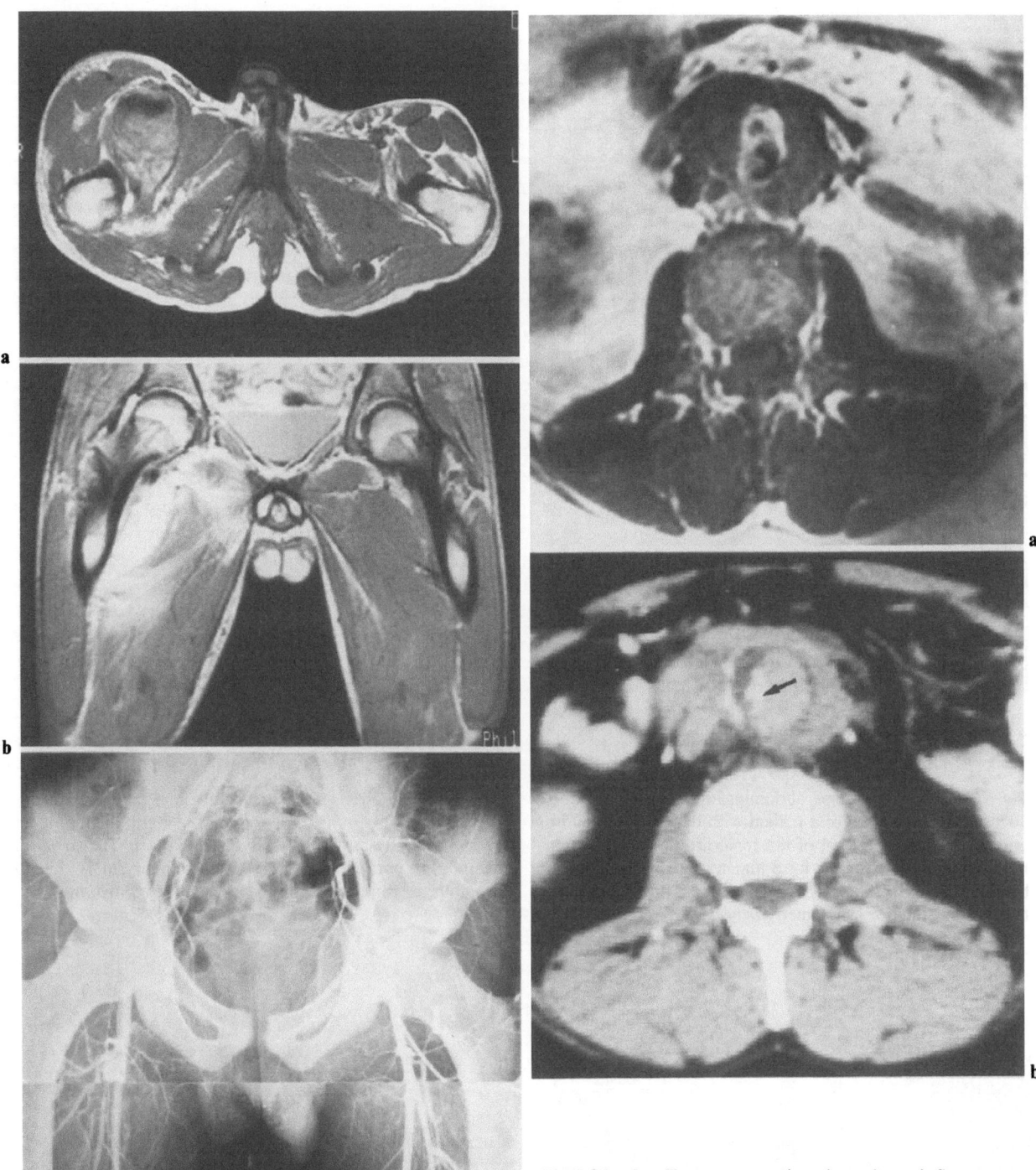

Fig. 5.26a, b. Transverse section through an inflammatory abdominal aneurysm. **a** MR image (SE ca. 600/30 ms, ECG triggered), showing the perfused lumen and the thrombotic layers. **b** Unlike the CT image, which shows the intimal calcifications to lie within the thrombotic material *(arrow)*, MRI cannot demonstrate this, and thus cannot make as specific a diagnosis as is possible with the CT in this case

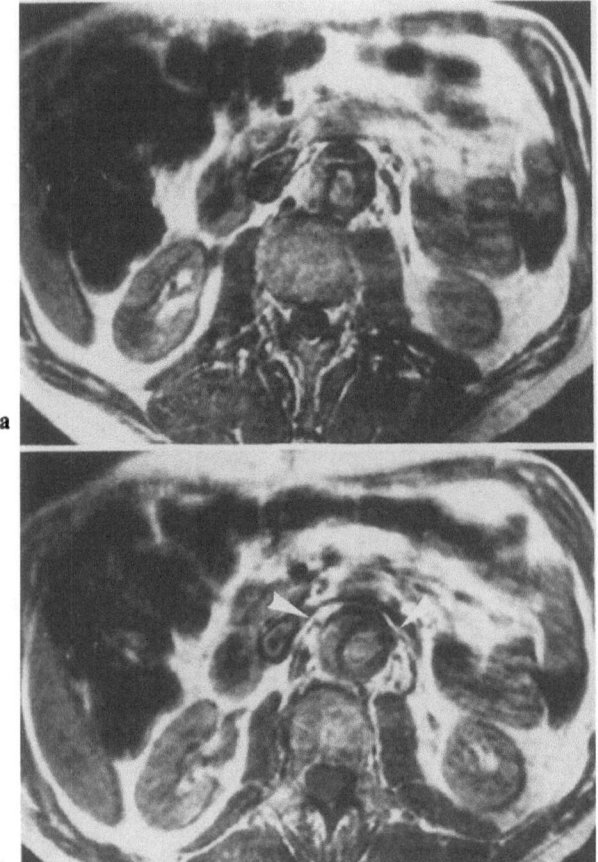

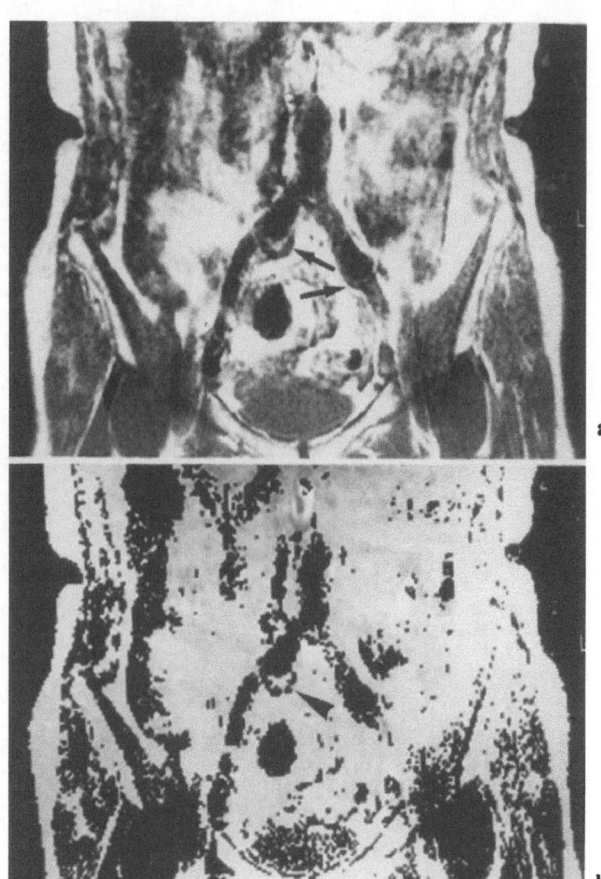

Fig. 5.27 a, b. Transverse abdominal images (SE ca. 750/ 30 ms, ECG triggered) of a patient with dissecting aortic aneurysm down to the level of the renal arteries. Note thrombotic material in posterior false lumen and dissection membrane coursing from left to right. Both renal arteries are seen to enter the anterior true lumen *(arrowheads)*

Fig. 5.28 a, b. Iliac artery aneurysms in a patient with implanted Y-graft *(arrows)*. **a** Note aneurysmatic dilatations at the site of graft anastomosis (SE 850/30 ms). **b** The signal in the inferior portion of the right-sided aneurysm is due to thrombus, as can be seen on the phase image *(arrowhead)*

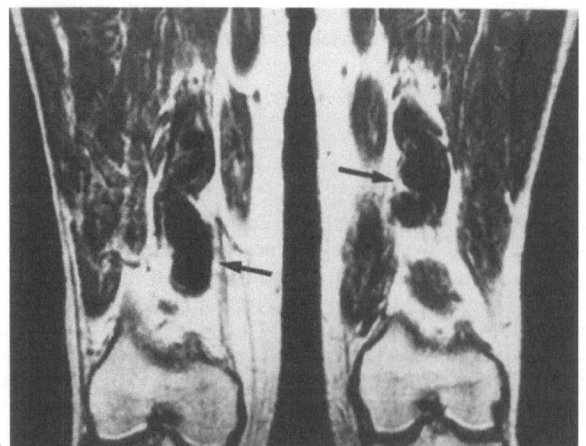

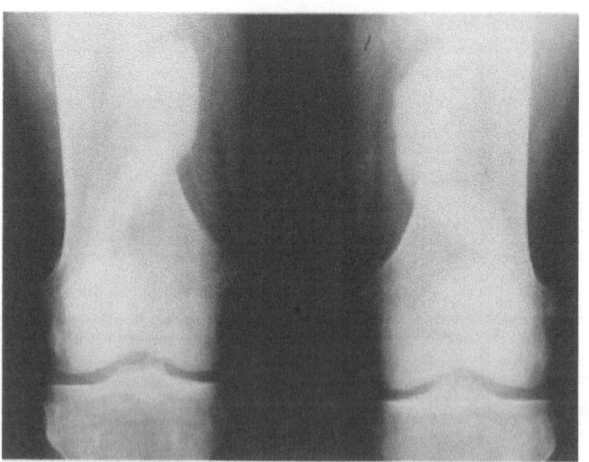

Fig. 29. a Enormously dilated popliteal arteries in a patient with the aneurysmatic form of atherosclerotic disease *(arrows;* SE 900/30 ms coronal image). **b** On angiography, the aneurysms can also be seen. However, an evaluation below

the popliteal level was not possible with angiography, since the contrast medium was too diluted to yield appropriate contrast, probably also layering in the posterior parts of the aneurysmatic dilatations

5.2.3 Arterial Stenoses and Thromboses

Peripheral arterial stenoses and thromboses have been evaluated with MRI [26]. Stenoses are seen in the aorta, but because of the inferior spatial resolution and the negative contrast on SE images compared with angiography, the results have been disappointing. High spatial resolution can be obtained only in the periphery, using surface coil technology, but with this no overview of the arterial system can be obtained. However, like CT, MRI can be more specific about the process causing the obstruction, as in the case of a patient with cystic degeneration of the adventitia shown in Fig. 5.30 [27], because information on the tissues surrounding the vessel are available with the tomographic methods. SE and gradient echo techniques have been evaluated in an angiography-like mode (Sect. 3.3). Impressive images of the lower extremities [2] and the head [28], obtained using such techniques, have been published, but since it is a subtraction technique, more difficulties arise in using the technique in the thorax and the abdomen because of motion artifacts. The inadequacy of MRI in evaluating stenoses caused by Takayasus disease has been documented [29]. Furthermore, bends in the vessel, and stenoses themselves, resulting in turbulent flow cause signal loss (Sect. 3.1.2), so that morphological information,

particularly on the extent of the lesion, thus far is difficult to obtain using MR angiography.

Several reports have appeared on the use of MRI to evaluate pulmonary embolism. Whereas central emboli can be seen well and differentiated from flowing blood [30] (Fig. 5.31), the role of MRI in detecting more peripheral emboli is not clear [31]. When a more centrally located embolus is detected, part of the signal may come from slowly flowing blood rather than from the embolus itself [32].

Function evaluation in cases of arterial obstruction is important, because it yields information on whether a vessel is only obstructed, resulting in proximal slow flow, or whether there is intraluminal thrombosis (Fig. 5.31). In a clinical study of 13 patients with intravascular signal (Table 5.3), von Schulthess and Augustiny demonstrated the usefulness of phase imaging to distinguish thrombus from slowly flowing blood on SE images and found that this method was superior to the calculation of T2 values (see Sect. 3.1.2). T2-value calculations have been advocated to distinguish pulmonary emboli from slow flow [30].

A special group of patients with pulmonary arterial hypertension has been analyzed in more detail, and the intravascular signal intensity has been found to correlate with the peripheral pulmonary vascular resistance (Fig. 5.16, Table 5.2).

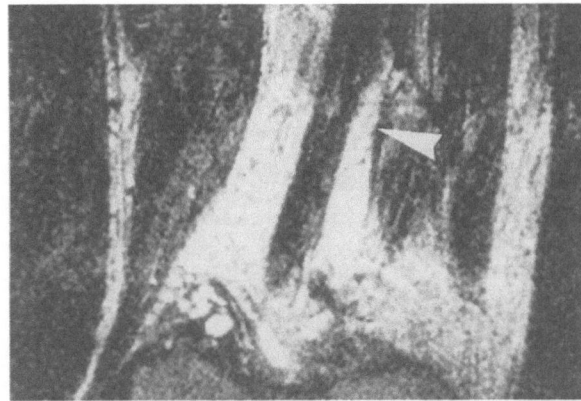

a

b

Table 5.3. Intravascular signal characteristics in 13 patients (With permission, from von Schulthess and Augustiny [22])

Diagnosis	Thrombus/ tumor T2 (ms)	Flow signal T2 (ms)
Dissecting aortic	...	68
aneurysm	44	339
	56	138.606
Art.-ven. fistula	35	100 (fistula)
		45 25 (femoral veins)
Thrombosis of inferior	44	135
vena cava	65	105
+ Budd-Chiari syndrome	55	...
Tumor thrombus IVC	46	...
Tumor compression IVC	...	105
	100	...
	86	...
	...	50
Leg swelling, normal		
iliac veins	44.111	...

◄ **Fig. 5.30a, b.** Cystic adventitial degeneration in a right popliteal artery. **a** T2-weighted coronal scan (SE 1500/100 ms) showing the cystic nature of the process. The vessel lumen itself does not present with signal void because of prestenotic slow flow *(arrowhead)*. **b** Angiogram showing the stenosis with a suggestive appearance

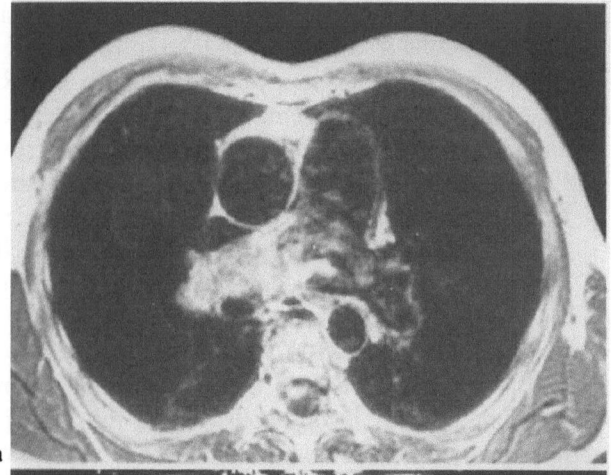

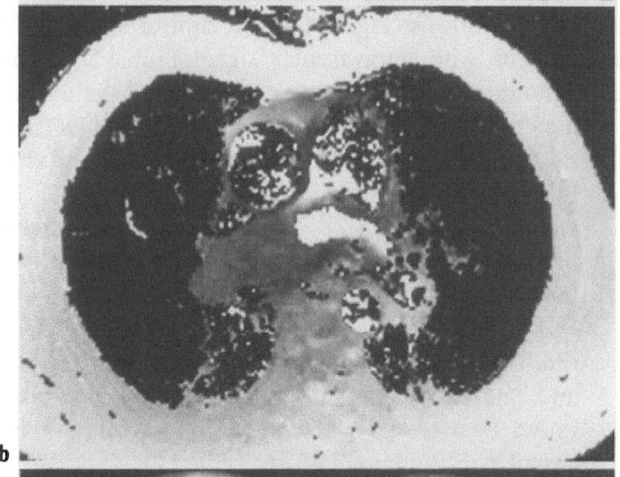

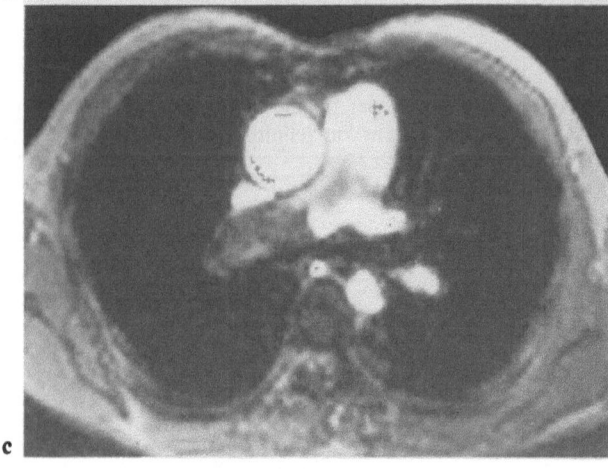

5.3 Venous Pathology

MRI is a useful tool for evaluating the venous system, particularly the larger veins. The pathology recognized in veins falls mainly into three groups: congenital malformations, thrombosis/stenosis/obstruction, and diseases of the portosplenic vessels. In all three groups it is important to recognize collateral pathways that open up when obstruction is present. The following section is thus devoted to a description of venous collateral circulations and their appearance on MR images.

5.3.1 Venous Collateral Circulation

A diagrammatic representation of collateral pathways is shown in Fig. 5.32 [33]. When obstruction of the superior vena cava occurs above the junction of the azygous vein, the lumbar, azygous, and hemiazygous veins will return the blood to the vena cava below the level of obstruction. If the obstruction is below the junction of the azygous vein with the vena cava superior, the collateral pathways go to the inferior vena cava using the internal mammaries,

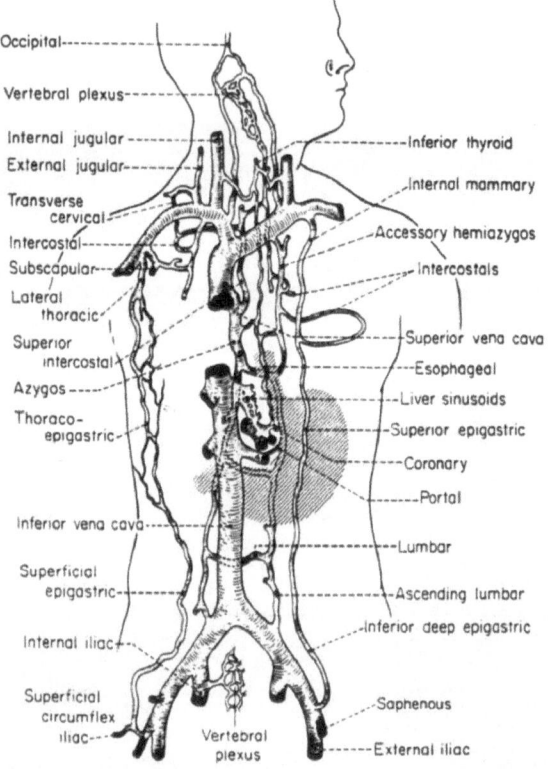

Fig. 5.31 a–c. Central pulmonary embolism. Transverse images taken at the level of the right pulmonary artery. **a** Magnitude image (SE ca. 700/30 ms, ECG triggered). On this image it is difficult to distinguish embolus from flowing blood. **b** The problem is resolved by phase imaging, where the sharp phase change in the area of the bifurcation of the main pulmonary artery indicates flow, whereas in the region of the embolus there is no phase change relative to the surrounding tissues. **c** On a gradient echo image (GFE, $\alpha = 40°$, 40/16 ms, ECG-triggered) embolus *(dark)* can be distinguished easily from flowing blood *(bright)*

Fig. 5.32. Main venous collateral channels by which blood may return to the heart in the event of either superior or inferior vena caval obstruction. (Reprinted with permission from Juergens et al. [33])

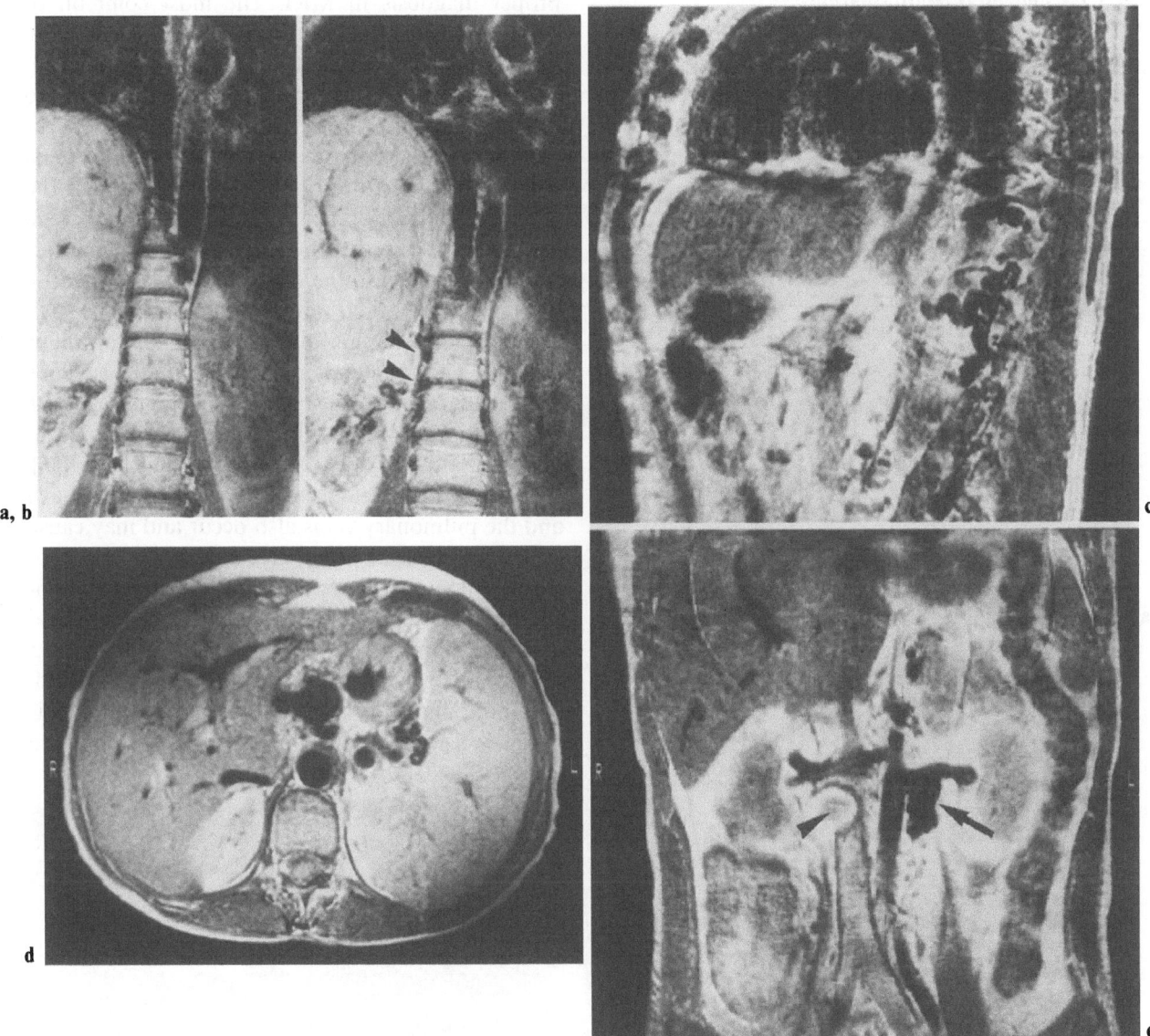

Fig. 5.33a-e. MRI SE images of collateral venous vessels. **a, b** Dilated azygous vein in a case of inferior vena cava obstruction. In addition to the dilated azygous vein, there is dilatation of the vertebral veins *(arrowheads).* **c** Ectatic and dilated vertebral and ascending lumbar veins. **d** Esophageal varices in a patient with portal hypertension. Note the enlarged spleen. **e** Dilated left spermatic vein *(arrow)* in a patient with IVC thrombosis and a paracaval hematoma *(arrowhead)*

epigastric, and thoracoepigastric veins as well as the veins of the vertebral pathways (azygous, hemiazygous, lumbar). The same collateral circulation with flow in the opposite, i.e., a cranial, direction is effective when there is obstruction of the inferior vena cava. Additional collateral pathways of the inferior vena cava involve the spermatic or ovarian veins and the ascending lumbars to the azygous and hemiazygous veins. Figure 5.33 shows such dilated collaterals in inferior vena caval obstruction. When the renal veins are involved the patient may suffer from the nephrotic syndrome. When thrombosis of the most proximal third of the inferior vena cava and hepatic veins occurs the Budd-Chiari syndrome develops, which leads to portal venous hypertension. The same is true with thrombosis of the portal vein. In this case, the pathways are through the gastric coronary veins and esophageal varices to the azygous system, as well as through recanalized umbilical veins [34] and superficial veins (Fig. 5.39).

5.3.2 Congenital Malformations

As with arterial congenital malformations, venous congenital malformations are most often of no clinical consequence. However, the existence and localization of such vessels has to be remembered for

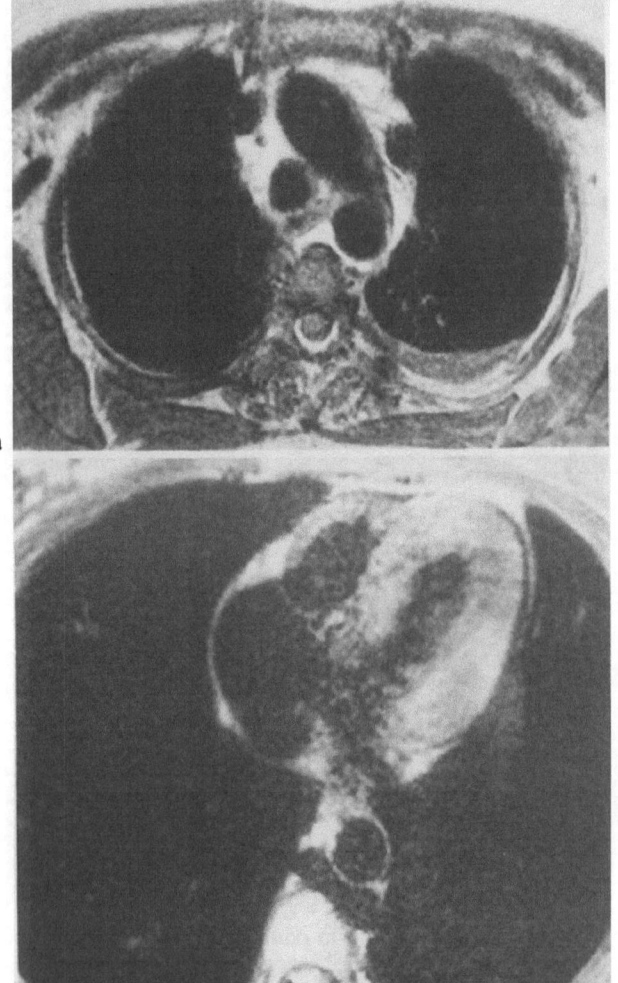

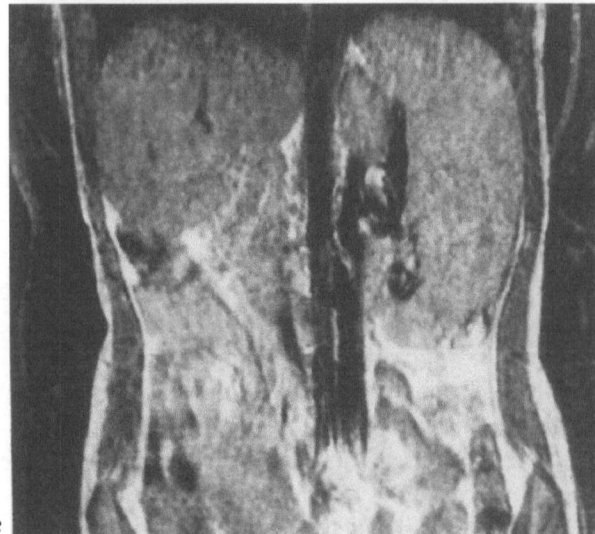

proper diagnosis in MRI. The most common of these anomalies is a persistent left subclavian vein, which runs anterior to the left main bronchus to enter the coronary sinus, thus bringing the blood to the right atrium (Fig. 5.34). Other common malformations are the persistence of a left inferior vena cava, which joins the right vena cava through the left renal vein [35]. There may be only a left vena cava inferior (Fig. 5.34). A fairly common malformation belonging to the same group is a retroaortic left renal vein. Much rarer are malformations such as a congenital absence of the suprarenal portion of the IVC. The collaterals in this case are the azygous and hemiazygous veins, hence the name azygous continuation syndrome. In rare cases there are apparently also collaterals through the liver [36]. Pathologic connections of the superior vena cava and the pulmonary veins also occur and may cause pathology, because they give rise to left-right or right-left shunts (Fig. 5.35). We were unable to image the pathologic pulmonary venous pathway and its connection to the IVC in a patient with scimitar syndrome, probably because of the thin vessel wall and intrapulmonary respiratory motion. In CT, this vessel was well visualized. Probably, gradient echo

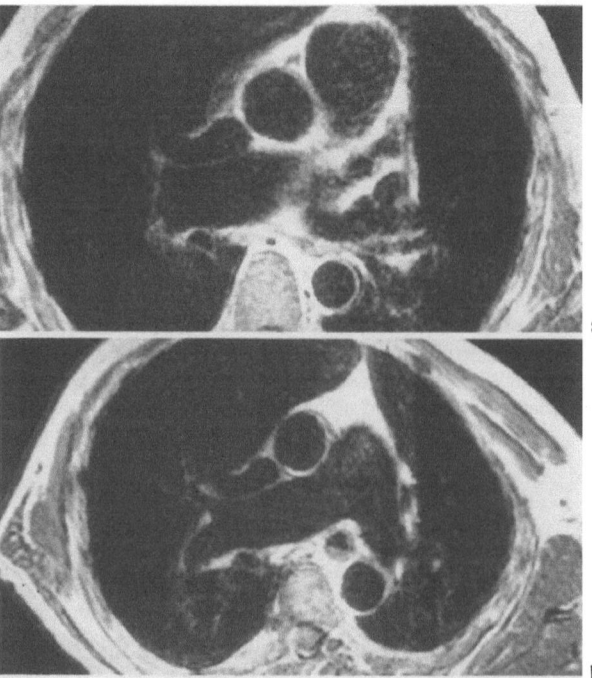

Fig. 5.35 a, b. Aberrant right superior pulmonary vein, which enters the superior vena cava just above the right atrium (SE ca. 850/30 ms, ECG-triggered)

◀ **Fig. 5.34.** **a** Transverse image at the level of the aortic arch, showing a left-sided vena cava superior. **b** Azygous/hemiazygous continuation syndrome with enlarged hemiazygous crossing behind descending aorta and **c** left-sided inferior vena cava (SE 700/30 ms)

imaging would have permitted proper imaging as well.

Function evaluation of blood flow in patients with congenital malformations is of limited interest. Intravascular signal on SE images points to and may help to identify areas of obstructed flow, and in shunt-producing malformations, shunt determination is of value and can be accomplished using the methods described in Sect. 4.2.2. But, as stated above, most of these malformations are found incidentally and are of no clinical consequence.

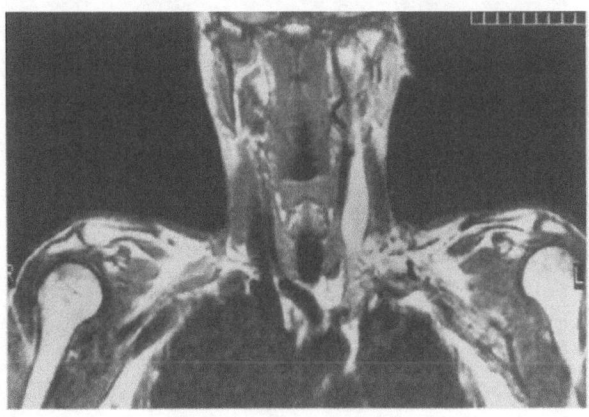

Fig. 5.36. Thrombosis of the jugular vein (coronal SE 650/30 ms) with a bright rim and central hypointense region corresponding to different hemoglobin breakdown states

5.3.3 Venous Thrombosis, Stenosis, and Obstruction

Obstructive disease represents the most comon venous pathology in the thorax and abdomen. Obstruction can be caused by extrinsic factors compressing a vein, such as a tumor, abscess, or hematoma, or by thrombus. When obstruction of a large vein is present, the collateral pathways described in Sect. 5.3.1 open up and the dilated collaterals will be seen in addition to the obstruction.

Thrombosis is seen on MR-SE images as an area in the anatomic confines of a vessel which is either dark or bright on T1- and T2-weighted images (Fig. 5.36). The signal intensity is a function of the age of the thrombus, fresh thrombosis usually being grayish in appearance, and older thrombosis being bright (Fig. 5.37). This is due to the variable paramagnetic relaxation enhancement effect of hemoglobin breakdown products (Sect. 1.3.3), and has to be contrasted with tumor thrombus, found in the IVC in some patients with renal cell carcinoma; this is dark on first and becomes brighter on second-echo images, which is typical for tumors (Fig. 5.38, Chap. 6). But differentiation between the two types of thrombi cannot always be made [37]. Thrombosis

Fig. 5.37 a–d. Patient with Budd-Chiari syndrome and thrombosis of the intrahepatic segment of the inferior vena cava (SE ca. 850/30 ms. ECG-triggered). **a** The initial T1-weighted scan showed the vena cava with a low signal intensity mass. **b** On repeat MRI, 2 weeks after unsuccessful thrombolytic therapy, the mass now appears bright with a somewhat decreased signal intensity, typical for an aging hematoma/thrombus. **c** A sagittal amplitude image shows the extent of the thrombus in the IVC and thrombosis of a liver vein *(arrow)*. **d** Distinction between thrombosis and slow flow in the liver vein can again be made on a phase image

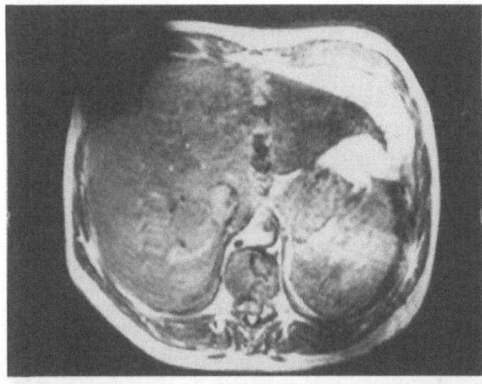

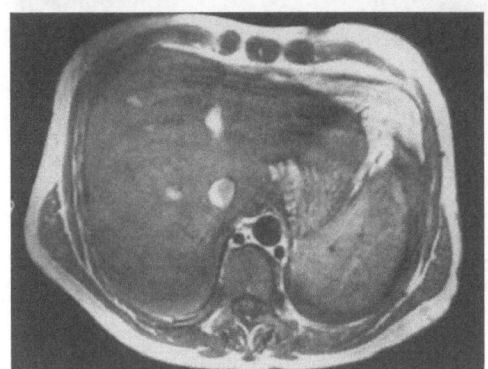

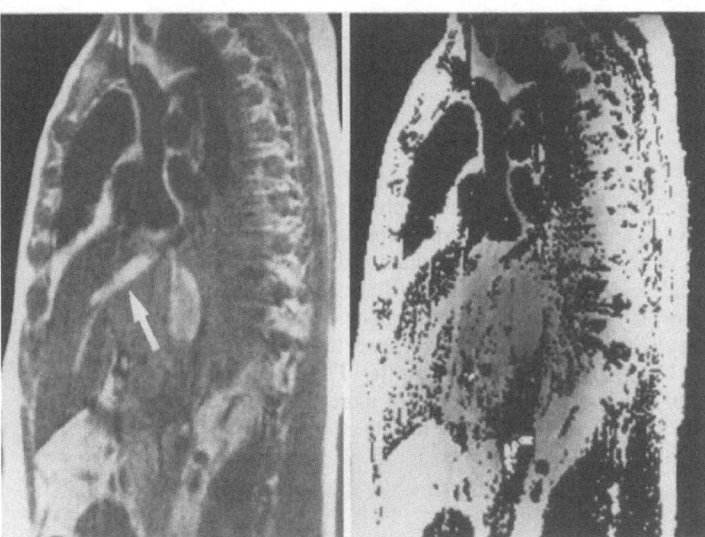

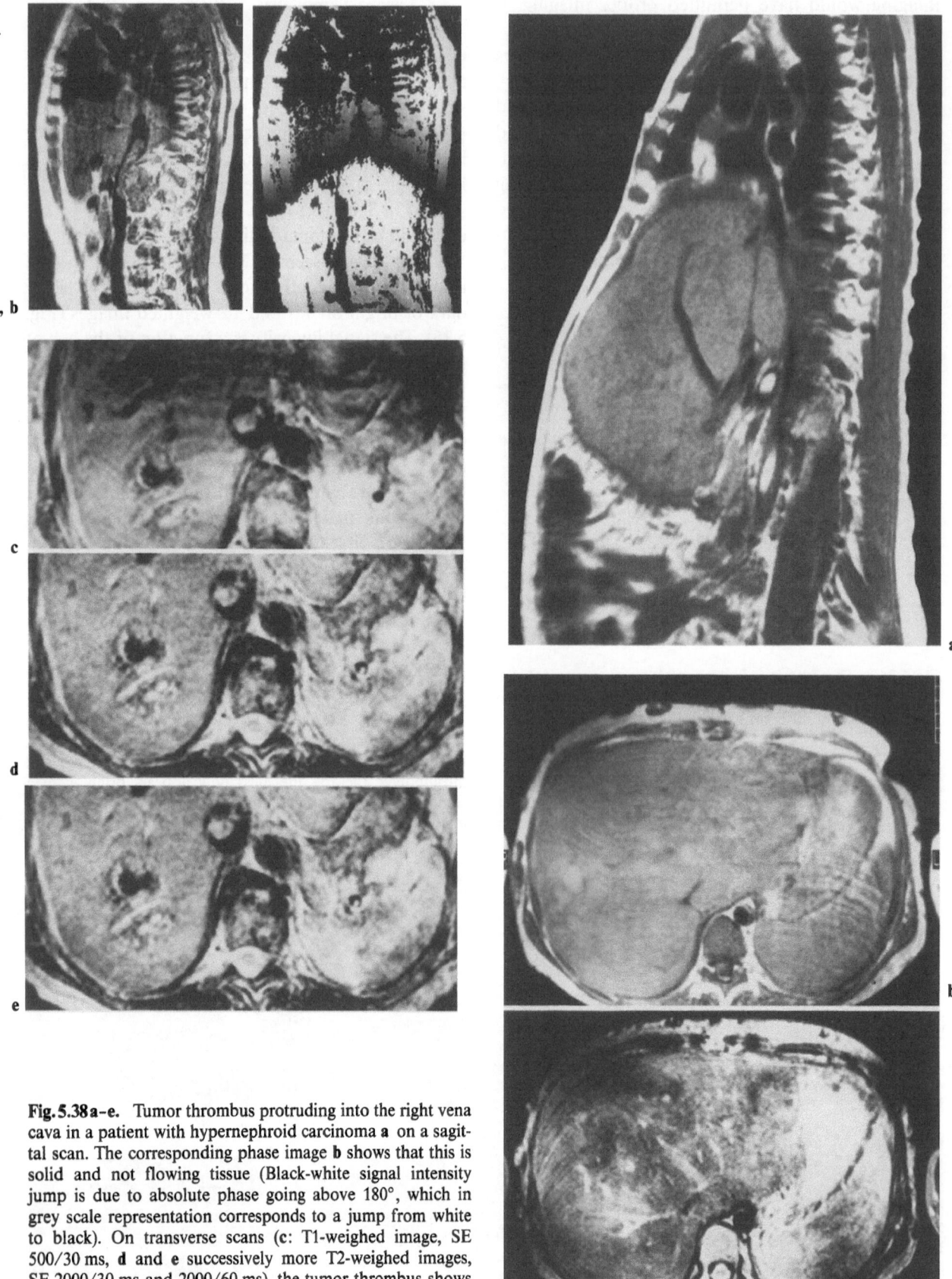

Fig. 5.38 a–e. Tumor thrombus protruding into the right vena cava in a patient with hypernephroid carcinoma **a** on a sagittal scan. The corresponding phase image **b** shows that this is solid and not flowing tissue (Black-white signal intensity jump is due to absolute phase going above 180°, which in grey scale representation corresponds to a jump from white to black). On transverse scans (**c**: T1-weighed image, SE 500/30 ms, **d** and **e** successively more T2-weighted images, SE 2000/30 ms and 2000/60 ms), the tumor thrombus shows increasing signal intensity

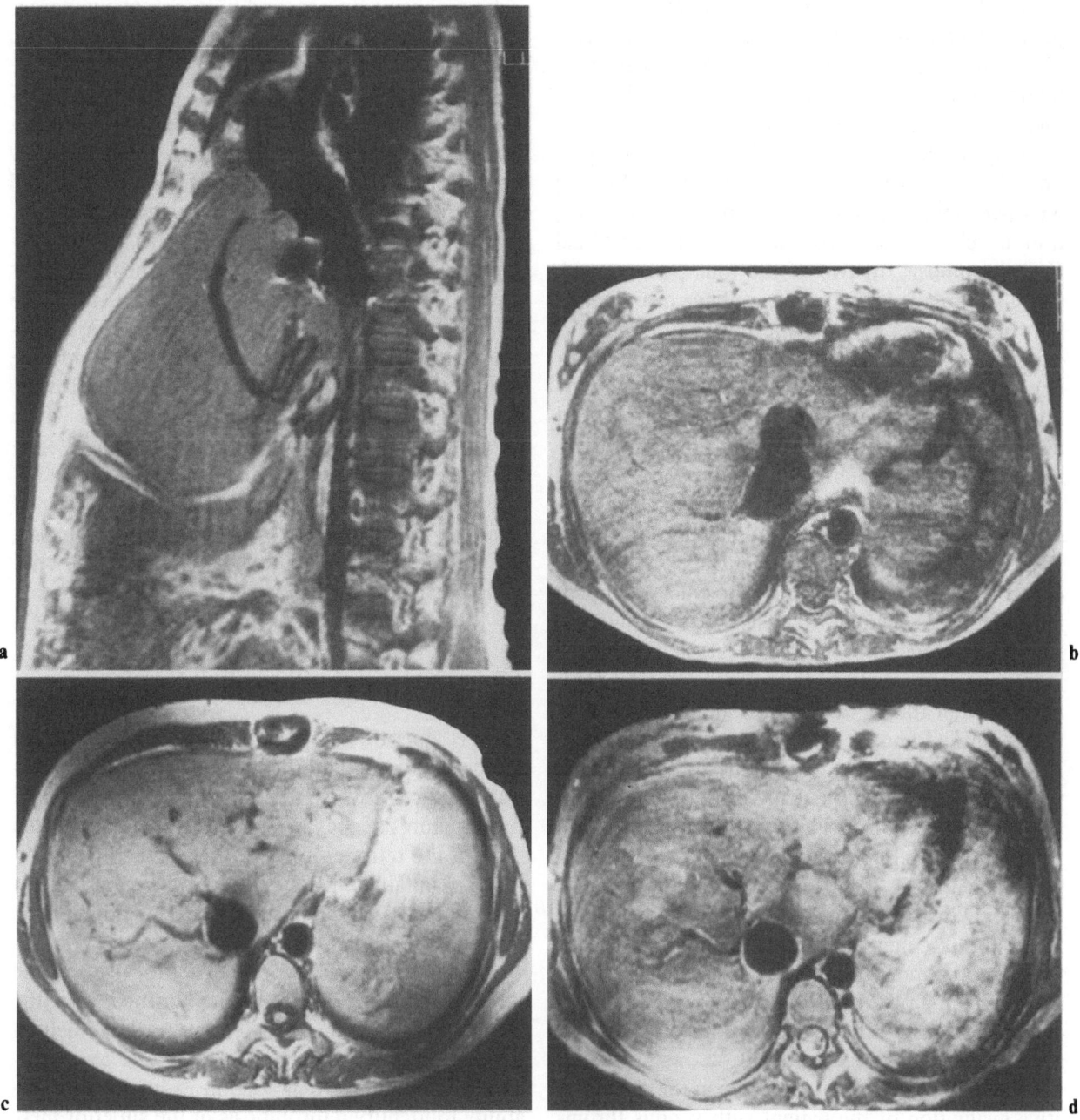

◄ Fig. 5.39. Narrow IVC on a sagittal scan **a** in a patient with Budd-Chiari syndrome. **b** Note the extremly narrow IVC on a transverse scan in another patient (SE 500/30 ms) and surface collaterals. Regenerating liver nodules appearing much like metastases are also seen. **c** Slow intrahepatic venous flow: T2-weighted scan with bright vessels showing rephasing (SE 2000/60 ms)

Fig. 5.40. **a** Patient after hepatoatrial anastomosis. Sagittal view shows signal void and some bright specks below the right atrium, corresponding to minimal artifacts from an implanted endoluminal stent (postoperative image corresponding to Fig. 5.39 a). **b** Another patient after hepatoatrial anastomosis. Note the signal void in the liver just below the right atrium, corresponding to the resected wedge-shaped liver portion, now belonging to the right atrium. **c, d** On transverse T1- (SE 700/30 ms) and T2- (SE 1260/60 ms) weighted scans no rephasing in the liver veins is seen, indicating reestablished adequate intrahepatic flow. Compare liver size with preoperative size on the transverse scans of Fig. 5.39 at the same level. The surface collaterals have disappeared

of the inferior [38] and superior vena cava [39], the renal, iliac (Fig. 3.22), femoral, subclavian, and jugular [40] veins is readily diagnosed with MRI, although sonography and CT provide similar information, at least in the abdomen, where motion artifacts often degrade MR image quality. MRI is particularly useful in evaluating the intrahepatic portion of the IVC when it is extremely narrow but still well perfused, as in the case of congenital obstruction or chronic vascular changes after proximal IVC thrombosis. In two of the four patients with Budd-Chiari syndrome whom we have examined, a narrow but open intrahepatic portion of the IVC was diagnosed on MRI (Fig. 5.39), but not on CT or angiography [41]. In anterograde cavography, only the collateral circulation was imaged by the contrast agent, as there was no caudocranial flow in the intrahepatic IVC segment, preventing contrast medium opacification. If IVC thrombosis involves the suprarenal as well as the infrarenal portion of the IVC, there is usually still communication at the level of the renal veins, permitting the collateral circulation from the kidneys to take place through the spermatic or ovarian veins (Fig. 5.33).

Function information using phase imaging plays an important role in the distinction between slowly flowing blood and venous thrombosis in spin-echo MRI. As discussed in Chap. 3, the two are not always readily distinguished on MR amplitude images, because thrombosis as well as slow flow can result in quite variable intravascular signal intensity [42]. As in arteries, thrombus and slow flow can also be distinguished by calculating T2 values (Table 5.3), but phase imaging is more reliable [22]. Identification of tumor thrombus is particularly important in the preoperative assessment of renal cell carcinoma, because thrombus extension into the right atrium requires bypass surgery.

MRI may play an important role in the postoperative evaluation of the patient with venous thrombosis. In an elegant surgical approach devised at our hospital by Senning [43], patients with Budd-Chiari syndrome can be helped by resection of the part of the liver residing above the hepatic veins, and anastomosis of the hepatic veins directly with the right atrium (Fig. 5.40). This operation, combined with intracaval stenting [44] often ameliorates the patients' symptoms drastically. Since these stents are made out of nonmagnetic stainless steel, MRI can still be performed with good results and the postoperative state of the IVC and the hepatic veins evaluated (Fig. 5.40). The effectivenes of venous drainage may be judged from the presence of intrahepatic dark vascular structures, which indicates good flow. Comparing the extent of second-echo rephasing on pre- and postoperative images is a qualitative measure of hepatic venous perfusion (Fig. 5.40), and thus indicative of function.

Like CT and sonography, MRI is useful in defining the cause of vascular obstruction and its effect on the perfusion of the vessel. Since the blood flow velocity profile in the stenosed region is high and the velocity profile steep, there is always total lack of signal in the stenosed segment (Sect. 3.1.2). Stenosis may be due to tumor (Fig. 3.2), hematoma, or any other type of mass adjacent to the vessel. The intrahepatic IVC may be compressed by the hypertrophied caudate lobe in Budd-Chiari syndrome (Fig. 5.39) or idiopathically (congenitally) narrowed. The SVC and the thoracic inlet are regions where good-quality MR images are obtained consistently and vascular obstruction diagnosed [45]. Flow signals present in the region proximal to the site of obstruction are indicative of the severity of the stenosis (Fig. 3.2), but quantitative analysis of flow velocities is of no particular interest.

5.3.4 Diseases of the Portosplenic Vessels

MRI is able to depict morphological alterations of the portal system and their sequelae. However, motion artifacts adversely affect the identification of the structures of the portal system much more often than of the retroperitoneal vessels. When good images are obtained. MRI of the portal venous system is particularly useful, because direct angiography is invasive.

Of our three cases studied so far with acute thrombosis in the region of the confluence of the splenic and superior mesenteric veins, MRI helped make a definitive diagnosis in only one case. Motion-induced image degradation resulted in the inability to identify a thrombosis of the superior mesenteric vein (Fig. 5.41), which was diagnosed by CT. If respiratory motion artifacts are not too strong, the intrahepatic portion of the portal vein and its major branches are well seen, and in a case of septic thrombosis of the portal system, MRI made the diagnosis first because of its sensitivity in detecting intrahepatic abscess formation (Fig. 5.42). Cavernous transformation of the portal vein may be diagnosed on MRI, and in slim patients, surface coil images can be used to improve resolution and minimize motion artifacts coming from the more anterior bowel loops (Fig. 5.43). Thrombosis of the portal vein is one of the causes of portal hypertension. In chronic portal hypertension, collaterals involving esophageal varices develop and are noted on MR images (Fig. 5.33). Surgical shunts for portal hypertension can be evaluated, but angiography appears superior [46]. In our experience with over 30 patients infected with *Echinococcus multilocularis*, MRI is a useful method and at least equivalent to CT and sonography in depicting the altered vascular morphology due to the disease itself, or due to surgery performed to control the disease [47]. Tumor compression of the portal system can also be assessed (Fig. 3.2), but sonography and CT are at present definitely the primary imaging modalities.

Flow studies to identify whether there is anterograde or retrograde flow in the portal system are very important for the assessment of the severity of portal hypertension. Even though flow direction can be identified on phase images (Fig. 3.2), and MRI should be very suitable to answer this question, the author is not aware of any clinical study evaluating this potential of MRI.

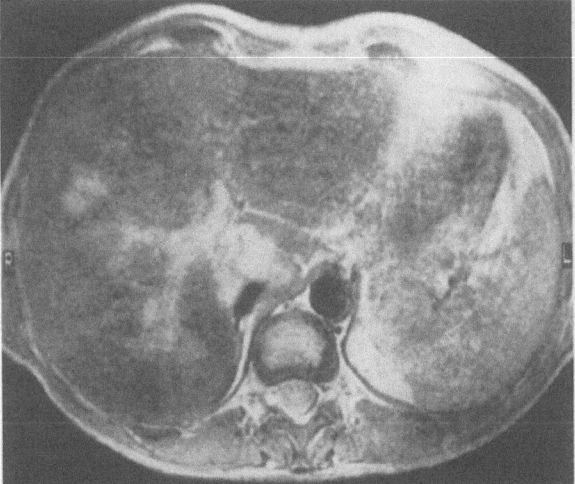
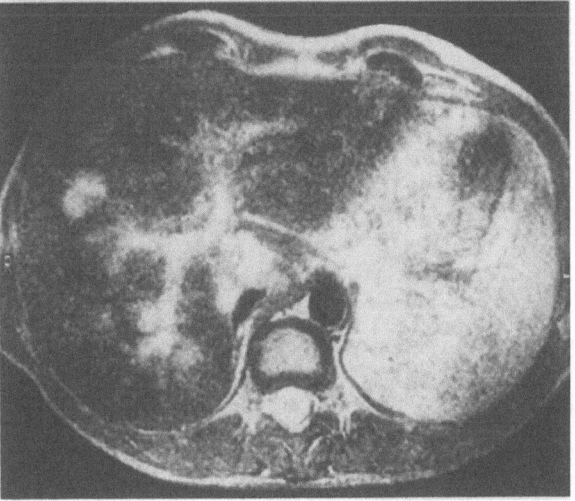

Fig. 42. a Transverse scan in a patient with septic thrombosis of the portal vein (SE 2000/30 ms). **b** Because of infection the thrombus signal intensity increases with increasing T2-weighting (SE 2000/60 ms). In addition, there are multiple foci of liver sepsis. These were first identified on MRI and seen neither on sonography nor on CT, both performed 1 day earlier

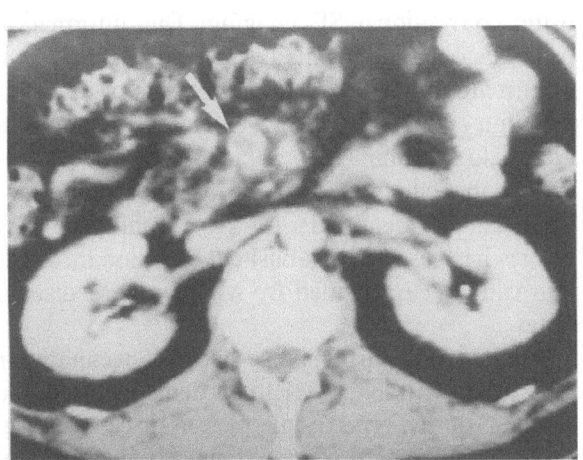
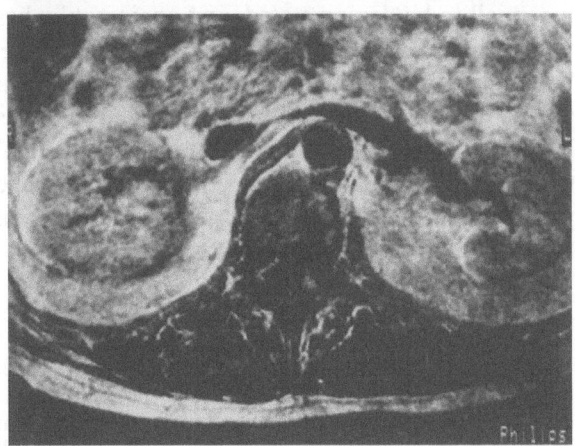

Fig. 5.41. a Thrombosis of the superior mesenteric vein, made with contrast-enhanced CT, showing the typical appearance of central hypodensity and rim enhancement *(arrow)*. **b** Because of motion artifacts on MRI, the mesenteric vessels were not adequately depicted (SE 500/30 ms)

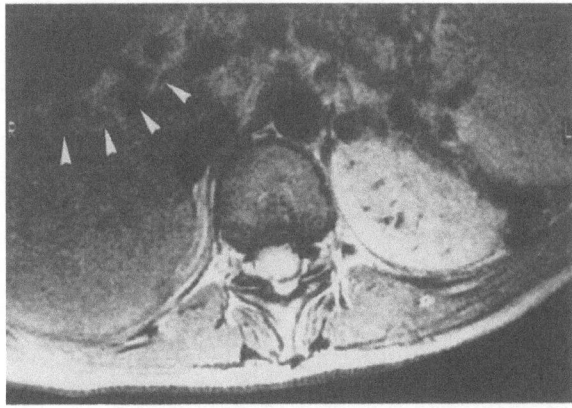

Fig. 5.43. Cavernous transformation of the portal vein showing beadlike appearance of recanalized portal vein *(arrowheads)* (SE 2000/30 ms). A surface coil placed posteriorly and 5-mm sections were used

5.4 Arteriovenous Malformations and Fistulas

As an imaging method with excellent soft-tissue contrast, MRI appears to be very useful in the evaluation of arteriovenous malformations, particularly in the lower extremities and the pelvis, where motion artifacts do not interfere with image quality. When surgery of such lesions is planned, the extent, and particularly the depth, of infiltration has to be established. Malformations confined to the subcutaneous fat can often be removed completely, whereas malformations infiltrating the underlying muscles are much more difficult to treat.

On MR images, malformations appear as regions containing multiple areas with high signal intensity on T2- and sometimes T1-weighted images, interspersed with tissue which has low signal intensity on T1-weighted images. They thus can be differentiated readily from fat and muscle, so extension into muscle groups can be defined and important information can be provided to the surgeon. However, the connection of the malformation to the deep arterial and venous structures cannot be established using conventional SE imaging. This information has to be obtained by angiographic methods, which in turn are not able to define the extent of tissue infiltration (Fig. 5.44). The two examination methods appear to be complementary [48]. Whether the vascular connections of the arteriovenous malformations can be identified on angiographic-type MR images has yet to be established. Function information cannot be provided by MRI in these disease states.

Arteriovenous fistulas may occur congenitally or be a result of trauma. MRI can demonstrate tissue changes of hyperperfusion of certain areas (Fig. 5.45), but the arteriovenous connection is usually too small to be demonstrated, and angiography has to be used. MR angiography may be useful here, but since this method is in its early investigational stages, no experience with arteriovenous fistulas has been accumulated. Since MRI has the potential to measure blood flow and is even able to image perfusion, it may provide important information on the magnitude of the shunt flow.

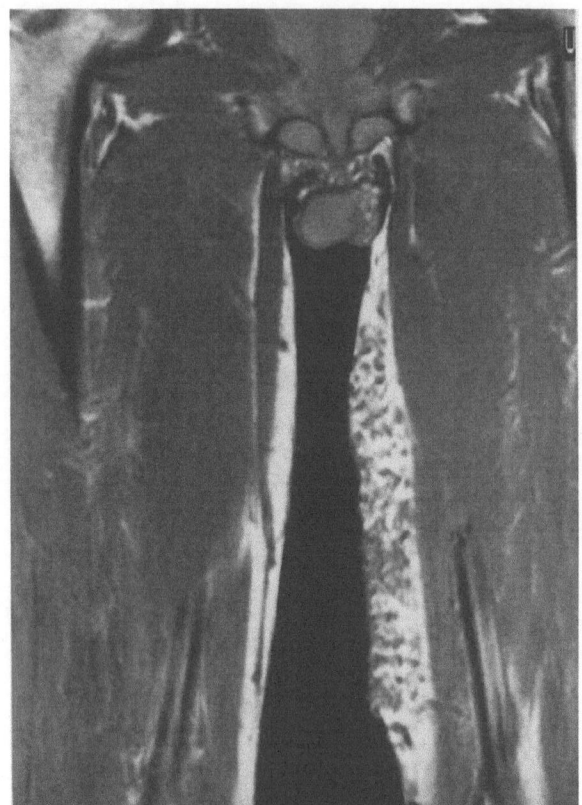

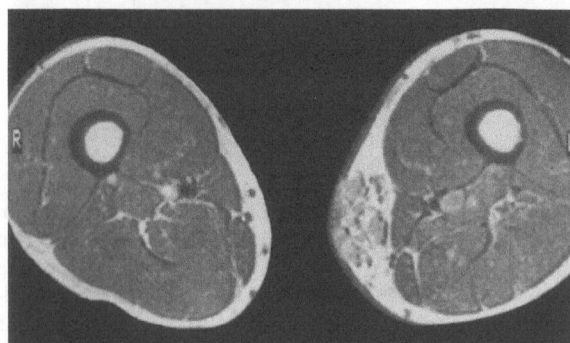

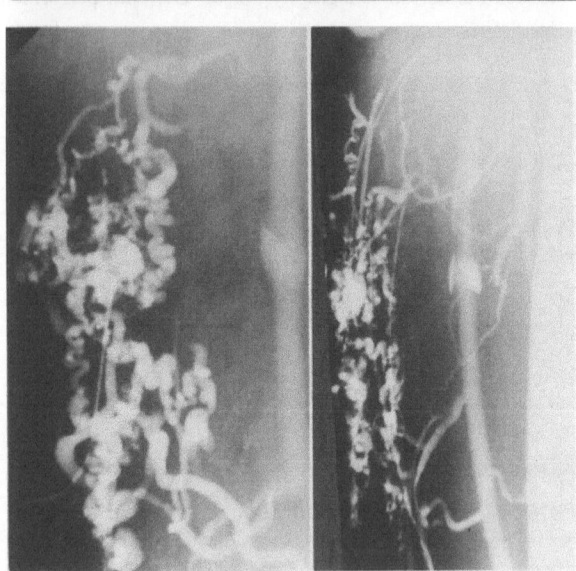

◄ **Fig. 5.44a–c.** Arteriovenous malformation of the left upper thigh. **a** MR scan (coronal SE 500/30 ms) showing multiple cystlike subcutaneous low-density regions, **b** but no muscular signal intensity increase on more T2-weighted scans (SE 2000/ 30 ms). **c** Angiography shows the hemangioma and its connection to the deep venous system, but cannot assess whether the muscle is affected

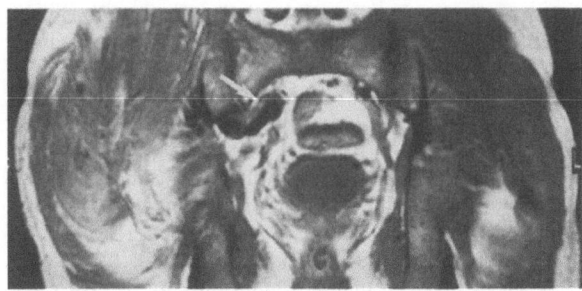

Fig. 5.45. Increased signal intensity in the right gluteal region on a coronal scan (SE 1100/30 ms) due to a hypercirculatory state resulting from an AV fistula in the region of the right internal iliac vessels *(arrow)*

5.5 Summary

MRI is very useful for imaging vascular structures and providing function information regarding vascular flow. This is a result of the intrinsically high soft-tissue/vessel contrast and the sensitivity of MRI to flow. The inferior spatial resolution of MRI compared with angiography makes MRI largely a tool for evaluating large vascular structures, but this may change with the introduction of MR-angiographic techniques. MRI has been found to be particularly useful in the evaluation of dissections and aneurysms, thrombosis, and obstruction, but its role compared with the other noninvasive imaging methods, CT and sonography, has yet to be established fully. It appears that in the mediastinum and thoracic inlet MR is at a slight advantage, whereas the motion artifacts which degrade images sometimes interfere with obtaining optimal information by MRI in the abdomen. Flow information is of interest in evaluating the severity of stenoses, establishing areas of turbulence, and distinguishing flow and thrombosis. Early results using flow-sensitive MRI are available, but the full potential of MR flow imaging has yet to be developed.

References

1. Paulin S, von Schulthess GK, Fossel E, Krayenbühl HP (1987) MR imaging of the aortic root and proximal coronary arteries. AJR 148: 665-670
2. Meuli RA, Wedeen VJ, Geller SC et al (1986) MR gated subtraction angiography: evaluation of lower extremities. Radiology 159: 411-418
3. von Schulthess GK, Fisher MR, Crooks LE, Higgins CB (1985) Gated MR imaging of the heart: intracardiac signals in patients and healthy subjects. Radiology 156: 125-132
4. von Schulthess GK, Fisher MR, Higgins CB (1985) Pathologic blood flow in pulmonary vascular disease as shown by gated magnetic resonance imaging. Ann Int Med 103: 317-323
5. Klipstein RH, Firmin DH, Underwood SR et al (1987) Colour display of quantitative blood flow and cardiac anatomy in a single magnetic resonance cine loop. Brit J Radiol 60: 105-111
6. Meier D, Maier S, Bösiger P, Moser U, Vieli G (1987) A comparative study of blood flow measurements with MR and Doppler ultrasound. SMRM, Book of abstracts, work in progress
7. von Schulthess GK, Higgins CB (1985) Blood-flow imaging with MR: spin-phase phenomena. Radiology 157: 687-695
8. Pettigrew RI, Dannels W, Galloway JR et al (1987) Quantitative phase-flow MR imaging in dogs using standard sequences. AJR 148: 411-414
9. Pettigrew RI, Dannels W (1987) Use of standard gradients with compound oblique angulation for optimal quantitative MR flow imaging in oblique vessels. AJR 148: 405-409
10. Moss AA, Gamsu G, Genant HK (1983) Computed tomography of the body. WB Saunders, Philadelphia
11. Fletcher BD, Jacobstein MD (1986) MRI of congenital abnormalities of the great arteries. AJR 146: 941-948
12. Kersting-Sommerhoff BA, Sechtem UP, Fisher MR, Higgins CB (1987) MR imaging of congenital anomalies of the aortic arch. AJR 149: 9-13
13. von Schulthess GK, Higashino SM, Higgins SS, Didier D, Fisher MR, Higgins CB (1986) Coarctation of the aorta: MR imaging. Radiology 158: 469-474
14. Formanek AG, Witcofski RL, D'Souza VJ, Link KM, Karstaedt N (1986) MR imaging of the central pulmonary arterial tree in conotruncal malformation. AJR 147: 1127-1131
15. Didier D, Higgins CB (1986) Estimation of pulmonary vascular resistance by MRI in patients with congenital cardiovascular shunt lesions. AJR 146: 919-924
16. Glazer HS, Gutierrez FR, Levitt RG, Lee JKT, Murphy WA (1985) The thoracic aorta studied by MR imaging. Radiology 157: 149-155
17. Moore EH, Webb WR, Verrier ED et al (1984) MRI of chronic post-traumatic false aneurysms of the thoracic aorta. AJR 143: 1195-1196
18. Geisinger MA, Risius B, O'Donnell JA et al (1985) Thoracic aortic dissections: magnetic resonance imaging. Radiology 155: 407-412
19. Amparo EG, Higgins CB, Hricak H, Sollitto R (1985) Aortic dissection: magnetic resonance imaging. Radiology 155: 399-406
20. Goldberg HI, Grossman RI, Gomori JM, Ashbury AK, Bilaniuk LT, Zimmerman RA (1986) Cervical internal carotid artery dissecting hemorrhage: diagnosis using MR. Radiology 158: 157-161
21. Dinsmore RE, Wedeen VJ, Miller SW et al (1986) MRI of dissection of the aorta: recognition of the intimal tear and differential flow velocities. AJR 146: 1286-1288
22. von Schulthess GK, Augustiny N (1987) Calculation of T2 values versus phase imaging for the distinction between flow and thrombus in MR imaging. Radiology 164: 549-554
23. Lee JTK, Ling D, Heiken JP et al (1984) Magnetic resonance imaging of abdominal aortic aneurysms. AJR 143: 1197-1202
24. Flak B, Li DKB, Ho BYB et al (1985) Magnetic resonance

imaging of aneurysms of the abdominal aorta. AJR 144: 991–996

25. Justich E, Amparo EG, Hricak H, Higgins CB (1985) Infected aortoiliofemoral grafts: magnetic resonance imaging. Radiology 154: 133–136

26. Wesbey GE, Higgins CB, Amparo EG, Hale JD, Kaufman L, Pogany AC (1985) Peripheral vascular disease: correlation of MR imaging and angiography. Radiology 156: 733–739

27. Augustiny N, von Schulthess GK, Meier D, Boesiger P (1987) MR imaging of large nonferromagnetic metallic implants at 1.5 T. J Comput Ass Tomogr 11: 678–683

28. Du Moulin CL, Hart HR jr (1986) Magnetic resonance angiography. Radiology 1161: 717–720

29. Miller DL, Reinig JW, Volkman DJ (1986) Vascular imaging with MRI: inadequacy in Takayasus arteritis compared with angiography. AJR 146: 949–954

30. Fisher MR, Higgins CB (1986) Central thrombi in pulmonary arterial hypertension detected by MR imaging. Radiology 158: 223–226

31. White RD, Winkler ML, Higgins CB (1987) MR imaging of pulmonary arterial hypertension and pulmonary emboli. AJR 149: 15–21

32. Stein MG, Crues III JV, Bradley WG et al (1986) MR imaging of pulmonary emboli: an experimental study in dogs. AJR 14: 1133–1137

33. Kazmier FJ, Juergens JL (1980) Venous thrombosis and obstructive diseases of the veins. In: Peripheral vascular diseases, 5th edn. Juergens JL, Spittel JA jr, Fairbairn JF II (eds). WB Saunders, Philadelphia, p 750

34. Weinreb JC, Hodges S, Garcia R (1985) Magnetic resonance imaging of patent umbilical veins. AJR 144: 747–748

35. Fisher MR, Hricak H, Higgins CB (1985) Magnetic resonance imaging of developmental venous anomalies. AJR 145: 705–707

36. Guinet C, Mathieu D, Métreau J-M, Dhumeaux D, Vasile N (1986) Unusual hepatic venous drainage in inferior vena cava obstruction: demonstration by MRI. AJR 147: 635–636

37. Hricak H, Amparo EG, Fisher MR, Crooks LE, Higgins CB (1985) Abdominal venous system: assessment using MR. Radiology 156: 415–422

38. Stark DD, Hahn PF, Trey C, Clouse ME, Ferrucci JT (1986) MRI of Budd-Chiari syndrome. AJR 146: 1141–1148

39. McMurdo KK, de Geer G, Webb WR, Gamsu G (1986) Normal and occluded mediastinal veins: MR imaging. Radiology 159: 33–38

40. Braun IF, Hoffman JC, Malko JA, Pettigrew RI, Dannels W, Davis C (1985) Jugular venous thrombosis: MR imaging. Radiology 157: 357–360

41. Duewell S, von Schulthess GK, Fuchs WA (1988) MR Venography, book of abstracts, EW Soc Mag Res Med and Biol, 189

42. Erdman WA, Weinreb JC, Cohen JM, Buja LM, Chaney C, Peshock R (1986) Venous thrombosis: clinical and experimental MR imaging. Radiology 161: 233–238

43. Senning A (1983) Transcaval posterocranial resection of the liver as treatment of the Budd-Chiari syndrome. World J Surg 7: 632–640

44. Maas D, Zollikofer CL, Largiader F, Senning A (1984) Radiological follow-up of transluminally inserted vascular endoprotheses: an experimental study using expanding spirals. Radiology 152: 659–663

45. Weinreb JC, Mootz A, Cohen JM (1986) MRI evaluation of mediastinal and thoracic inlet venous obstruction. AJR 146: 679–684

46. Bernardino ME, Steinberg HV, Pearson TC, Gedgaudas RK, Torres WE, Henderson JM (1986) Shunts for portal hypertension: MR and angiography for determination of patency. Radiology 158: 57–61

47. Duewell S, von Schulthess GK, Goebel N, Tschudi S, Ammann R (1987) 1.5 Tesla MRI of patients with echinococcosis: prospective comparison with CT. SMRM, New York, book of abstracts, 681

48. Cohen JM, Weinreb JC, Redman HC (1986) Arteriovenous malformations of the extremities: MR imaging. Radiology 158: 475–479

Chapter 6 Renal Morphology and Function in Magnetic Resonance Imaging

6.1 Renal Anatomy and Physiology Pertinent to MRI

6.1.1 Renal Morphology

The kidneys are located in the retroperitoneum, the left in a somewhat more caudal position than the right. They are surrounded by fat, and the space surrounding the kidneys is divided into fascial compartments. As in CT, these compartments can be recognized in MRI, provided that the patient is not too thin and that motion artifacts of the images are not too prominent.

The space surrounding the kidneys is divided into the anterior and posterior pararenal compartments and the perirenal spaces by the anterior and the posterior layers of the renal facia (Fig. 6.1). Between the kidneys themselves and the fascial planes there is a variable amount of fat, which, due to its high signal intensity, separates the kidneys from the surroundings, particularly on T1-weighted scans, where the kidneys themselves are of low signal in-

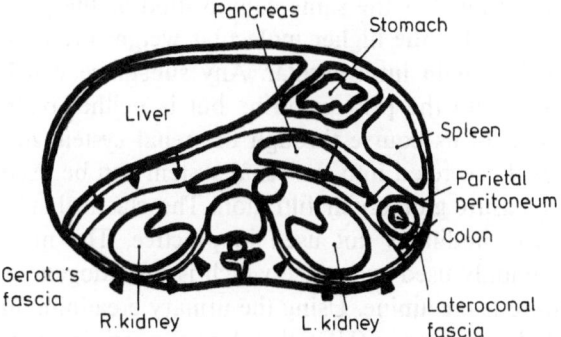

Fig. 6.1 Transverse sectional anatomy at the level of the kidneys. Note the separation of the retroperitoneum from the peritoneal space by the peritoneal fascia. Zuckerkandl's fascia separates the perirenal from the anterior pararenal space *(arrows)*. In this anterior pararenal space the pancreas, the ascending and descending colon, and the duodenum are found. The posterior pararenal space is separated from the perirenal space by Gerota's fascia *(arrowheads)* and contains mainly fat. The perirenal space contains the kidneys, adrenal glands, vessels, lymph nodes, and fat

tensity. The anterior pararenal compartment contains the pancreas, the ascending and descending colon, pars I and II of the duodenum, and the vessels supplying the liver, spleen, pancreas, and colon.

Separated by the anterior renal fascia, the right kidney is in the immediate vicinity of the vertebral column and the muscle layers of the back. Anteriorly and superiorly, it abutts the liver, and in the inferior portion the anterior renal fascia separates it from the right colon. The C-loop of the duodenum also lies in the immediate vicinity of the right kidney. The left kidney approaches the spleen antero-superiorly and is close to the left colonic flexure and the tail of the pancreas. As on the right, it is also close to the muscles of the back and the vertebral column. In the lower portions, both kidneys lie lateral to the psoas muscle, which originates from the vertebral column. The renal vessels enter and leave the renal hili to join the great vessels. The right renal artery courses posterior to the inferior vena cava, and the left renal vein swings over the aorta (Fig. 3.21). In general, the vessels follow a horizontal or slightly ascending course towards the vena cava and the descending aorta. The ureters leave the hili of the kidney to run caudally, just anterior to the psoas muscles. They are joined by the spermatic or ovarian vessels, the left vein entering the left renal vein and the right one the IVC. These veins are commonly prominent in the presence of a collateral circulation (Fig. 5.33).

The kidneys themselves are divided into a cortex, a renal medulla, and a pelvis. These structures are best appreciated on long axis cuts through the kidney, something which can in fact be done with MRI in contradistinction to CT. The cortex in adult human beings has a thickness of approximately 1 cm. The medulla is divided into 8–18 pyramids [1] whose bases abut the cortex and whose apices are in contact with the renal pelvis (Fig. 6.2). The cortex forms caps over the pyramids, resulting in the so-called renal columns of Bertin, which insert themselves between the pyramids. The glomeruli are contained in the cortex, whereas the medulla, which

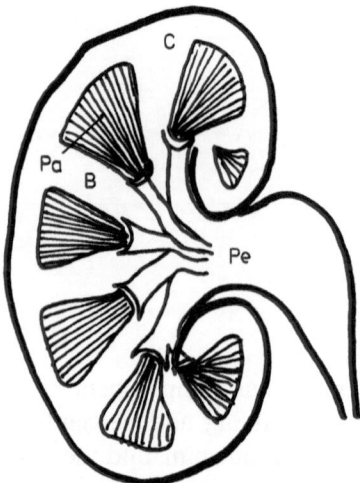

Fig. 6.2. Long-axis cut through a human kidney. The cortex touches the bases of the medullary pyramids. The cortex *(C)* also inserts itself between the pyramids *(Pa)*, forming the columns of Bertin *(B)*. The apices of the pyramids are in contact with the minor calices of the renal pelvis *(Pe)*, which in turn originate from the two to three major calices arising from the renal pelvis

can be separated into an outer and an inner zone, contain the countercurrent loops of Henle and the collecting ducts. The renal pelvis is formed by a central portion with usually three outpouchings, the major calices. From these main calices, several minor calices extend towards the renal pyramids. The renal vascular supply is as follows: The renal arteries divide into segmental arteries, which are end arteries; thus, their occlusion leads to infarction of the tissues supplied by them. In 20%–30% of cases the lower pole of each kidney is supplied by an accessory renal artery, which originates from the aorta. These main arteries give rise to segmental arteries, which in turn give rise to the interlobular arteries located along the columns of Bertin. The branches of the interlobular arteries are the arcuate arteries, which tend to lie parallel to the kidney surface at the border between cortex and outer medulla. The venous drainage occurs through arcuate and interlobular veins which run parallel to the arteries. They drain through several main trunks into the renal vein.

6.1.2 Renal Physiology

The main function of the kidneys is the filtration of the plasma and the excretion of "waste" molecules in the form of urine. The smallest functional unit of the kidney is the nephron. It consists of the glomerulus, the descending and ascending limbs of the

loops of Henle, the proximal and distal convoluted tubules, and the collecting ducts. Whereas the glomeruli and the proximal and distal convoluted tubules are located in the renal cortex, the ascending and descending loops of Henle and the collecting ducts are located in the medulla. The medullary configuration of these structures and the surrounding vasa recta are necessary for the function of the well-recognized renal "countercurrent loop" system. This permits the kidney to concentrate the urine in a wide range of osmolarities and up to 1200 mosmol in human beings. In MR imaging, the mechanisms of glomerular filtration and renal secretion are of relevance, as it is these processes which can be evaluated by injecting exogenous paramagnetic molecules into a patient and thus help to assess renal function. In order to understand the renal filtration and secretion processes, we briefly describe the fate of a substance in the blood arriving at the kidneys.

The total blood flow through the kidneys is about 1200 ml/min in the adult [2], that is, approximately one fifth of the cardiac output. The kidneys themselves weigh together about 300 g. Thus, they are by far the most highly perfused organs in the body. Most of the blood entering the kidneys remains in the cortex, and only 1% reaches the inner medulla. With a total blood flow of 1200 ml/min the renal plasma flow (RPF) is 600 ml/min, if a hematocrit of 50% is assumed. Part of this plasma is filtered by the glomeruli, with essentially all solutes with a molecular weight of <70000 daltons passing the glomerular "sieve". The filtration ratio is 20%–25% thus, the glomerular filtration rate (GFR) is approximately 120–150 ml/min. This ultrafiltrate, the primary urine, has the same composition as the plasma, save for the higher molecular weight proteins, which remain intravascular. Any substance which passes into the primary urine but is neither reabsorbed in its course through the renal system nor actively secreted into the renal system can be used to measure glomerular filtration. The classical substance, inulin, is not used in practice. The most commonly used substance which is of endogenous nature is creatinine. Using the urinary creatinine in a 24-h urine in mg (UC), the plasma creatinine concentration in mg/100 ml, and the fact that 1440 is the number of minutes in 24 h, the creatinine clearance C_{creat} is given by:

$$C_{creat} = (UC \times 100)/(P \times 1440) \qquad (6.1)$$

which has the dimensions of ml/min. Other substances which are glomerularly filtered are the iodinated contrast compounds used in roentgenographic diagnostic procedures, the chelates of metal ions, such as technetium-EDTA or DTPA used in nuclear medicine, and Gd-DTPA, Gd-DOTA, and ferrioxamine derivatives, which are all used in various stages of trials as "contrast" agents for MRI.

Volume, concentration, and composition of the primary urine are altered in the tubules and collecting ducts by reabsorption and secretion of solutes. Schematically, this is represented in Fig. 6.3. It is seen that in the descending limb, water and sodium ions diffuse freely into the medulla and the urine, respectively, to remain in equilibrium with the concentrations in the environment of the outer and then inner parts of the medulla. This hyperosmolar environment of up to 1200 mosmol in humans is generated by the active process of sodium secretion in the ascending limb of the loop of Henle. The result is that by the time the urine has passed through the descending and ascending loops of Henle it has been concentrated by a factor of 8, and by the time it enters the collecting ducts, by a factor of 20. Further passive reabsorption of water occurs during the passage down the collecting ducts, such that the final concentration of glomerularly filtered substances in urine is on the order of 200 times that of primary urine. It may vary depending on the concentration of antidiuretic hormone, which regulates the amount of water reabsorption.

Substances which are actively excreted on first pass can be used to measure the clearance of secreted substances. Bilirubin is actively secreted. Exogenous substances also undergoing this fate are penicillin and Hippuran. A radiolabelled analog of this later substance, orthoiodo-hippuric acid, is used in nuclear medicine for the assessment of renal secretion. This compound is secreted to approximately 90% on first pass.

Very valuable substances such as amino acids and glucose are also present in the primary urine. They are reabsorbed to practically 100% in normals (but not in diabetics, where the reabsorption mechanism is overwhelmed!). This reabsorption process is of no further importance if one is interested in understanding the renal handling of glomerularly filtered substances such as Gd-DTPA, Gd-DOTA, another gadolinium chelator, and ferrioxamine compounds, which are chelators highly specific for iron. A bolus of contrast agent passing through the kidney is first glomerularly filtered, then concentrated in the medulla as it passes through the tubules and loops of Henle. Thus, the concentrated "bolus" travels through the nephrons with a typical transit time. From renal function studies with Tc-

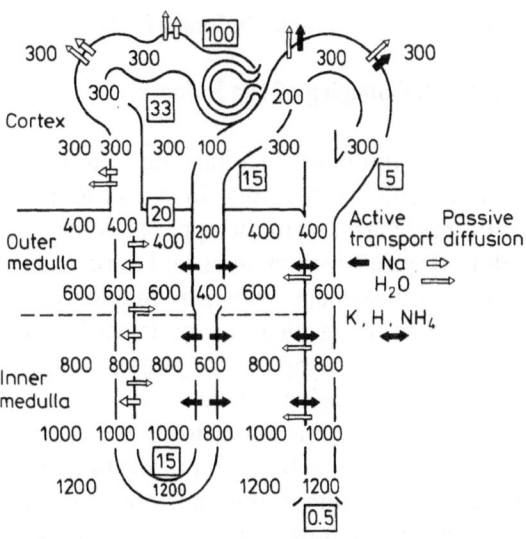

Fig. 6.3. The countercurrent scheme of urine concentration and preservation of water, extending from the cortex into the outer and inner medulla. The numbers give osmolalities in milliosmols, showing the concentrated environment in the inner medulla. The boxed numbers give urine concentration along its pathway, relative to the primary urine coming from the glomerulus and taken to be 100 (arbitrary number). (Reprinted with permission from Scheitlin and Buehlmann [2])

DTPA it is known that this transit time through the nephrons is on the order of 3-6 min. After bolus injection, such a substance is expected to attain its peak concentration in the kidney within 3 to 6 min, whereas the initial perfusion phase of the kidney after venous injection lasts only about 30 s. Close to total clearance of a glomerularly filtered substance takes on the order of an hour. Hence, the renal excretion and filtration obey grossly a 30″-3′-30′ or 60″-6′60′ rule for the times during which mainly perfusion, then perfusion plus filtration/secretion, and finally urinary elimination as well as filtration/secretion and perfusion take place.

Various disease states interfere with normal handling of glomerularly filtered substances. In prerenal pathologies, the perfusion pressure of the kidneys may become so low that filtration is no longer possible. This occurs typically if the pressure drops below 60 mmHg in patients with cardiac failure, renal arterial thrombosis, and stenosis. Renal parenchymal diseases lead to various forms of renal dysfunction. Finally, postrenal obstruction can cause renal dysfunction. In this disease, the pressure in the renal pelvis rises, thus reducing the concentrating ability of the kidneys and eventually damaging them.

6.2 Technical Considerations in Renal MRI

6.2.1 Spin-Echo Imaging of the Kidneys

Unfortunately, spin-echo (SE) imaging in apnea is not possible. This often results in a considerable number of image artifacts in the upper abdomen [3], due both to respiratory excursions and to peristaltic motion of the bowel loops, which are in close vicinity to the kidneys. Image degradation is particularly strong at high field strengths. Respiratory motion leads to marked excursions of the kidneys, which, depending on the respiratory state of the patient, can vary in their position by 1–2 cm. The basic motion of the kidneys with respiration is one of sliding up and down on the psoas muscles. Since the kidneys are fixed by the hilar vessels and ureters, they also perform a slight rotatory motion during respiration. As a result of these motions, the kidneys are among the most difficult organs to image in MRI [4].

In addition to the technical limitations, standard use of MR contrast media for imaging the kidneys is not yet established, further reducing the diagnostic information obtainable from a renal MRI exam compared with that from CT. There is thus rarely an indication to perform MRI in the early stages of a diagnostic renal workup [5].

The imaging coil used in MRI of the kidneys is usually the body coil, with its high field of view but its relatively poor signal to noise ratio. If a patient is slim and the examination can be limited to the region of the kidney, a posteriorly applied surface coil, such as a transversely positioned spine coil or round surface coil, may be of use (Fig. 5.43). For renal transplants, surface coil imaging with the patient in prone or supine position is preferable.

Fig. 6.4a–f. Normal coronal scans through the kidneys **a–c** Spin-echo images using a TR of 500 and 2000 ms, respectively, and echo times of 30 and 60 ms. **a** SE 500/30 ms; **b** 2000/30 ms; **c** 2000/60 ms. Note the corticomedullary differentiation on the T1-weighted image, which often does not appear as clearly as in renal transplants (Fig. 6.27) because of the more severe motion artifacts in the upper abdomen. **d–f** Gradient echo images taken in the same patient, again during apnea and with more T1- and T2-weighted parameter settings (**d** GFE 50/16.1 ms, α = 70°; **e** 50/30.3, and **f** 50/60.6 ms; α = 20°). **e** Note the absence of motion artifacts due to apnea scanning and anatomic detail not much inferior to that in SE scanning

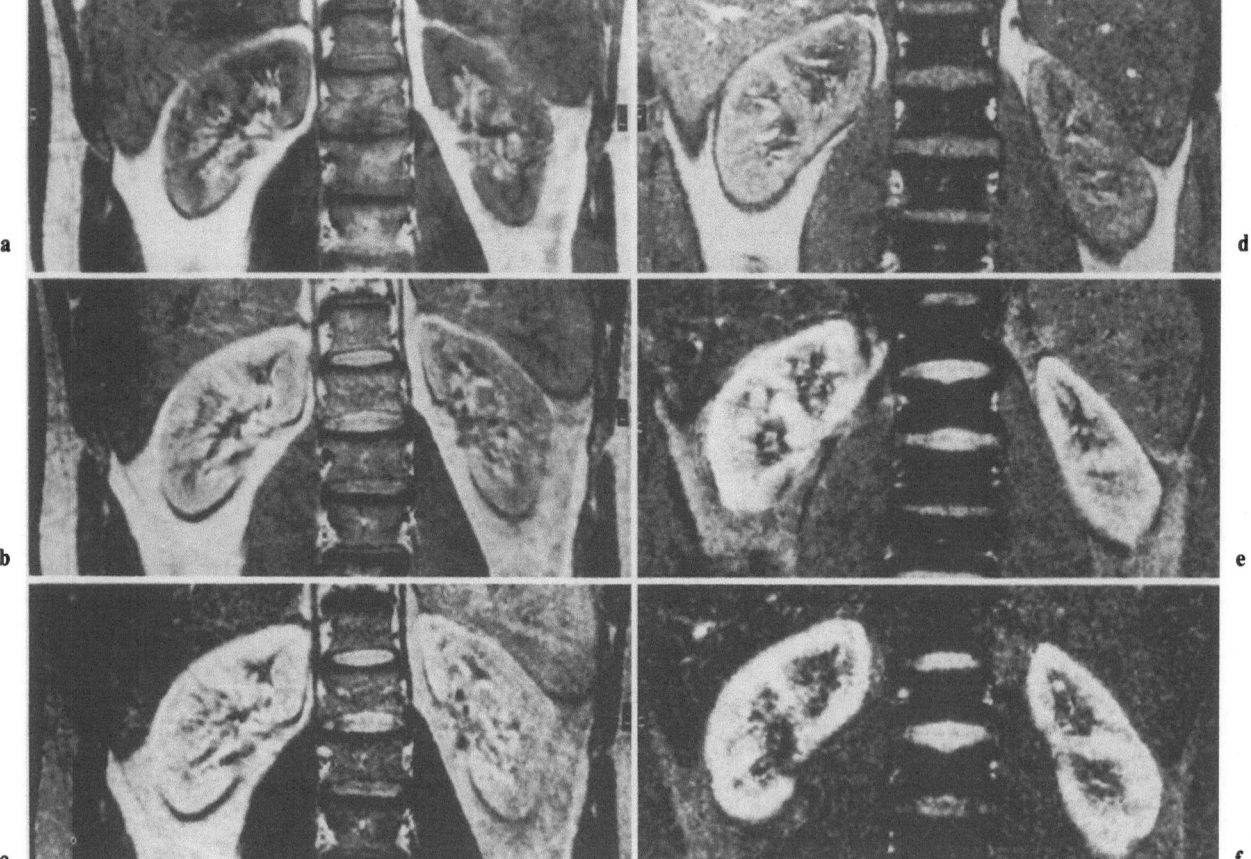

The pulse sequences used in MR examinations of the kidneys do not differ substantially from the pulse sequences used in other organs [3, 6], and imaging strategies have been clearly defined. In most situations, acquisition of T1- and T2-weighted sequences is necessary. On T1-weighted images, the corticomedullary differentiation between renal cortex and medulla can be appreciated. This differentiation is lost on more T2-weighted images, where the kidneys with their high fluid content become very bright structures (Fig. 6.4). In fact, they become so bright that the differentiation of tumor tissue from renal tissue often is possible only by the resulting contour abnormalities [7]. Loss of corticomedullary differentiation is a nonspecific finding associated with many disease states, such as infection and renal transplant rejection [3].

The imaging planes to be used are transverse or coronal in most instances. Transverse scans clearly demonstrate the relation of the kidneys to the psoas muscle, the fascial planes of the perirenal space, the vessels, and the more lateral parts of the liver and spleen. However, infiltration of these two organs and the psoas muscles by tumor is often better assessed using coronal and, rarely, sagittal scans. The coronal scans (Fig. 6.4) have the further advantage of yielding a larger field of view, at times permitting imaging of the entire abdomen and pelvis. Unfortunately, peristaltic motion and respiration artifacts make image quality in coronal planes anterior to the great abdominal vessels poor.

6.2.2 Gradient Echo Imaging of the Kidneys

Gradient echo imaging of the kidneys has two distinct advantages over spin-echo imaging. First, apnea imaging is possible, as good images may be obtained in a few seconds, typically 10–15 s with a 256×256 matrix resolution (Fig. 6.4d–e). Imaging time may be further shortened by reducing the number of phase-encode steps, thereby lowering the resolution in one spatial dimension. Second, the imaging time, which may be chosen as short as 2–3 s, is sufficiently short to temporally resolve the renal transit of a glomerularly filtered substance such as Gd-DTPA [8]. Since the same imaging plane may be examined many times without exposure to ionizing radiation, MR function studies to examine the handling of glomerularly filtered substances become possible [9]. MR studies evaluating renal secretion are not possible at present because of the lack of a paramagnetic agent to label the secretion process.

Static gradient echo imaging yields images of good quality (Fig. 6.4). T1- and T2-weighting are accomplished by chosing large flip angles ($\approx > 70°$) and short echo times (< 20 ms) and small flip angles ($10°$–$20°$) and longer echo times (30–60 ms, for example) respectively. The influence of proton density is more marked in such gradient echo images that in spin-echo images.

6.2.3 Dynamic Gradient Echo Imaging Using Contrast Agents

For dynamic scanning, imaging protocols combining either 5- or 10-s apnea scanning, interleaved with 5- or 10-s respiratory pauses, have been successfully tested and are tolerated well by all patients but those with severe respiratory disease [10]. The flip angles used in these studies are between $40°$ and $50°$, approximately corresponding to the Ernst angle, which optimizes the signal obtained in gradient echo imaging (Sect. 1.4.8). T1- or T2-weighting is not necessary in such studies, because plenty of contrast is achieved with the injected contrast medium and the main goal is to obtain as much signal as possible. Care has to be taken in chosing the proper echo time. It is extremely useful to acquire opposed-phase images (Sects. 1.4.7 and 1.5.5), because a dark line usually appears around the kidneys (Fig. 1.35), corresponding to pixels which contain the watery renal parenchyma as well as perirenal fat, and which make automatic edge detection relatively easy. For magnets operating at 1.5 Tesla (63.9 MHz), the time for which water and fat spins are out of phase by $180°$ is 2.33 ms. Echo times corresponding to odd multiples of this time, e.g., 16.3 ms, should thus be used. Long axis cuts through both kidneys can be obtained by moderate anterior angulation of coronal imaging planes after appropriate sagittal localizing scans through both kidneys have been acquired. The coronal angulated scans offer the most information, as they show large portions of the renal parenchyma as well as the renal pelves. These planes intersect the great abdominal vessels, usually in their caudal portion, and because of the high intravascular signal intensity (Sect. 3.1.2) and the phase-encode artifacts (Sect. 3.5.1) resulting from the pulsatile aortic flow, image quality in the lower portions of the image can be degraded with the usual right-left phase-encode direction. Alternatively, coronal imaging with a large field of view and craniocaudal phase encoding can be done to project the artifacts away from the lower parts of the kidney and in a craniocaudal direction. In order to cover most of the filtration and excretion time course, imaging should be done over the first 15 min after bolus injection; thus, two or three dynamic sequences containing 15–30 images, each lasting 3–5 min overall should be acquired.

Typically, a dynamic sequence is started with the bolus injection of a contrast medium into the antecubital vein with the patient in his final position in the magnet. For Gd-DTPA [11] and Gd-DOTA the recommended standard doses are 0.1 mmol/kg body weight. There is a saline flush immediately following contrast medium injection.

In order to extract quantitative information from the dynamic sequences, region of interest (ROI) analysis of the renal parenchymal components and the pelves has to be performed, similar to the procedures in nuclear medicine. The difficulty in doing this is that the images obtained are of much higher spatial resolution than scintigraphic images. The slightly different inspiratory or expiratory apnea levels which occur during the course of a dynamic

scan sequence result in a variable position of the kidneys on different images. This prohibits the use on subsequent images of an ROI defined on the first image. Either the ROI has to be adjusted manually in its position in each image [10] or computer algorithms adjusting subsequent images relative to the starting one have to be used [12]. In our algorithm developed for this purpose, significant edges in the images are first extracted on the starting image of the dynamic sequence (Fig. 6.5). The best-matching edges are then found on subsequent im-

Fig. 6.5a–d. Automatic edge detection in MRI. **a** On a starting image, the **b** regions of interest (ROIs) for the kidneys are identified. **c** Significant contours are then extracted on the other images of the dynamic sequence. **d** Using a so-called Hough transformation, the best match between the starting ROI and the contour map of the other images is identified. This best match defines the distances by which each kidney has to be shifted on all the other images relative to the first one for optimal positional readjustment. Once this readjustment has been done, an ROI placed on the starting image will fall into the same anatomic region for all subsequent images

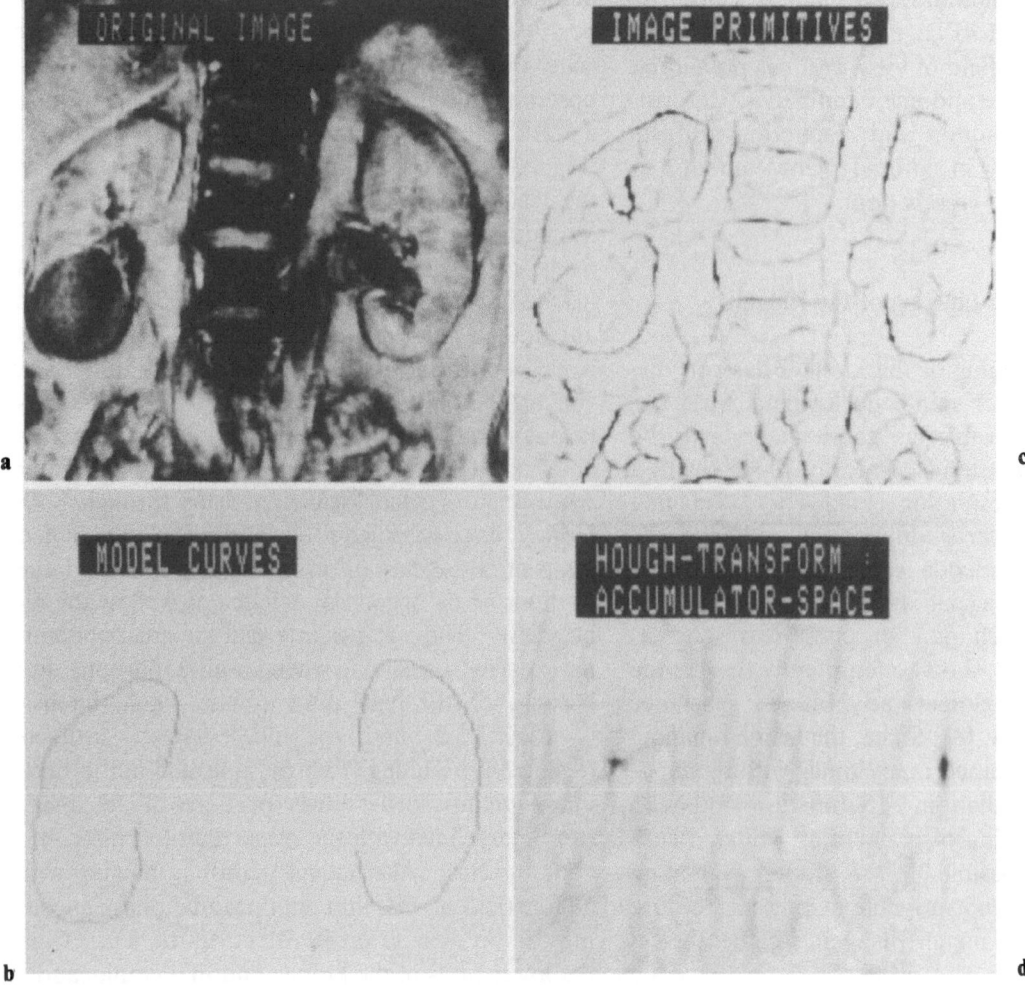

ages using a Hough transformation [13]. Each kidney is positionally readjusted such that renal ROIs placed on the starting image cover the same anatomic region on the subsequent images [13]. From such readjusted dynamic sequences, signal intensity versus time curves can then be extracted.

6.3 Normal Morphology and Function of the Kidneys in MRI

6.3.1 Normal Renal Morphology in MRI

The present technical limitations in imaging the kidneys with MRI have been discussed above. On T1-weighted images, particularly on coronal and sagittal scans, the cortex and the medullary pyramids can be distinguished: normal kidneys show corticomedullary differentiation on T1-weighted images (Figs. 6.4 and 6.26). The renal pelvis, if it contains any significant amount of urine, is dark, and the normal ureters usually cannot be identified. The kidneys can be well separated from the perirenal fat, but less well from the liver and the surrounding muscles. On T2-weighted images the corticomedullary differentiation is lost and the renal parenchyma appear homogeneous (Figs. 6.4 and 6.26). Urine, like any other fluid, becomes very bright, and the kidney is not clearly distinguishable from the perirenal fat. However, differentiation from the liver and the surrounding muscles is clear. The renal veins are seen in their entire course from the kidneys to the vena cava in most instances (Fig. 5.5). Imaging of the renal arteries is sometimes more difficult, and thin transverse slices of 5 mm have to be used, particularly if the origins of the renal arteries have to be identified relative to an aortic aneurysm (Fig. 5.27). Common imaging artifacts on SE images are the chemical shift effect (Fig. 3.21) and spatial misregistration phenomena (Sect. 3.5.3).

The appearance of renal morphology on gradient echo images is similar (Fig. 6.4) to that on SE images, except for the fact that vascular structures appear bright.

6.3.2 Normal Renal Function Studies with MRI

The signal intensity changes in renal dynamic scanning are interesting and initially somewhat difficult to understand, because the relation between signal intensity and concentration of a paramagnetic contrast medium in the tissue of interest is nonlinear

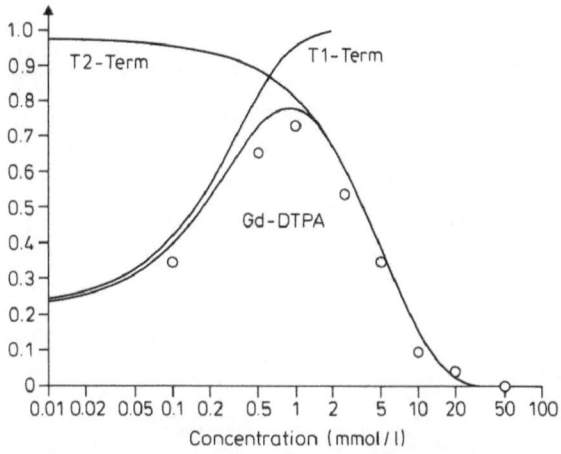

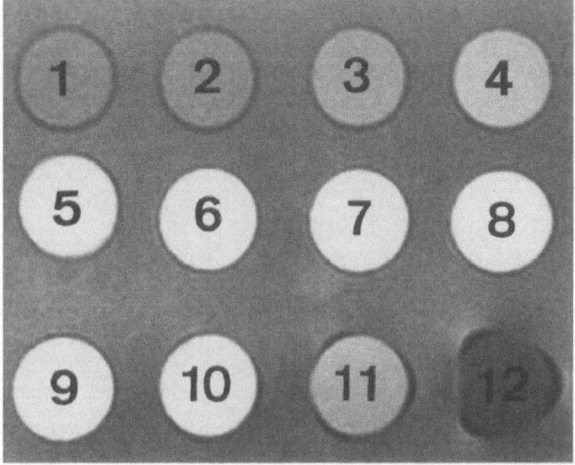

Fig. 6.6. a Signal intensity versus concentration curve for Gd-DTPA (SE 500/28 ms, 15 MHz, after Grodd and Brasch [14]). Note the nonlinear behavior. The initial rise in signal intensity is due to T1-shortening. At higher concentration of the contrast medium, T2-shortening effects start to supervene, leading eventually to a signal drop at higher concentration. **b** This can also be seen in the dilution series. (SE 500/30 ms) At the highest concentration, susceptibility effects lead to triangular distortions of the test tube image (1 = 40, 2 = 80, 3 = 160, 4 = 320, 5 = 640 µmol/l, 6 = 1.03, 7 = 1.75, 8 = 2.0, 9 = 6.5, 10 = 12.5, 11 = 25, 12 = 50 mmol/l)

[14]. Figure 6.6 shows data for various paramagnetic compounds and images of a dilution series of ferrioxamine B in test tubes. Whereas in standard applications of paramagnetic agents the tissue concentrations of these compounds are in the ascending limb of the Gd-DTPA curve of Fig. 6.6a, this is not necessarily the case in renal imaging. This is a result of the renal concentrating ability for glomerularly filtered substances such as Gd-DTPA, and in fact, a simple calculation makes this clear. It was stated in Sect. 6.1.2 that normal kidneys concentrate the primary urine by a factor of approximately 200. If a standard dose of 0.1 mmol/kg body weight of Gd-DTPA is injected into a patient of 70 kg, the extracellular volume, which corresponds roughly to the

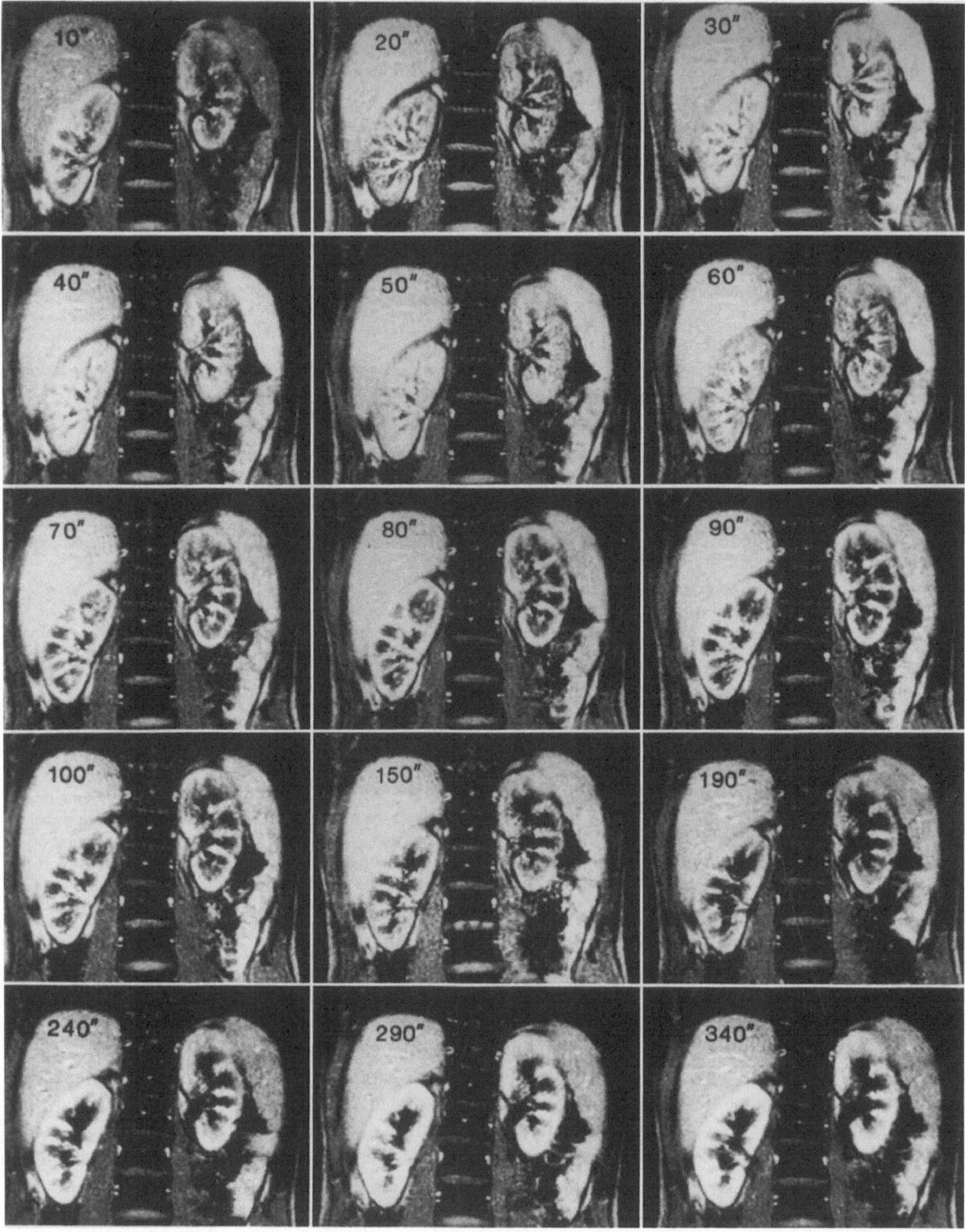

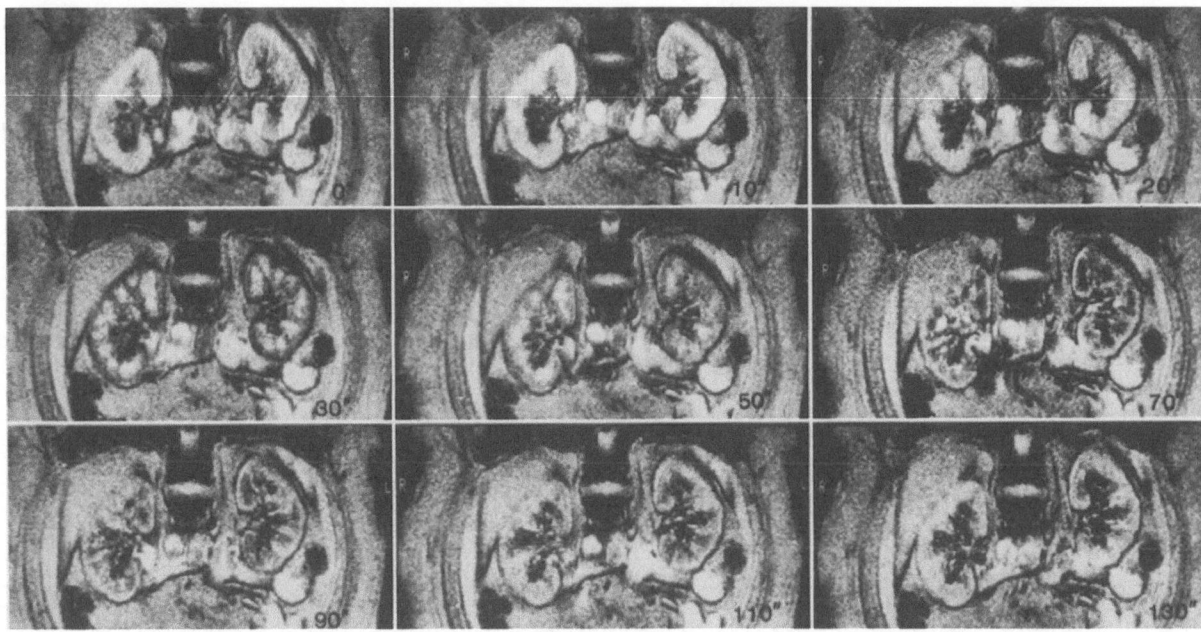

Fig. 6.8. Same imaging parameters as in Fig. 6.7 in a patient with normal renal parenchyma after shock wave lithotripsy. Presumably, the bolus quality during Gd-DTPA injection was very good. The result is seen in the nine images of a dynamic scan presented here. In distinction to Fig. 6.7, there is a signal drop in the cortex after an initial rise (30″), occurring somewhat earlier than in the medulla (70″). Other signal intensity changes are similar to the ones in Fig. 6.7

◀ **Fig. 6.7.** Fifteen dynamic images through the long axis of the kidneys in a normal volunteer. Imaging parameters were TR = 30 ms, TE = 16.1 ms, α = 40°, ca. 170 phase-encode steps, one measurement, scan time per image ca. 5 s. The time elapsed since the bolus injection of 0.1 mmol Gd-DTPA/kg body weight is found on each image. Note initial signal intensity rise in the cortex (30″) and more prominently in the medulla (40″). Whereas the cortex in this subject stays more or less isointense, there is a marked papillary signal drop after approximately 70 s. This makes the papillae sharply contrasted against the other renal structures and reflects their ability to concentrate Gd-DTPA. In later images, after several 100 s, the renal pelvis, which was small and void of signal in the early images, appears to grow in size. This is probably an artifact due to susceptibility change-induced signal dropout in the structures surrounding the urine in the pelvis, which now has a very high Gd-DTPA concentration

distribution volume of Gd-DTPA, is 14 liters. Thus, a concentration of about 0.5 mmol/liter is an estimation of the lowest initial concentration of Gd-DTPA. This is concentrated by 200 to about 100 mmol/liter in the medullary pyramids and the urine, a concentration which is definitely in a region where signal loss due to T2 effects dominates the signal behavior of the urine [10]. As a result, one expects the renal signal intensity to drop in the kidneys after an initial rise.

This behavior has indeed been observed using Gd-DTPA [10] and is demonstrated in a dynamic sequence in normal patients in Figs. 6.7 and 6.8. In an image without contrast medium, the renal cortex is somewhat brighter than the medulla and appears gray, comparable to the liver. In the earliest phase after contrast medium injection there is an increase in cortical signal (perfusion phase in the first 30–60 s), followed by an increase in medullary signal. After an initial period of about 1 min, there is a variable drop in cortical signal and then a marked drop in the signal of the medullary pyramids. The strength of cortical signal drop probably depends on the quality of the contrast medium bolus. This signal drop migrates from the pyramidal bases to the apices (glomerular filtration phase between 60 and about 300 s), and its strength is an expression of renal concentrating ability. Finally, the renal pelvis turns dark (excretion phase). A signal intensity versus time curve for a normal renal cortex and pyramid are plotted in Fig. 6.9. The curve clearly demonstrates a signal drop and subsequent rise of sig-

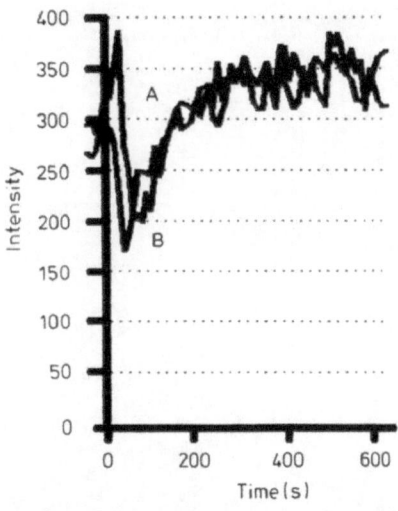

◀ **Fig. 6.9.** Signal intensity versus time curves of cortex and medulla in the patient imaged Fig. 6.8. The signal behavior described in the images above is clearly seen. The medullary signal intensity *(A)* drops after the cortical signal intensity *(B)* by approxiately 30 s as a result of renal transit time from the glomeruli into the papillae

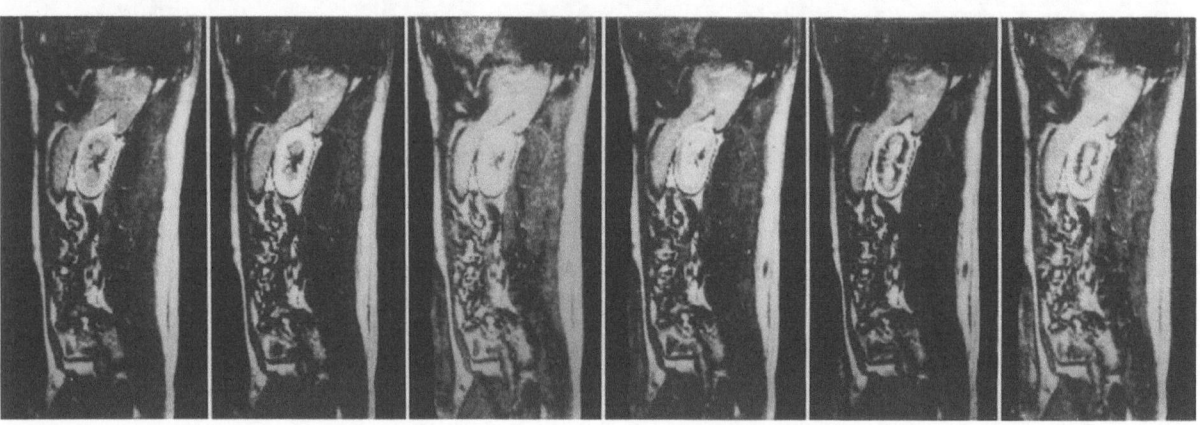

Fig. 6.10. Six images of a dynamic sequence (sagittal, GFE 40/16.1 ms, α = 40°) through the left kidney of a dog after bolus injection with a derivative of ferrioxamine B, showing the migration of a dark band of highly concentrated contrast agent from the renal cortex across the pyramids towards the pelvis as time progresses. This occurs in a manner completely analogous to the behavior of Gd-DTPA seen in Figs. 6.7 and 6.8

nal in the expected time scales. This latter effect is a result of the dilution of the contrast agent in the kidney by glomerular filtrate, containing less and less paramagnetic agent as the clearance of the substance progresses. Identical behavior can be seen with a derivative of ferrioxamine B (Fig. 6.10). Thus, the dynamic signal intensity behavior of the various renal portions after injection of paramagnetic agents can be readily explained with the nonlinear signal intensity versus contrast medium curve found in vitro.

6.4 Pathologic Morphology and Function of the Kidneys in MRI

As stated above, MRI of morphological renal abnormalities offers no striking advantages over CT imaging, aside from its multiplanar imaging capability. The almost standard use of contrast media in renal CT, apnea scanning, a higher spatial resolution, and the ability of CT to detect renal calculi as very hyperdense structures ar all advantages which have to be weighted before MRI is chosen over CT to image a patient. Nevertheless, MRI of various renal disease entities will be discussed, because fast apnea scanning using contrast media as well as flow artifact suppression methods are around the corner and promise to make renal MRI much more competitive very soon.

Congenital anomalies involving the morphology or position of the kidneys can be examined with MRI. Congenital anomalies of the ureters are best evaluated using intravenous urograms (IVUs) and are difficult to identify on MRI unless they are dilated. Our attention will focus on acquired disease.

6.4.1 Renal Obstruction

The morphology of renal obstruction is best examined with T1-weighted images, because on these images urine has a very low signal intensity and is clearly separable from the renal parenchyma and the surrounding fat, showing a dilated renal pelvis or ureter (Fig. 6.11). The site of obstruction can be located on either transverse or coronal images. Differentiation of causes of obstruction is possible [15]. Tumors can be differentiated from retroperitoneal fibrosis as the cause, because retroperitoneal fibrosis, in contradistinction to tumors, has low signal intensity on T2-weighed images as well [15]. Hematomas usually can also be identified (see Sect. 6.4.3). Even though renal calculi appear as structures without signal, they are much more difficult to detect on MRI than on CT, where they appear bright. There is a distinct difference in the appearance of acutely obstructed (<7 days) and chronically obstructed kidneys. Whereas the former show corticomedullary differentiation on T1-weighted images, this is lost in the latter situation [16]. In addition to loss of the corticomedullary differentiation in chronic

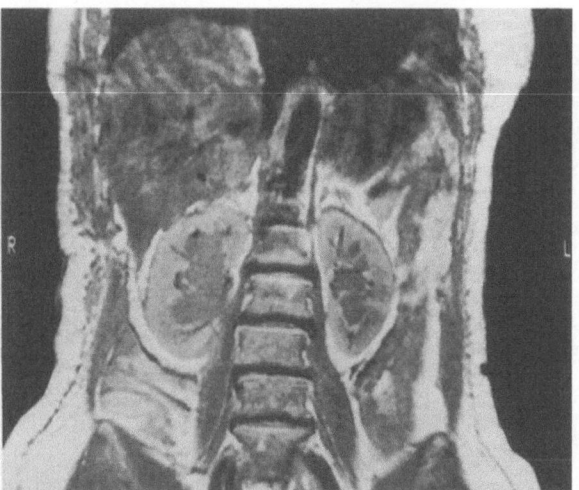

Fig. 6.11. Coronal SE image (1100/30 ms) in which the obstructed pelvis, containing low signal intensity urine is clearly outlined against the renal parenchyma. Parenchymal thickness is maintained excluding long-standing obstruction

obstruction, there is also loss of renal parenchyma (Fig. 6.12).

Renal obstruction results in decreased renal excretory function and, if present for too long, re-

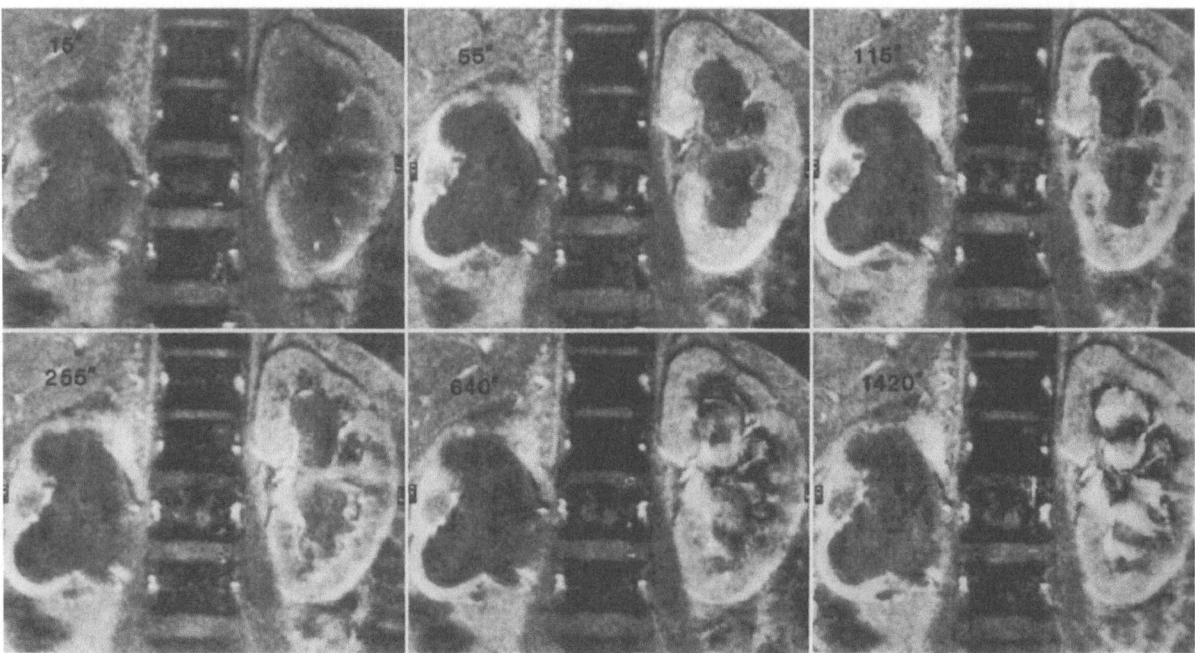

Fig. 6.12. Six dynamic scans post Gd-DTPA injection in a patient with bilateral hydronephrosis due to tumorous obstruction in the pelvis (GFE 40/16.1 ms, $\alpha = 40°$). Note the right kidney, which is small and consists of very few parenchyma surrouding an extremly dilated pelvis. The pelvis on the left is dilated as well, but the parenchyma seem intact. Compared with the normal dynamic contrast scans, two intersting features are noted. First, the papillae in the two kidneys do not turn dark some 100 s after injection, but compared with the right, the left kidney seems to enhance more in the time course of the scan. Second, the left pelvis enhances in the late images, showing that, despite its impaired function, it is still able to excrete the contrast medium, albeit at a lower than normal concentration, where we would expect opacification of the renal pelvis. This is a result of the impaired renal concentrating ability. The reduced amount of parenchyma in the right kidney and the lack of pelvic enhancement together suggest a virtually nonfunctioning kidney

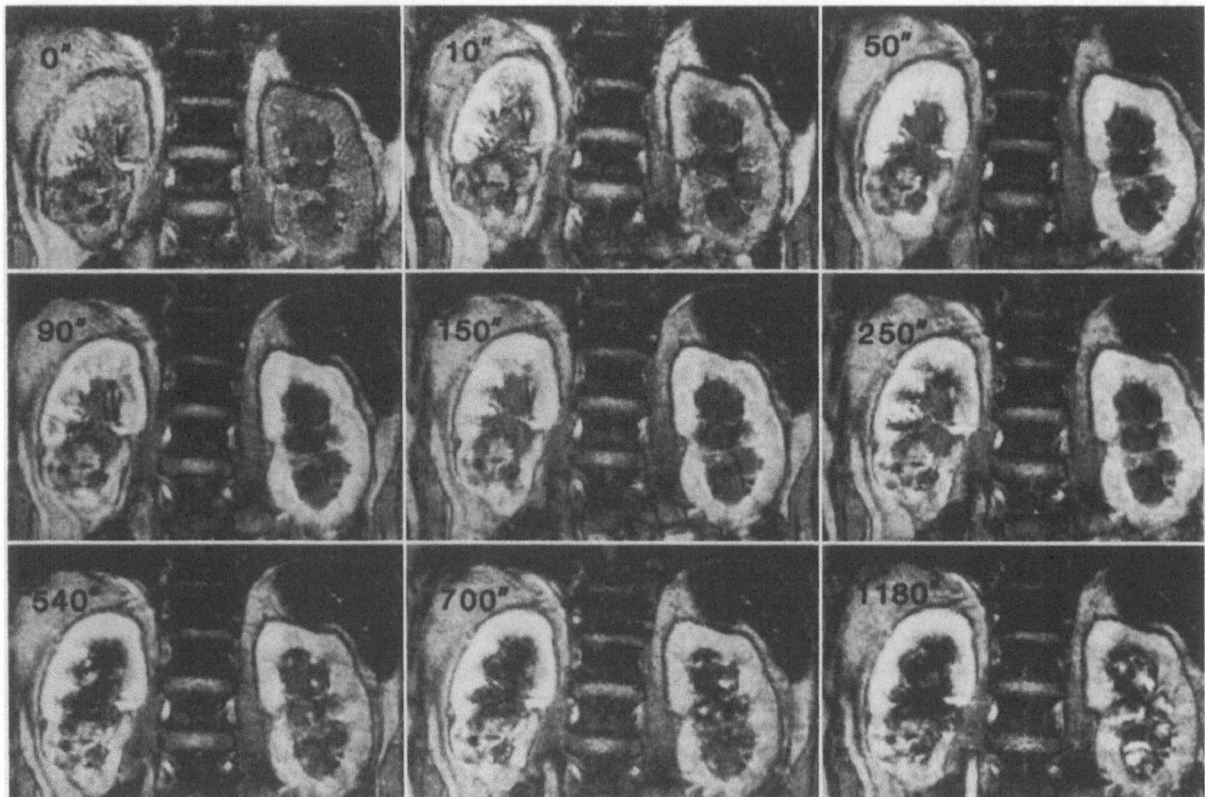

Fig. 6.13. Nine sequential images in a patient with right lower pole renal hypernephroma and left hydronephrosis (GFE 40/16.1 ms, $\alpha = 40°$). Whereas the normal portions of the right kidney show darkening of the pyramids, as expected with normal function, this is absent in the hydronephrotic left kidney. The left kidney shows pelvic increase in signal intensity over the time course of the examintion, whereas the right renal pelvis remains dark. The tumor in the right kidney shows enhancement (Sect. 6.4.5)

sults in damage and eventually loss of renal function. The transit of paramagnetic contrast agents in obstructed kidneys has been evaluated recently in humans [10]. There is cortical and medullary enhancement after injection of contrast medium, as can be seen in the representative images of the dynamic sequences in Figs. 6.12 and 6.13. However, the obstructed kidneys show no clear decrease in medullary signal intensity during the time of expected maximum contrast medium concentration, 3–6 min after Gd-DTPA injection, which is in contradistinction to normals. The renal pelvis, initially showing little or no signal on more T1-weighted gradient echo images, becomes more and more intense as the time after injection increases (Figs. 6.12 and 6.13). This is simply the result of a decreased renal concentrating ability, and it has been suggested that this phenomenon may be used to semiquantitatively assess renal function [10]. Corresponding function curves are shown in Fig. 6.14.

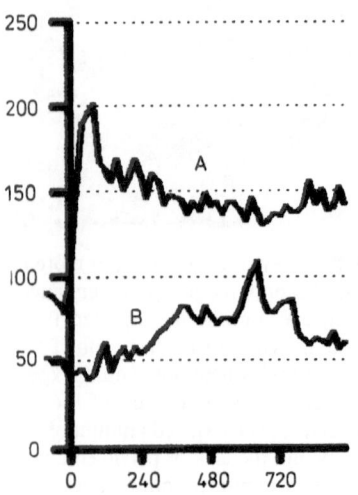

◀ **Fig. 6.14.** Function curves in renal obstruction from the left kidney in Fig. 6.13 *(A)* The renal medulla shows contrast enhancement after injection of Gd-DTPA, but due to impaired function, the signal drop expected in normals after the first 100 s and the subsequent rise are not present. *(B)* The renal pelvic function curve of the left kidney shows a gradual increase in signal intensity due to obstruction

6.4.2 Infectious and Noninfectious Renal Parenchymal Disease

Renal infectious disease is primarily diagnosed on clinical presentation and laboratory findings [17]. There is rarely a need to use imaging beyond ultrasonography. Usually, one finds renal parenchymal enlargement due to edema, and infections present as wedge-shaped cortical phlegmons or frank abscesses. The latter often extend into the perirenal tissue and even into the posterior chest wall (Fig. 6.15). The signal intensity changes are nonspecific, with a loss of corticomedullary differentiation on T1-weighted images in the afflicted renal portions. On T2-weighted images, simple edematous portions cannot be differentiated from normal kidney portions, which are also bright on T2-weighted images. Thus, diagnosis has to rely mostly on anatomical alterations. If an abscess is present, its signal intensity is usually lower than that of normal kidneys on T1-weighted images.

Noninfectious parenchymal disease may be due to glomerulonephritis, interstitial nephritis, radiation-induced nephritis, and therapy-induced nephritis. The changes on MR images are again nonspecific with loss of corticomedullary differentiation on T1-weighted images [3]. In the case of a nephrotic syndrome, MRI is of value in excluding thrombosis of renal veins. As stated in Chap. 5, the renal veins are readily seen on transaxial MR scans, and, if they to appear as structures void of signal, or intravascular signal is suggestive of slow flow (Sect. 3.6), renal vein thrombosis as a cause of the nephrotic syndrome can be excluded. On the other hand, renal enlargement and intravascular signal suggest thrombosis (Fig. 6.16). As in acute obstruction, corticomedullary differentiation may be present in some cases of renal medical disease, such as acute tubular necrosis or cyclosporin nephrotoxicity. In end-stage renal disease, the kidneys appear small, and there is usually abundant perihilar fat. If there is a long-standing transfusion history, the papillae may appear hypointense even on T2-weighted images, presumably due to the deposition of paramagnetic iron compounds. Cortical iron deposits have been found in paroxysmal nocturnal hemoglobinuria [18].

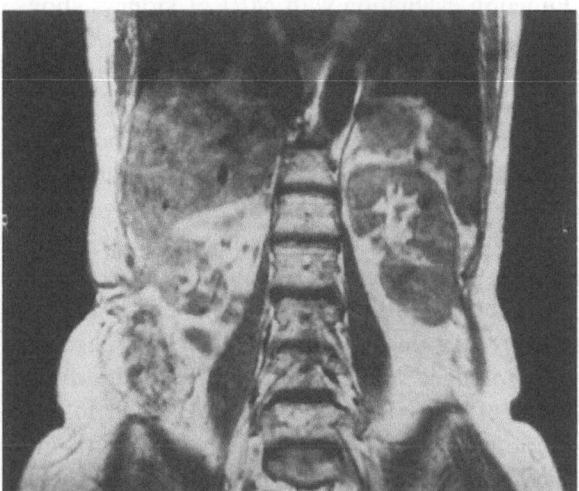

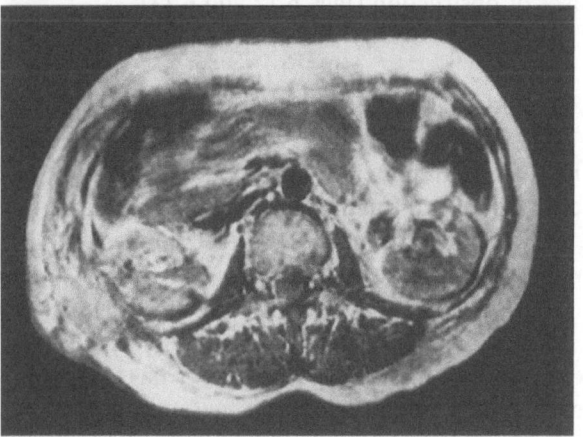

Fig. 6.15a, b. Right renal abscess extending into the flank. **a** Coronal image (SE 1100/30 ms) and **b** sagittal image (SE 2000/30 ms) showing involvement of the kidney as well as the right flank. Infected renal tissues cannot be differentiated from normal tissue on the images

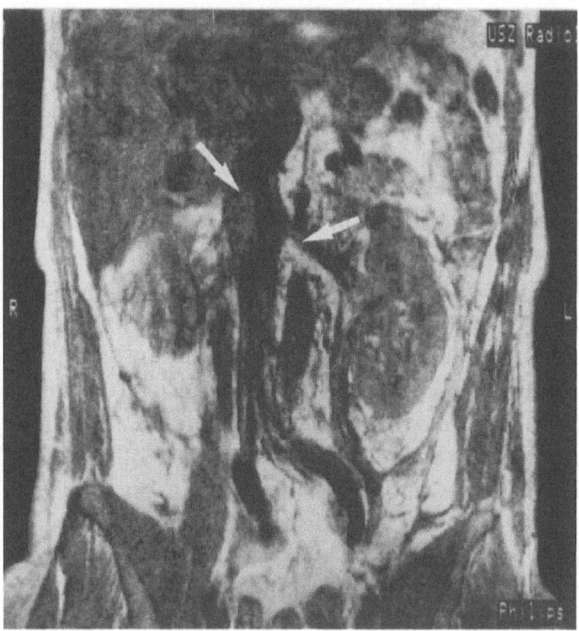

Fig. 6.16. Coronal scan (SE 500/30 ms) in a patient with ► nephrotic syndrome showing mostly the left kidney. It is enlarged, and thrombus is seen in the renal vein as well as in the inferior vena cava *(arrows)*. In addition, we find an enlarged right spermatic vein, which serves as a pathway for the collateral circulation

Function evaluation with MRI of kidneys showing infectious or noninfectious renal parenchymal
disease has been done only in the animal model of
acute glomerulonephritis [19]. The results of the dynamic sequences following a Gd-DTPA bolus are
interesting. Apparently, the concentration ability of
the kidney, characterized by the zone of signal loss
migrating from the corticomedullary junction towards the pelvis (Figs. 6.7, 6.8, and 6.10) observed in
normals after Gd-DTPA injection persists for the
first few days during injury, and in fact becomes
more prolonged and accentuated. With the development of renal failure and the resulting loss of
concentrating ability of the kidneys, the dark medullary zones are no longer present, similar to the
cases of obstruction (Figs. 6.12 and 6.13).

6.4.3 Perirenal Fluid Collection

There are multiple causes of perirenal fluid collections. Abscess formation has been discussed (Fig.
6.15), and other frequently observed entities are hematoma and urinoma.

Renal hematomas occur as a result of trauma, be
it accidental or iatrogenic. If it arises without evi-
dent cause, an underlying malignancy has to be suspected. Morphologically, the hematomas are either
subcapsular, and then take a lentiform shape compressing the renal parenchyma (Fig. 6.17), or they
are perirenal and then are more rounded in appearance. In this location they may compress adjacent
structures such as the inferior vena cava.

Functional aspects are the assessment of renal
impairment due to the hematoma/urinoma or to
compression of the adjacent vessels. Being confined
in their extent, renal and perirenal collections of
fluid usually affect only the kidney function in the
region of parenchymal affliction. The author is not
aware of studies analyzing renal function with MR
contrast media, except in the case of shock-wave
lithotripsy, for which hematoma and urinoma formation are well-known complications. Shock-wave
lithotripsy is discussed in Sect. 6.4.6. Another aspect
of more functional nature is the time course of the
MR appearance of a hematoma in organization. It
is intimately linked with the mechanisms responsible for the breakdown of hemoglobin. As in other
regions of the body, the MR appearance of a hematoma is quite variable and depends on its age.
Acute hematomas tend to show low signal intensity
on T1- as well as on T2-weighted images (Fig. 5.37).
After a few days, the hematoma becomes bright on
T1-weighted images and stays so on T2-weighted

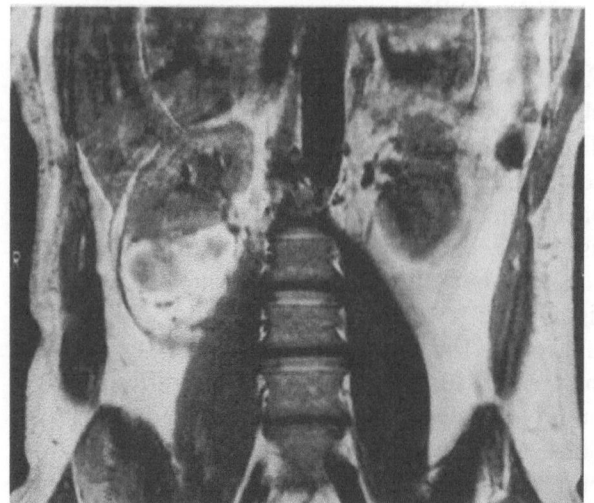

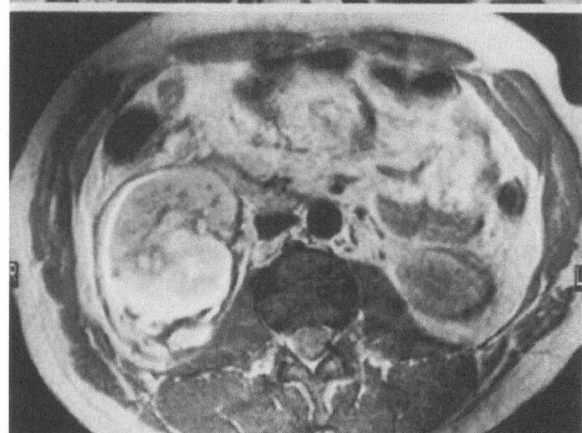

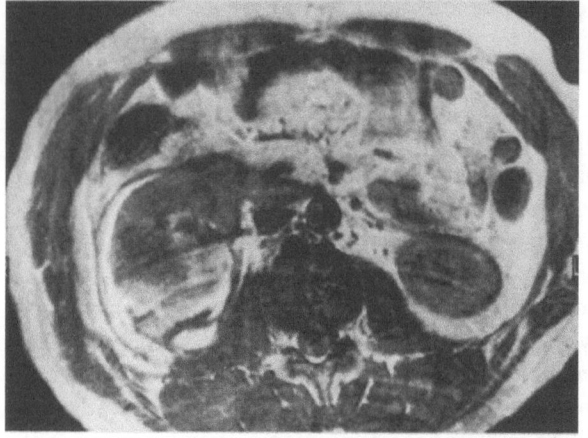

Fig. 6.17 a–c. Posttraumatic subcapsular hematoma of the
right kidney. **a** On coronal imaging (SE 1100/30 ms) the
hematoma is seen to lie in the region of the inferior pole.
b Transverse T1-weighted image (SE 500/30 ms) shows high
signal intensity with interspersed areas of lower signal, typical
ob subacute hematoma. **c** More T2-weighted images show
persisting bright, inhomogeneous appearance

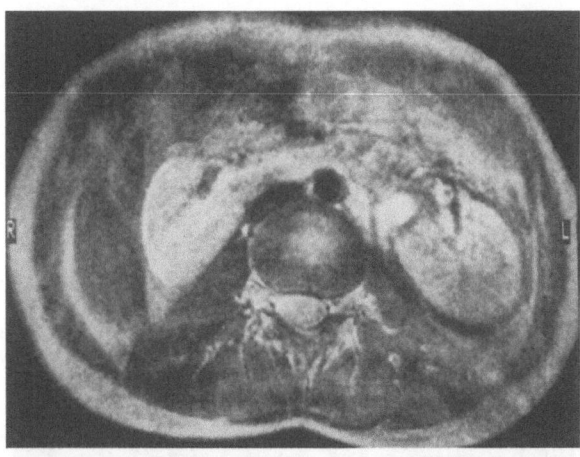

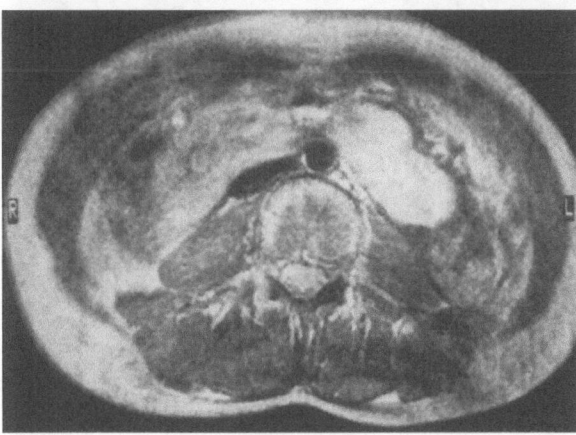

Fig. 6.18 a, b. Urinoma in a patient with traumatic renal rupture and horseshoe kidney. **a** A small fluid collection lies anterior to the left lower portions of the horseshoe kidney and is bright on T2-weighted images (SE 2000/60 ms). **b** A few centimeters lower, the urinoma is seen to extend anteriorly

images. Usually, there is a somewhat darker central zone (Figs. 5.36, 5.37 and 6.17), which is due to a different stage of hemoglobin breakdown compared with the surrounding zone. The same appearance is noted in vascular thrombi. Finally, chronic hematomas most often show a dark rim corresponding to hemosiderin, which is formed in the macrophages involved in the organization of the hematoma. The central part of the now-liquefied hematoma contains little paramagnetic iron; thus, there is an increase in signal intensity on T2-weighted images of chronic hematomas. This description of the appearance of aging hematomas in MRI applies for high field imagers only, and has been given in detail for cerebral hematomas [20]. It probably also applies to hematomas in other parts of the body, except that the organizing processes involved in the breakdown of hemoglobin take different time courses, depending on the location of the hematoma.

Urinomas have the same signal behavior as urine in the bladder, and are thus of very low signal intensity on T1-weighted images. On these they are often best identified, unless the patient is very slim, because of their good contrast to renal parenchyma and perirenal fat. On T2-weighted images, they exhibit very high signal intensity (Fig. 6.18). When identifying a small urinoma on T1-weighted images, one has to be aware of the always existing chemical shift artifact between kidneys and perirenal fat (Fig. 3.21) and should not mistake it for an urinoma. If small, they resolve in a few days, but larger urinomas may dissect retroperitoneally as far down as the perineum.

6.4.4 Cystic Renal Disease

Renal cysts are quite common and are present in more than 50% of patients over 50 years of age [21]. They are simple or multiple and can grow to an enormous size (Figs. 6.19 and 5.24 c). The etiology of these cysts is unknown, but they may arise due to tubular obstruction or vascular compromise. They are rounded and thin walled, containing amber-colored fluid but usually no hemoglobin. As such, they exhibit low signal intensity on T1-weighted images, which increases strongly on T2-weighted images like any other type of clear fluid. Their signal intensity remains homogeneous throughout [22]. Hemorrhagic and infected cysts, on the other hand, are inhomogeneous in appearance on T1- and T2-weighted images [23], because there may have been intracystic hemorrhage, and in fact, fluid levels containing differing concentrations of iron have been observed within cysts [24]. Calcifications sometimes contained in the cyst walls cannot be identified with MRI. Differentiation of complex, hemorrhagic, or infected cysts from solid benign and malignant lesions is not possible at present [25].

A step towards clearer distinction between these disease entities may well be imaging with MR contrast agents. Function imaging of renal cysts shows that there is no uptake of Gd-DTPA into the cyst, as evidenced by a lack of variation in a signal intensity (Fig. 6.19). This is true for parenchymal as well as for parapelvic cysts. Function curves of the kidneys depicted in Fig. 6.19 are shown in Fig. 6.20. There is no loss of function of the adjacent parenchyma. An apparent loss of cystic signal close to the renal pelvis in later images of the function scan is the result of susceptibility-induced signal loss occurring adjacent to the very high Gd-DTPA urinary concentration in the renal pelvis.

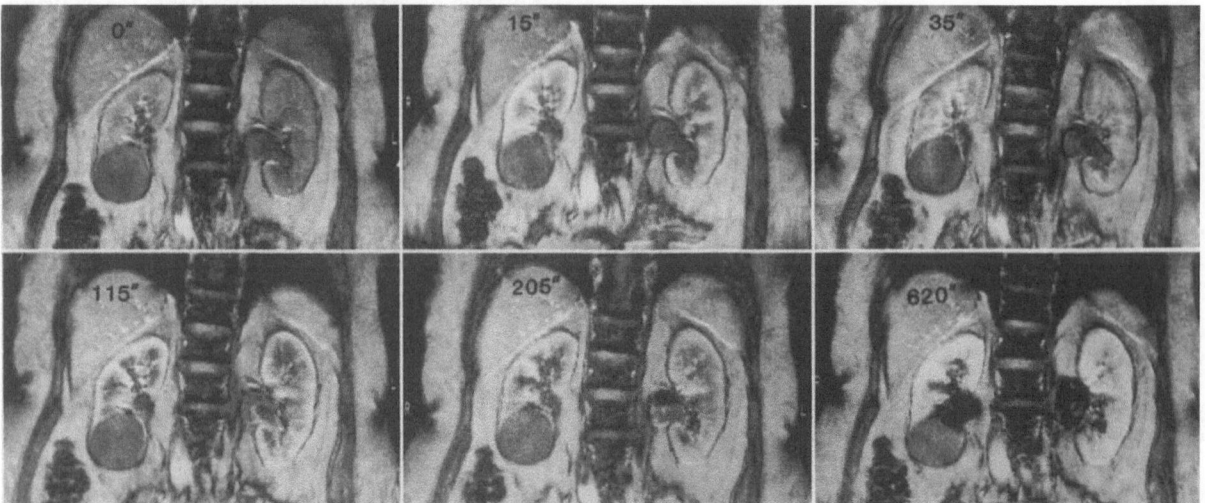

Fig. 6.19. Six scans of a dynamic Gd-DTPA sequence (GFE 40/16.1 ms, α = 40°) in a patient with a right parenchymal and a left parapelvic renal cyst. Note the normal function of the renal parenchyma with early papillary signal drop. No signal variation is noted in the cysts over the course of the ex-amination. In the late phases, when concentrated contrast medium has reached the renal pelves, the cysts exhibit eaten-out regions corresponding to susceptibility artifact-induced signal loss (Sect. 1.4.8)

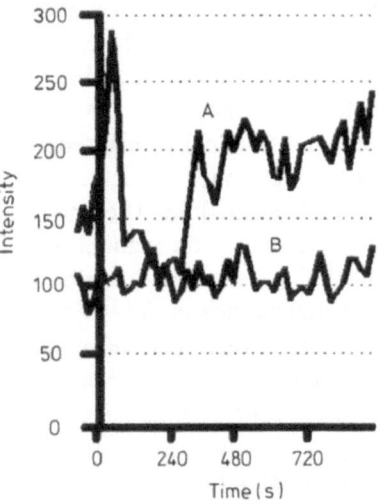

Fig. 6.20. Renal function curves of a papilla *(A)* and the large renal parenchymal cyst *(B)* in the patient shown in Fig. 6.19. Note normal function of the unaffected parenchyma and no signal change in the cyst during the course of the examination

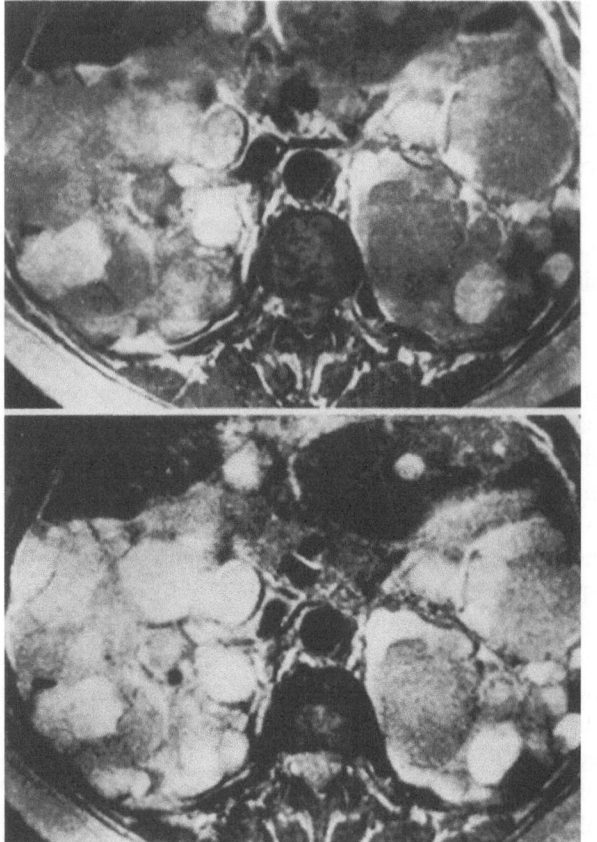

Fig. 6.21. **a** T1-weighted and **b** T2-weighted scans (SE 500/30 ms and 2000/60 ms) in a patient with polycystic kidney disease. Note cystic structures throughout the region of both kidneys with quite variable signal intensity. This corresponds to various concentrations of hemoglobin inside these cysts

In polycycstic kidney disease all renal parenchyma are interspersed with multiple cysts of variable size (Fig. 6.21). These cysts contain fluid with a very variable concentration of hemoglobin or hemoglobin breakdown products. As a result, they appear quite "colorful" in MRI. No MR function data from such patients are available, but it is known that patients suffering from the adult form of this disease eventually develop renal failure.

6.4.5 Neoplasms

The most common, but still rare, benign neoplasms of the kidneys are hamartomas and angiomyolipomas. Little experience in imaging these tumors has been accumulated. Both tumors contain significant amounts of fat and blood, which makes them appear bright even on T1-weighted images. Therefore, it is difficult to differentiate them from hemorrhagic cysts and sometimes even from necrotic solid tumors, and a specific diagnosis is rarely possible.

Malignant neoplasms have been studied much more extensively in MRI, because renal cell carcinoma is a common disease entity, accounting for roughly 3% of all tumors. In addition to renal cell carcinoma, Wilms' tumors occurring in neonates and children have been studied [26]. Other tumors include tumors of the renal capsule, metastases to the kidneys, and lymphomas and leukemic infiltrates. Our discussion will focus on renal cell carcinoma, because all tumors have similar appearances and cannot be differentiated from each other.

Renal cell carcinoma is grossly a very inhomogeneous tumor, containing in addition to tumor tissue areas of sclerosis, fibrosis, and hemorrhage. For tumors that were larger than 3 cm in diameter, a recent series reported a detection rate of 96% with MRI [27]. However, below this diameter, the detection rate dropped to 89%. This is due to the poor contrast between tumor and renal parenchyma on T1- as well as on T2-weighted imates (Fig. 6.22). Because the kidney is a structure with a high fluid content, relaxation times are similar to those for tumorous tissue. Thus, diagnosis of a tumorous mass lesion has to be made based primarily on the finding of a morphological contour abnormality. This, together with the enhanced motion sensitivity of high field strength imagers, means that there are few clinical indications for MRI in detecting renal tumors.

The appearance of all tumors on MR images is alike, with an increase in signal intensity from T1- to T2-weighted images. Areas of hemorrhage appear like hemorrhagic cysts with increased signal intensity even on T1-weighted images. Tumorous lymph nodes are similar in appearance, but staging is difficult, because larger regions of the body still

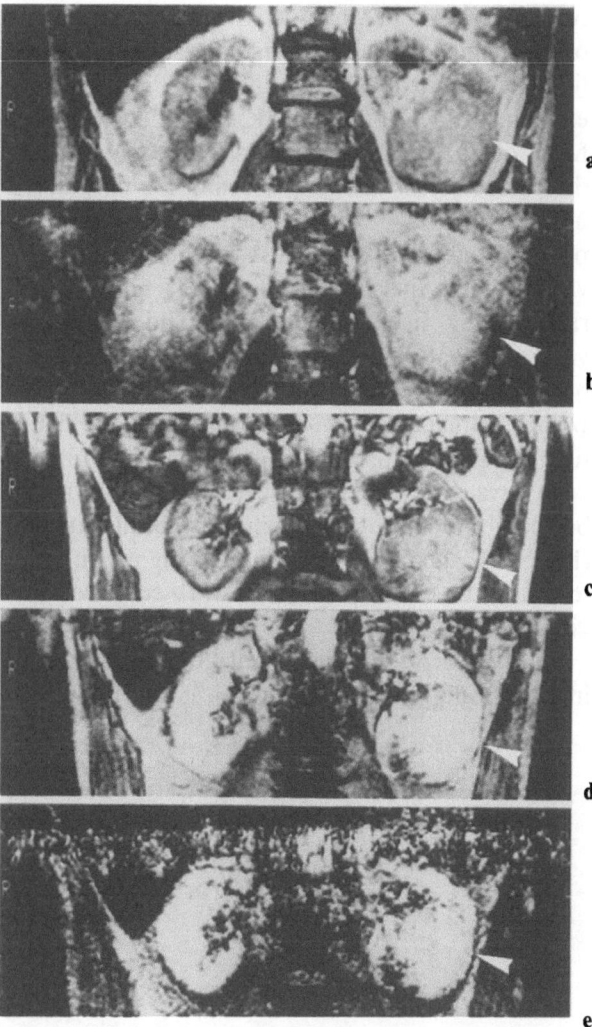

Fig. 6.22a–e. Hypernephroid carcinoma of the left lower pole of the kidney, coronal scans. **a** SE 500/30 ms, **b** SE 2000/60 ms. Note the similar appearance of normal renal parenchyma and tumor *(arrowhead)* on all images. The same is true for gradient echo images: **c** 75/16.1 ms, α = 70°; **d** 75/30.3 ms and **e** 75/60.6 ms, α = 20° for both

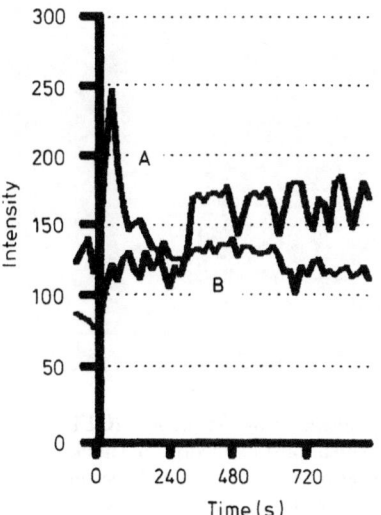

Fig. 6.23. Signal intensity versus time curve taken from the ▶ sequence shown in Fig. 6.13. Papillary parenchymal signal behavior *(A)* has to be contrasted with the initial increase in tumor signal intensity *(B)*, reaching a nearly constant level after 100–200 s

require an unduly long examination time. There are two indications in which MRI may be superior to other imaging modalities. First, invasion of adjacent tissues on horizontal tissue interfaces is difficult to examine with CT but can be examined well with MRI, due to its multiplanar imaging capability and the possibility of always projecting the partial volume effect in a direction where it least hinders a proper diagnosis. This is the case when assessing invasion of the liver by an upper pole tumor of the right kidney. In the case of liver (and muscle) invasion, the additional advantage of high contrast between tumor and invaded tissue exists on T2-weighted images. A second advantage is the detection of tumor thrombus extending into the inferior vena cava. The extension of such a thrombus can be readily identified on sagittal or coronal images (Fig. 5.38). Therefore, MRI appears slightly superior to CT for assessing stage-III and -IV renal cell carcinoma [27].

Gradient echo imaging of renal tumors is promising, particularly if combined with intravenous contrast agent injection and thus dynamic scan function studies. This is because static imaging also shows little contrast between tumor and renal parenchyma. It seems, that as in CT, renal parenchyma and the tumor can be differentiated better using intravenous contrast medium. Depending on the dose administered the renal papillae and the pelvis can be made dark, whereas the uptake of administered contrast medium into tumors is such that only enhancement is possible (Fig. 6.13). This behavior is illustrated by the signal intensity versus time curve of Fig. 6.23. Further experience with this method of imaging renal tumors must be accumulated, but it is likely that, as in CT, the use of contrast medium for renal scanning will be beneficial.

6.4.6 Trauma, Including Extracorporeal Shock-Wave Lithotripsy

In more severe cases, renal trauma results in parenchymal damage with hematoma or urinoma forma-

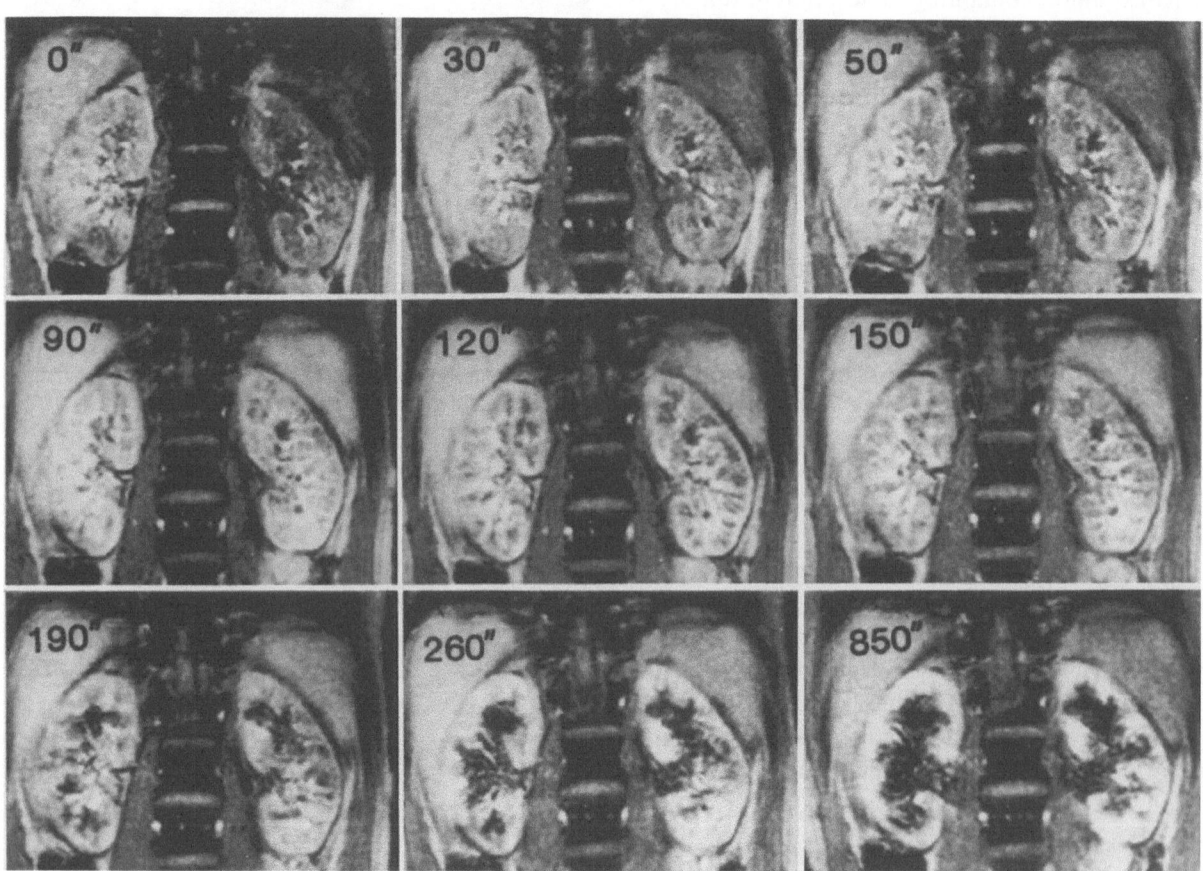

Fig. 6.24. Dynamic gradient echo sequence (GFE 34/16.1 ms, α = 40°) in a patient post extracorporal shock-wave lithotripsy to the left lower pole of the kidney. Persistence of high signal intensity in this region of the left kidney is noted, whereas the other renal parenchymal parts show the normal behavior of medullary signal loss shortly after injection of contrast medium

tion or vascular lesions. MRI is not the method of choice for evaluating acute trauma, but it may play some role in more chronic situations in distinguishing hematomas from other entities, such as urinoma and abscess. Perirenal fluid collections were discussed in Sect.6.4.3. No experience exists regarding function evaluation of traumatized kidneys. However, it is well recognized that extracorporeal shock-wave lithotripsy (ESWL) [28] can result in renal trauma [29, 30]. It thus will be considered under this heading.

A small initial study of renal morphology and function in 14 patients after ESWL with MRI has appeared in the literature [31]. Minimal morphological abnormalities were found. In particular, no subcapsular hematomas, a well-recognized complication of ESWL, were noted in this series. The only changes were a loss of corticomedullary differentiation in one quarter of the patients and an increase in size in almost half the treated kidneys. No alterations in renal function were found. A study using excretory urography, radionuclide renography, and morphological MRI detected similar morphological changes and, in addition, some decrease in effective renal plasma flow, which was atributed to the traumatization of parts of a kidney by the shock waves [32]. That such localized trauma can also be recognized by function MRI is shown in Fig.6.24 and the corresponding function curve in Fig.6.25, where a persistence of high signal intensity in the lower pole region over the entire scan period is observed. This

is in contradistinction to the papillae of the upper pole and suggests that there is a reduction in renal concentrating ability, preventing the contrast medium concentration from exceeding the level at which T2-effects start to dominate. Whether this effect is due to parenchymal damage or partial obstruction cannot be stated at present, and more experience with the method has to be gained.

6.4.7 Renal Transplants

As there is a continuing need for a noninvasive evaluation of renal transplant function, it is not surprising that MRI of kidney transplants has received considerable attention in the literature [2, 33-36].

The appearance of normal renal transplants is identical to that of normal kidneys, save for the dif-

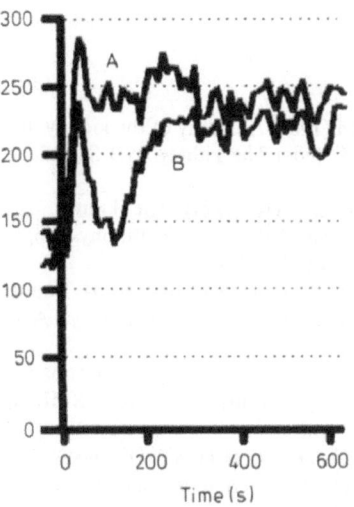

Fig. 6.25. Function curve corresponding to sequence in Fig.6.24, comparing a papillary region in the left upper with one in the left lower pole of the kidney. Whereas there is the characteristic signal drop in the upper pole papilla *(B)*, the region in the lower pole shows signal increase but no early signal drop *(A)*

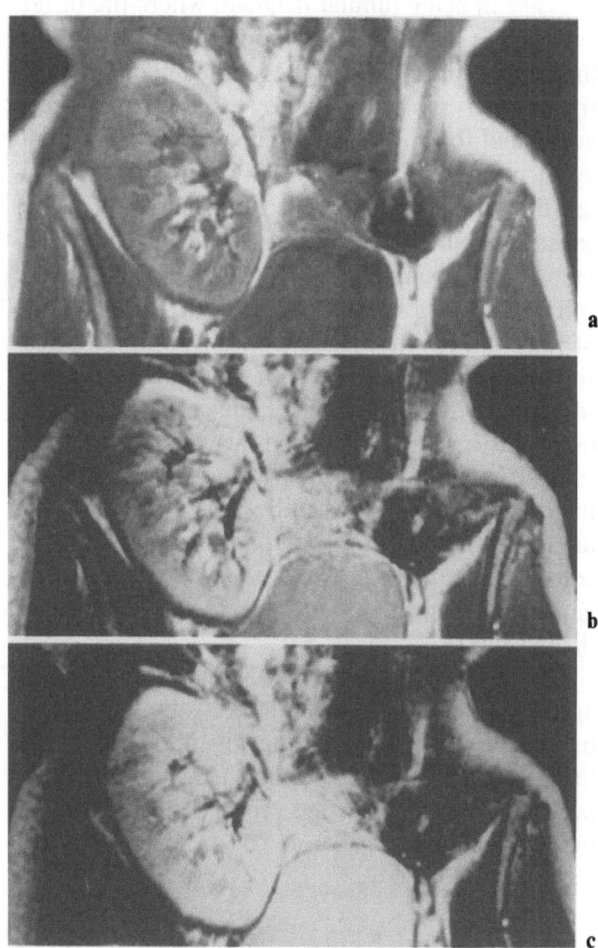

Fig. 6.26a–c. Normal renal transplant in a coronal scan, **a** showing the well-preserved corticomedullary differentiation with the lower signal intensity medulla on a T1-weighted image (SE 500/30 ms), confirming appropriate function. On more T2-weighted scans this differentiation is lost. **b** SE 2000/30 ms; **c** SE 2000/60 ms

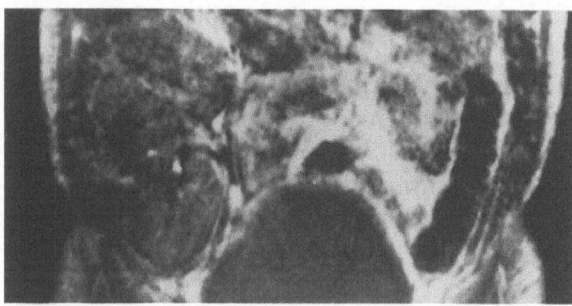

Fig. 6.27. Chronic transplant rejection. The T1-weighted image (SE 500/30 ms) shows loss of corticomedullary differentiation. There is image degradation due to peristaltic motion

ferent anatomic position and the vascular supply (Fig. 6.26). Because of their more pelvic location, respiratory motions do not degrade renal transplant images as much. Rejection results in loss of corticomedullary differentiation (Fig. 6.27). This is not the case in acute tubular necrosis, where the differentiation is usually preserved. Furthermore, in cyclosporin nephrotoxicity, the corticomedullary differentiation remains intact, and MRI has been advocated for differentiating between rejection and cyclosporin nephrotoxicity. However, in our hospital, the latter problem does not seem to arise because combination drug regimes are used for immune suppression, for which the cyclosporin dose can be kept below the toxicity level. The diagnosis of rejection is often made clinically, and no extensive imaging is necessary. If imaging is needed, sonography is at an advantage due to its lower cost, but in cases where questions remain, MRI is a good second imaging choice, particularly if contrast-enhanced CT cannot be used because of impaired renal function. It has to be emphasized that there are considerable differences voiced in the literature regarding the sensitivity and specificity of MRI for diagnosing rejection [36, 37].

Function imaging using paramagnetic contrast agents has not been attempted, to our knowledge, because if renal function is heavily impaired, excretion of Gd-DTPA is so much delayed that there may be some adverse effects from deposition of the toxic gadolinium ion.

6.4.8 Summary

Spin-echo imaging to detect morphological abnormalities in the kidneys, particularly with high field imagers, at present has limited significance. This is due to the generally suboptimal image quality,

which is a result of respiratory and peristaltic motion, but is less of a consideration in renal transplant imaging because the pelvic location of renal transplants results in fewer image artifacts. Indications are primarily the evaluation of unknown masses, where MRI may add some specificity, particularly if there is a question of hematoma, which in high field imagers often has a quite characteristic appearance. For tumor staging MRI may have a role in stage-III and -IV disease, where invasion of adjacent tissues can be evaluated using the multiplanar imaging capacity and the fact that on T2-weighted images tumors become bright, whereas liver and muscle tissues remain dark. Compared with CT, the definite disadvantage of MRI has been that no intravenous contrast media are used.

With the advent of gradient echo imaging, good-quality high-resolution dynamic renal images with a temporal resolution of 2–5 s have become a reality, and image acquisition in apnea is possible. Such scanning can be done parallel to the long renal axes, thus including major portions of the renal parenchyma. This is superior to dynamic transaxial CT scanning. Furthermore, multiple scans through the same slice are of no concern in MRI. The dynamic scan sequences shown in this chapter and the function curves derived from them suggest that MRI will have an important role in the assessment of renal disease, because it has the ability to demonstrate morphology and function jointly with high-resolution, high-contrast images.

References

1. Tisher CC, Madsen MM (1986) Anatomy of the kidney. In: Brenner BM, Rector FC (eds) The kidney. WB Saunders, Philadelphia
2. Scheitlin WA, Buehlmann AA (1979) The kidney. In: Buehlmann AA, Froesch ER (eds) Pathophysiology. Springer, Berlin Heidelberg New York
3. Leung AW-L, Bydder GM, Steiner RE, Bryant DJ, Young IR (1984) Magnetic resonance imaging of the kidneys. AJR 143: 1215–1227
4. Spritzer CE (1987) An overview of magnetic resonance imaging of the pelvis and genito-urinary systems. SMRM, book of abstracts, New York
5. Fein AB, Lee JKT, Balfe DM et al (1987) Diagnosis and staging of renal cell carcinoma: a comparison of MR imaging and CT. AJR 148: 749–754
6. Hricak H, Williams RD, Moon KL jr et al (1983) Nuclear magnetic resonance imaging of the kidney. Radiology 147: 765–772
7. Demas BE, Hricak H, Williams RD (1985) Magnetic resonance imaging in the evaluation of urologic malignancies. Sem Urol 3: 27–33

8. Pettigrew RI, Aruch L, Dannels W, Coumans J, Bernardino ME (1986) Fast-field-echo MR imaging with Gd-DTPA: physiologic evaluation of the kidney and liver. Radiology 160: 561–563

9. Haase A, Matthaei D, Hänicke W, Rahm J (1986) Dynamic digital subtraction imaging using fast low-angle shot MR movie sequences. Radiology 160: 537–541

10. Kikinis R, von Schulthess GK, Jäger P, Bino M, Kuoni W (1987) Normal and hydronephrotic kidney: evaluation of renal function with contrast-enhanced MR imaging. Radiology 165: 837–842

11. Weinmann HJ, Brasch RC, Press WR, Wesbey GE (1984) Characteristics of gadolinium-DTPA complex: a potential NMR contrast agent. AJR 142: 619–624

12. Gehrig G (1987) Linking feature space and accumulator space. A new approach to object recognition. Proc. of 1. Int Conf on Computer Vision (ICCV 87), London 112–117

13. Gehrig G, Wüthrich R, von Schulthess GK, Kikinis R, Kübler O (1987) Computer-assisted ROI analysis of 1.5 T MRI renal function studies with gradient echo sequences and Gd-DTPA. SMRM, Book of abstracts, works in progress, p 43

14. Grodd W, Brasch RC (1986) Magnetopharmazeutische Kontrastveränderungen in der Kernspintomographie. Fortschr Röntgenstr 145: 130–139

15. Demas B, Thurnher, Hricak H (1987) The kidney, adrenal gland, and retroperitoneum. In: Higgins CB, Hricak H (eds) Magnetic resonance imaging of the body. Raven press, New York

16. Thickman D, Kundel H, Biery D (1984) Magnetic resonance evaluation of hydronephrosis in the dog. Radiology 152: 113–116

17. Raynaud C, Tran-Dinh S, Bourguignon et al (1987) Acute pyelonephritis in children: preliminary results obtained with MR imaging. Contr Nephrol 56: 129–134. Karger, Basel

18. Mulopulos GP, Turner DA, Schwartz MM, Murakami ME, Clark JW (1986) MRI of the kidneys in paroxysmal nocturnal hemoglobinuria. AJR 146: 51–52

19. Carvlin MJ, Arger PH, Kundel HL et al (1987) Dynamic renal MR imaging to investigate antiglomerular basement membrane antibody-induced glomerulonephritis (abstract). Radiology 165 (P): 85

20. Gomori JM, Grossman RI, Goldberg HI et al (1986) Intracranial hematomas: imaging by high-field MR. Radiology 158: 707–713

21. Love L, Reynes CJ, Churchill R, Moncada R (1979) Third-generation CT scanning in renal disease. Radiol Clin North Am 17: 77–102

22. Hricak H, Crooks L, Sheldon O, Kaufman L (1983) Nuclear magnetic resonance imaging of the kidney. Radiology 146: 425–432

23. Marotti M, Hricak H, Fritzsche P, Crooks L, Hedgcock MW, Tanagho EA (1987) Complex and simple renal cysts: comparative evaluation by magnetic resonance imaging. Radiology 162: 679–684

24. Hilpert PL, Freidman AC, Radineck PD et al (1986) MRI of hemorrhagic renal cysts in polycycstic kidney disease. AJR 146: 1167–1172

25. Choyke PL, Kressel HY, Pollack HM, Arger PM, Axel L, Mamourain AC (1984) Focal renal masses: magnetic resonance imaging. Radiology 152: 471–477

26. Bett TG, Cohen MD, Smith JA, Cory DA, McKenna S, Weetman R (1986) MRI of Wilms' tumor: promise as the primary imaging method. AJR 146: 955–961

27. Hricak H, Thoeni RF, Carroll P, Marotti M, Tanagho EA (1987) MRI in the detection and staging of renal neoplasms. Radiology

28. Chaussy C, Schmiedt E, Jocham D, Brendel W, Forssmann B, Walter V (1982) First clinical experiences with extracorporeally induced destruction of kidney stones by shock waves. J Urol 127: 417–420

29. Chaussy C, Schiedt E, Jocham D, Schuller J, Brandl H, Liedl B (1984) Extracorporeal shock-wave lithotropsy (EDWL) for treatment of urolithiasis. Urology 23: 59–66

30. Rubin JI, Arger PH, Pollack HM et al (1987) Kidney changes after extracorporeal shock-wave lithotripsy: CT evaluation. Radiology 162: 21–24

31. Foerster EC, Bino M, Jäger P, von Schulthess GK (1987) Renal morphology and function before and after shock-wave lithotripsy at 1.5 T with gadolinium-DTPA. In: Bischof A, Blaufox D (eds) Progress in nephrourology. Karger, Basel

32. Kaude JV, Williams CN, Millner MR, Scott KN, Finlayson B (1985) Renal morphology and function immediately after extracorporeal shock-wave lithotripsy. AJR 145: 305–313

33. Geisinger MA, Risius B, Jordan ML, Zelch MG, Novick AC, George CR (1984) Magnetic resonance imaging of renal transplants. AJR 143: 1229–1234

34. Baumgartner BR, Nelson RC, Ball TI et al (1986) MR imaging of renal transplants. AJR 147: 949–953

35. Hricak H, Terrier F, Demas BE (1986) Renal allografts: evaluation by MR imaging. Radiology 159: 435–441

36. Steinberg HV, Nelson RC, Murphy FB et al (1987) Renal allograft rejection: evaluation by Doppler US and MR imaging. Radiology 162: 337–342

37. Hricak H, Terrier F, Marotti M et al (1987) Post-transplant renal rejection: comparison of quantitative scintigraphy, ultrasonography, and magnetic resonance imaging. Radiology 162: 685–688

Appendices

Appendix A: Taylor Series Expansions

A function $y = f(x)$, which is continuous and for which all derivatives at the point $x = x_o$ exist, can be written as a power series. It can be obtained according to the Taylor formula:

$$f(x) = f(x_o) + f'(x_o)(x - x_o)/1! + f''(x_o)(x - x_o)^2/2! +$$

$$+ f^{(n)}(x_o)(x - x_o)^n/n! + \ldots \qquad (A1)$$

Here $f^{(n)}$ is the n-th derivative of f with respect to x, taken at position x_o, i.e.

$$f^{(n)}(x_o) = \partial^n f/\partial x^n \, | \, x = x_o$$

In some situations, the higher-order terms can be neglected, and only the first (few) terms have to be included into the series to obtain a value of $f(x)$ which is very close to its actual value. This is the case when the higher-order terms become progressively smaller, such that the series expansion is convergent. Rather than defining the conditions of convergency here, we give a few examples of important series expansions.

1. Exponential function

$$e^{\pm x} = 1 \pm x/1! + x^2/2! \pm x^3/3! + \ldots + (-x)^n/n! +$$

For $x \ll 1$, this expansion reduces to

$$e^{\pm x} \approx 1 \pm x$$

Typical examples of where such an expansion is useful to simplify the mathematical expressions occur in the text. The Boltzmann factor, containing the ratio of the transition energy between spin up and down states, and the thermal energy, which is much smaller than 1, may be Taylor-series expanded (Eq. 1.2). Similarly, an expansion can be used to simplify the expression for the magnetization in T1- and T2-weighted spin-echo experiments (Eqs. 1.30 and 1.31). In writing down these expressions the equation $1 - e^x \simeq 1 - 1 + x = x$ was used.

2. Sine and cosine functions

$$\sin x = x - x^3/3! + x^5/5! - \ldots$$

$$+ (-1)^n x^{2n+1}/(2n+1)! \pm$$

$$\cos x = 1 - x^2/2! + x^4/4! - x^6/6! + \ldots$$

$$+ (-1)^n x^{2n}/(2n)! \pm$$

Other such expansions can be found in mathematical handbooks [1].

If the spatial position vector is expanded, we assume that the temporal change of the position is not very drastic, thereby justifying a termination of the series after its third or forth term (Eq. 1.42).

Appendix B: Vector Manipulations

A vector in an orthogonal coordinate system is an entity characterized by its coordinates. Typical vectors are the position, velocity, and acceleration vectors. Other vectors are the magnetic field H or the magnetic gradient field G. The position vector r in three-dimensional space can be written as

$$r = (x_o, y_o, z_o)$$

Addition and subtraction of vectors is done by adding or subtracting the coordinates of the different vectors individually; i.e., if vectors $A = (5,3,-2)$ and $B = (-1,4,2)$ are added, the sum vector C is given by $C = (4,7,0)$.

In the case of intravoxel incoherence, where the magnetization vectors of individual spins point in all spatial directions within a voxel, it is important to understand the concept of vector addition. Here, the magnetization vectors are spread over the phase circle to a variable degree. Once they are spread over the entire circle, the sum which is the net magnetization in a voxel approaches zero for the following reason. For each vector pointing in the $+x$ direction there is one pointing in the $-x$ direction, and the same holds true for the y direction. Thus, the vector sum can be thought of as a sum of vectors which approximately cancel pairwise. The net result is often total signal loss.

The multiplication of a vector r with a constant c is simple. The rule is:

$$cr = c(x_o, y_o, z_o) = (cx_o, cy_o, cz_o).$$

The multiplication of two vectors is conceptually more difficult. In fact, there are two ways to multiply vectors. The first is called "inner product formation". For example, the inner product of the position vector r and the gradient vector G is obtained by performing the following operation:

$$Inner\ Product\ (r.G) = (x_oG_x + y_oG_y + z_oG_z).$$

The inner product simply corresponds to the sum of the product of the projections of one vector onto the other. In two dimensions, the simplest case of the use of the inner product is Pythagoras' rule, by which the length of a vector is obtained. In general, the length of a vector is defined as:

$$length\ (r) = \sqrt{(r.r)} = \sqrt{(x_o^2 + y_o^2 + z_o^2)}.$$

There is a second way by which vectors can be multiplied, called "vectorial product". It has to be used, for example, when the torque of the magnetic radiofrequency field on the magnetization vectors of the spins is to be computed. Details will not be given here, but this product is used when the Bloch equations are analyzed.

Appendix C: More About the Fourier Transformation

A function f(t) defined on a finite interval T (period) can be approximated by a series of sine and cosine functions (Fourier series):

$$f(t) = a_o/2 + a_1\cos\omega t + a_2\cos 2\omega t + + a_n\cos n\omega t +$$

$$+ b_1\sin\omega t + b_2\sin 2\omega xt + \ldots + b_n\sin n\omega t +.$$

where $\omega = 2\pi/T$. The Fourier coefficents a_k and b_k are obtained through the formulae

$$a_k = 2/T \int_0^T f(t) \cos k\omega t\ dt$$

$$b_k = 2/T \int_0^T f(t) \sin k\omega t\ dt$$

If the interval on which the Fourier expansion has to be obtained is the entire t-axis, the situation is more complicated. In this case, there are no longer discrete values k, but the coefficients a become a continuous function of k. It can be shown that the Fourier coefficients for the series expansions of some well-known functions are given by some other well-known functions. These pairs of functions are called Fourier pairs. The graphic representation of some ot these pairs is given in Fig. 1.22. Typical examples are the sine wave, whose counterpart is the δ-function, the (sine x)/x or sinc x function, whose conunterpart is the square function, and the symmetrical exponential, whose counterpart is the Lorentzian function, given by $x^2/(1+x^2)$. To give further information is beyond the aim of this appendix, and the interested reader is referred to the textbooks [2].

Appendix D: Phase Calculations

If an ensemble of spins, called an isochromat, moves in a magnetic gradient field, the phase angle of the xy-plane magnetization of these isochromats changes relative to the phase angle of stationary isochromats according to Eq. D1

$$\partial\Phi/\partial t = \gamma(G.r) \tag{D1}$$

where γ is the gyromagnetic ratio, G the vector of the magnetic gradient field, r the position vector, and $\partial\Phi/\partial t$ the temporal change of these phase angle. (G.r) is the inner product between gradient and position vector (Appendix B), i.e., the sum of the projections of the gradient vector onto the position vector. The position vector can be written as a sum of motion terms (in the form of so-called Taylor series expansion, Appendix A):

$$r = x_o + v_ot + a_ot^2/2 + (higher-order\ terms) \tag{D2}$$

Here x_o is the position, v_o the velocity, and a_o the acceleration of the isochromats. In general, r also depends on the higher-order terms in the series expansion (D2), but depending on the problem considered, higher-order terms may be neglected. Because the changes in cardiac-induced motions occur over periods of time on the order of 50-100 ms, and a typical spin-echo sequence acquisition takes on the order of 30-50 ms only, the first three terms in the expansion will be dominant, however. The acceleration term is particularly important, because of the arterial pulsations and the changes in spatial orientation of the vessels, which induce accelerations as well.

It is the purpose of this appendix to calculate the values of the phase angle Φ for a multi-spin-echo sequence and to evaluate for which echoes constant velocity and acceleration terms will affect MR spin-echo images. In our analysis we shall limit ourselves to motion along the x-axis, without much loss in generality, as spin phase-angle changes due to motion along the other axes are calculated in analogy to the analysis given below. We shall denote here as "z-axis" the axis parallel to the bore of the imager, as "x-axis" the horizontal, and as "y-axis" the vertical axis in a plane perpendicular to the axis of symmetry of the imager.

The spin phase angles incurred by an isochromat at the 180° pulses and the echoes is calculated with the use of Eq. D1. For constant velocity motion the phase change Φ_v is found by integration of Eq. D1 as

$$\Phi_v(nT) = \gamma G_x v_o \int t\,dt = \gamma G_x v_o t^2/2, \qquad (D3a)$$

and for motion with constant acceleration we have

$$\Phi_a(nT) = \gamma G_x a_o \int t^2 dt = \gamma G_x a_o t^3/6. \qquad (D3b)$$

The integrals have to be evaluated over the time spans during which the gradient fields are turned on. Assuming that the gradient in the x-direction is the readout gradient (Fig. 1.20), we note that this gradient is turned on for a time t_p right after the 90° pulse, then for t_p just prior to the echoes and for t_p just after the echoes, which occur at $2nT$ ($n = 1,2,3,\ldots$) Hence, the integration limits are $2nT - t_p$ and $2nT$ for the phase changes incurred at the echoes, and $2nT - t_p$ and $2nT + t_p$ for the phase changes incurred when the 180° refocusing pulses are applied (at times $(2n+1)T$). The refocusing pulses change the phase angle by changing its sign, so that at $(2n+1)T$ the instantaneous value of the phase angle Φ changes from Φ to $-\Phi$. Thus, we find that

$$\Phi_v[(2n+1)T] = ct^2\Big|_{2nT-t_p}^{2nT+t_p} - \Phi_v[(2n-1)T] =$$

$$= 8cnTt_p - \Phi_v[(2n-1)T] \qquad (D4a)$$

just prior to the 180° refocusing pulses at $(2n+1)T$, and

$$\Phi_v(2nT) = ct^2\Big|_{2nT-t_p}^{2nT} - \Phi_v[(2n-1)T] =$$

$$= c(4nTt_p - t_p^2) - \Phi_v[(2n-1)T], \qquad (D4b)$$

where $c = \gamma G_x v_o/2$. In analogy we find

$\Phi_a[(2n+1)T]$ and $\Phi_a[(2n-1)T]$ to be

$$\Phi_a[(2n+1)T] =$$
$$= d(24n^2T^2t_p + 2t_p^3) - \Phi_a[(2n-1)T] \qquad (D5a)$$

and

$$\Phi_a(2nT) =$$
$$= d(12n^2T^2t_p - 3nTt_p^2 + t_p^3) - \Phi_a[(2n-1)T] \qquad (D5b)$$

with $d = \gamma G_x a_o/6$.

These recursive equations can be solved as follows. We shall do this for the acceleration terms. The velocity terms are found in analogy. Taking Eq. D5a, we note that

$$\{\Phi_a[(2n+1)T] + \Phi_a[(2n-1)T]\}/d =$$

$$= 24n^2T^2t_p + 2t_p^3 + \{-\Phi_a[(2n-1)T]$$
$$- \Phi_a[(2n-3)T]\}/d =$$

$$= 24(n-1)^2T^2t_p - 2t_p^3 + \{\Phi_a[(2n-3)T]$$
$$+ \Phi_a[(2n-5)T]\}/d = \text{etc.,} \qquad (D6)$$

Thus, by summing the expressions above, we obtain on the right hand side $\Phi_a[(2n+1)T] - \Phi_a(T)$ for even n and $\Phi_a[(2n+T] + \Phi_a(T)$ for odd n, with $\Phi_a(T) = d\,t_p^3$ being the phase angle just prior to the first 180° pulse. For even n we obtain:

$$\{\Phi_a[(2n+1)T] - \Phi_a(T)\}/d =$$

$$\sum_{i=1}^{n} (-1^i)\{24i^2T^2t_p + 2it_p^3\} \qquad (D7)$$

$$= 24T^2t_p^2\{\sum_{i=1}^{n} i^2 - 2\sum_{i=1}^{n/2} (2i-1)^2\} + t_p^3\{\sum_{i=1}^{n} (-1)_i\}.$$

The last term is zero, and the values of the sums in the first and second terms are found in standard texts [1]:

$$\sum_{i=1}^{n} i^2 = n(n+1)(2n+1)/6$$

and $2\sum_{i=1}^{n/2} (2i-1)^2 = 2n(n^2-1)/6$

Thus, the phase angles just prior to the 180° refocusing pulses are found as

$$\Phi_a[(2n+1)T] = \gamma G_x a_o\{/2(n^2+n)T^2 t_p + t_p^2\}/6 \quad (D8)$$

For odd n the second sum in Eq. D7 has to be evaluated at $(n+1)/2$ rather than at n, and the third sum equals -1, whereas the left-hand side of Eq. D7 is $\Phi_a[(2n+1)T] + \Phi_a(T)$. With these changes, Eq. D7 is found to yield the same result as in the case of even n, hence Eq. D8 is valid for even and odd n. By combining Eq. D8 with Eq. D5b we also find the expression for $\Phi_a(2nT)$, i.e., the phase angle incurred at the echoes:

$$\Phi_a(2nT) = \gamma G_x a_o\{12nT^2t_p - 3nTt_p^2\}/6. \quad (D9)$$

A completely analogous procedure, using Eq. D4 as the starting point, yields the expressions for $\Phi_v[(2n+1)T]$ and $\Phi_v(2nT)$:

$$\Phi_v[(2n+1)T] =$$
$$= \gamma G_x v_o\{4nTt_p + t_p^2\}/2 \qquad \text{n even} \qquad (D10)$$

$$= \gamma G_x v_o\{4(n+1)Tt_p - t_p^2\}/2 \qquad \text{n odd}$$

$$\Phi_v(2nT)$$
$$= 0 \qquad \text{n even}$$

$$= \gamma G_x v_o\{4Tt_p - 2t_p^2\}/2 \qquad \text{n odd} \qquad (D11)$$

The expressions resulting from these equations are summarized in Table 1.3 for n up to 8, i.e., up to the fourth echo. It is important to note that Φ_v is zero for even echoes, a phenomenon which is known as even-echo refocusing or rephasing. Thus, isochromats moving at a constant velocity will have a phase angle of zero at even echoes, independent of their velocity. For isochromats undergoing constant acceleration, the phase angle is dependent on acceleration at all echoes and increases linearly with increasing echo number 2n. Thus, although even echoes are insensitive to isochromat motion at constant speed, they are sensitive to motion at constant acceleration.

References

1. e.g. Bronstein IN, Semendjajew KA (1969) Taschenbuch der Mathematik, 9. Aufl. Verlag Harri Deutsch, Zürich und Frankfurt a. Main
2. Champeney M (1973) Fourier transforms and their physical applications. Academic Press, New York

Abbreviations

		SI units
$A_{xyo}(t)$	Time varying signal	
a	Distance in random walk	m(eter)
$a_{xo, yo, zo}$	Acceleration along the x-, y-, z-direction	ms (econd)$^{-2}$
arccos	Inverse of the cosine function ($\{arccos\{cos\alpha\}\}=\alpha$)	
arctan	Inverse of the tangent function ($\{arctan\{tan\alpha\}\}=\alpha$)	
B	Magnetic induction or flux density	Tesla
B_o	of magnetic induction Amplitude	
$B(t)$	Amplitude of incoming RF wave	
BSA	Body surface area	m^2
b	$=\gamma G_x x_o$, abbreviation in phase-angle expression	
C_{creat}	Creatinine clearance	ml min^{-1}
CI	Cardiac index	ml min^{-1} m^{-2}
c	$=\gamma G_x v_{xo}/2$, abbreviation in phase-angle expression	
D	Translational diffusion constant//vessel diameter	m^2 s^{-1}/m
D_{rot}	Rotational diffusion constant	rad^2 s^{-1}
d	$=\gamma G_x a_{xo}/6$, abbreviation in phase-angle expression	
d...	Derivative	
EDL	End-diastolic length of the heart	cm
EDV	End-diastolic volume	ml
EF	Ejection fraction	
ESL	End-systolic length of the heart	cm
ESV	End-systolic volume	ml
ΔE	Energy difference	Joule
F	Proportionality factor, containing flow effects, etc.	
F_b	Fraction of protein-bound water	

		SI units
F_f	Fraction of free water	
f(.)	function of (.)	
%FS	Percent fiber shortening	
G	Magnetic gradient field vector	Tesla/m
G_{xyz}	Components of magnetic gradient field vector	Tesla/m
g_n	Fraction of blood leaving slice until n-th echo	
g_{TR}	Fraction of blood replaced during a repetition time TR	
H	Proton density	m^{-3}
H_o	Magnetic field	Tesla
H_{eff}	Effective magnetic field at nucleus	Tesla
$H_{mx,y,z}$	Components of molecular magnetic field	Tesla
ΔH_o	Variation due to field inhomogeneities	Tesla
HR	Heart rate	min^{-1}
h	Planck's constant ($=6.62620\times10^{-34}$)	Joule s
I	In-phase signal	
i	Number of steps in one-dimensional random walk	
$J(\omega)$	Spectral density function	s
k	Phase-encoding gradient step increase	
k_B	Boltzmann constant ($=1.3807\times10^{-23}$)	Joule Kelvin^{-1}
L	Length of a tube	m
M	Magnetization	Tesla
M_o	Equilibrium magnetization	Tesla
$M_{x,y,z}$	x-, y-, z-components of magnetization	Tesla
$M_{xo,yo,zo}$	x-,y-,z-components of equilibrium magnetization	Tesla
$M_{xy'}$	xy-plane magnetization in rotating frame	Tesla
M_{xyo}	Initial xy-plane magnetization	Tesla

		SI units				SI units
N	Number of protons with spin antiparallel to field per unit volume//number of particles	m^{-3}	$v_{xo,yo,zo}$	Velocity (of spin) along x-, y-, z-axis	ms^{-1}
N_o	Number of protons with spin parallel to field per unit volume//number of particles	m^{-3}	$<v>$	Average velocity	ms^{-1}
			v_{max}	Maximum velocity	ms^{-1}
n	Number of pixels in a row or column//echo number		W+	Transition probability from low- to high-energy state	s^{-1}
n(t)	Number of spins in excess of spins in state N_o	m^{-3}	W−	Transition probability from high- to low-energy state	s^{-1}
n_o	Number of spins in excess of spins in thermal equilibrium state N_o at saturation	m^{-3}	WT_{ED}	End-diastolic wall thickness	m
			WT_{ES}	End-systolic wall thickness	m
NEX	Number of excitations with the same phaseencode gradient		w_x	Displacement of vascular signal along the read direction	m
O	Opposed-phase signal		w_{xy}	distance a spin moves between phase encode and read gradient	m
P	Collision probability per unit time//plasma creatinine conc.	mg// 100 ml	X_i	Position after i bumps	
			$<X_i>$	Positional expection value after i bumps	
P_1	Pressure at one end of tube	Newton m^{-2}	$<X_i2>$	Mean square distance of one-dimension random walk	m^2
P_2	Pressure at other end of tube	Newton m^{-2}	$<x^2>$	Mean square distance	m^2
PCFS	Peak circumferential fiber shortening	$cm\ s^{-1}$	x,y,z	Coordinates in laboratory frame	m
Q	Flow	mls^{-1}	x',y',z'	coordinates in rotating frame	m
R	Radius of a vessel	m	x_o, y_o, z_o	Initial position/distance along x-, y-, z-axis	m
Re	Reynolds number		α	Flip (nutation) angle	rad
ΔR	Change in vessel radius	m	α_E	signal optimizing flip angle in gradient echo imaging (so-called Ernst angle)	rad
r	Radius of a molecule// position vector//radius variable	m			
r_{IS}	Distance between protons I and S on a molecule	m	β	Angle between read direction and direction of blood vessel	
SV	Stroke volume	ml	γ_p	Proton magnetogyric ratio $(=2.6752 \times 10^8)$	$rad\ s^{-1}$ $Tesla^{-1}$
s	Slice thickness	m	Δ	Time between first and second gradient field pulse	s
T	Absolute temperature	(degree) Kelvin	Δ_c	Critical time in restricted diffusion	s
T1	Splin-lattice relaxation time	s	δ	Chemical shift constant (given in parts per million) /duration of gradient field pulse	//s
T2	Spin-spin relaxation time	s			
T2*	Effective T2 relaxation time	s			
TE	Echo time	s			
TR	Repetition time	s	Φ	Phase angle	radians
t	Time	s	η	Viscosity coefficient $(=0.8904 \times 10^{-3}$ @ 298 Kelvin)	$kg\ s^{-1}m^{-1}$
U	Water signal				
UC	Urinary creatinine	mg/24 h			
V	Fat signal//ventricular volume	$//m^3$	μ	Magnetic moment of proton//viscosity coefficient	
v	Velocity	ms^{-1}			

		SI units
ν_o	Larmor frequency	Hertz$=$s^{-1}
π	Constant	3.1415
σ	Screening constant//wall or shear stress	
ρ	Density of fluid	
χ	Magnetic susceptibility	
χ_C	Curie susceptibility	
τ_c	Correlation time	s
τ_{cR}	Correlation time for rotational diffusion	s
τ_{cs}	Correlation time for electron spin relaxation	s
τ_{ce}	Correlation time for molecular exchange	s
Θ	Angle	rad
ω_o	Angular Larmor frequency	rad s^{-1}
ω_I	Proton Larmor frequency	rad s^{-1}
ω_S	Electron Larmor frequency	
$\Delta\omega_o$	Variation in Larmor frequency due to field inhomogeneities	rad s^{-1}
$\Delta\omega$	Frequency range	rad s^{-1}
ω_s	Angular Larmor frequency of sample	rad s^{-1}
ω_r	Angular Larmor frequency of reference compound	rad s^{-1}

Subject Index